MOSBY'S REVIEW QUESTIONS FOR THE

National Board Dental Hygiene Examination

Edited and Contributed by

Barbara L. Bennett, CDA, RDH, MS
Associate Vice President
Office of Student Learning
Instructor, Department of Dental Hygiene
Allied Health Division
Texas State Technical College
Harlingen, Texas

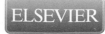

ELSEVIER
MOSBY

3251 Riverport Lane
St. Louis, Missouri 63043

MOSBY'S REVIEW QUESTIONS FOR THE NATIONAL   ISBN: 978-0-323-10172-1
BOARD DENTAL HYGIENE EXAMINATION

Copyright © 2014 by Mosby, an imprint of Elsevier Inc.

Notices

Knowledge and best practice in this field are constantly changing. As new research and experience broaden our understanding, changes in research methods, professional practices, or medical treatment may become necessary.

Practitioners and researchers must always rely on their own experience and knowledge in evaluating and using any information, methods, compounds, or experiments described herein. In using such information or methods they should be mindful of their own safety and the safety of others, including parties for whom they have a professional responsibility.

With respect to any drug or pharmaceutical products identified, readers are advised to check the most current information provided (i) on procedures featured or (ii) by the manufacturer of each product to be administered, to verify the recommended dose or formula, the method and duration of administration, and contraindications. It is the responsibility of practitioners, relying on their own experience and knowledge of their patients, to make diagnoses, to determine dosages and the best treatment for each individual patient, and to take all appropriate safety precautions.

To the fullest extent of the law, neither the Publisher nor the authors, contributors, or editors, assume any liability for any injury and/or damage to persons or property as a matter of products liability, negligence or otherwise, or from any use or operation of any methods, products, instructions, or ideas contained in the material herein.

ISBN: 978-0-323-10172-1

Vice President and Publisher: Linda Duncan
Content Strategist: Kristin Wilhelm
Senior Content Development Specialist: Courtney Sprehe
Publishing Services Manager: Julie Eddy
Project Manager: Jan Waters
Design Direction: Paula Catalano

Printed in United States of America

Last digit is the print number: 9   8   7   6   5   4   3   2

Working together
to grow libraries in
developing countries

www.elsevier.com • www.bookaid.org

Contributors

Debra K. Arver, LDA, RDH, MAEd, RF
Program Chair
Dental Hygiene Program
Argosy University
Eagan, Minnesota

Christine French Beatty, RDH, PhD
Professor Emeritus
Dental Hygiene Program
Texas Woman's University
Denton, Texas

Connie E. Beatty, RDH, BS, MSDH(c)
Adjunct Clinical Instructor
Dental Hygiene Program
Texas Woman's University
Denton, Texas

Phyllis L. Beemsterboer, RDH, MS, EdD
Professor and Associate Dean for Academic Affairs
School of Dentistry
Oregon Health & Science University
Portland, Oregon

Joanna Campbell, RDH, MA, MA
Academic Department Chair and Professor
Dental Hygiene
Bergen Community College
Paramus, New Jersey

Gina Cano-Monreal, PhD
Senior Instructor
Nursing Preparatory/Biology Department
Texas State Technical College
Harlingen, Texas

Elizabeth Odom Carr, MDH, RDH
Assistant Professor
Department of Dental Hygiene
The University of Mississippi Medical Center
Jackson, Mississippi

Jamie Collins, CDA, RDH
Instructor
Dental Assisting Program
College of Western Idaho
Eagle, Idaho

Mary Cooper, RDH, MSEd
Associate Dean and Professor
College of Health and Human Services
Indiana University-Purdue University
Fort Wayne, Indiana

Frank J. Dowd, DDS, PhD
Professor Emeritus of Pharmacology
School of Dentistry
Creighton University
Omaha, Nebraska

Gwen Essex, RDH, EdD
Health Sciences Clinical Professor
Department of Preventive and Restorative
    Dental Sciences
School of Dentistry
University of California, San Francisco
San Francisco, California

Jean Frahm, RDH, MSEd
Instructor
Dental Hygiene Program
Argosy University
Eagan, Minnesota

Danielle Furgeson, RDH, MS
Clinical Assistant Professor
Division of Dental Hygiene
Department of Periodontics and
    Oral Medicine
School of Dentistry
University of Michigan
Ann Arbor, Michigan

Vicki Gianopoulos, RDH, MS
Assistant Professor
Division of Dental Hygiene
College of Health Sciences
The University of New Mexico
Albuquerque, New Mexico

Ashley Martin Hale, RDH, MS
Manager, Professional Education,
    Southeast
Philips Oral Healthcare
Raleigh, North Carolina

Elena Bablenis Haveles, BS, PharmD
Adjunct Associate Professor of Pharmacology
Gene W. Hirschfeld School of Dental Hygiene
Old Dominion University
Norfolk, Virginia

Sandra Horne, RDH, MHSA
Associate Professor and Clinical Director
Department of Dental Hygiene
School of Health-Related Professions
University of Mississippi Medical Center
Jackson, Mississippi

Olga A.C. Ibsen, RDH, MS
Adjunct Professor
Department of Oral and Maxillofacial
    Pathology, Radiology, and Medicine
College of Dentistry
New York University
New York, New York;
Adjunct Professor
Fones School of Dental Hygiene
University of Bridgeport
Bridgeport, Connecticut

Leslie Koberna, RDH, BSDH, MPH/HSA, PhD
Clinical Associate Professor
Dental Hygiene Program
Texas Woman's University
Denton, Texas

Demetra Daskalos Logothetis, RDH, MS
Professor
Graduate Program Director
Division of Dental Hygiene
University of New Mexico
Albuquerque, New Mexico

Jodi L. Olmsted, RDH, PhD
Assistant Professor
School of Health Care Professions
University of Wisconsin–Stevens Point
Stevens Point, Wisconsin

Dorothy A. Perry, RDH, PhD, MS
Professor and Associate Dean for Education
    and Student Affairs
School of Dentistry
University of California, San Francisco
San Francisco, California

Frieda Atherton Pickett, RDH, MS
Author, Educator, Lecturer
Pickett Professional Presentations
Butler, Tennessee

Joseph W. Robertson, DDS
Dentist in Private Practice
Troy Michigan;
Co-Director and Instructor
Dental Hygiene Program
Oakland Community College
Waterford, Michigan

Cynthia A. Stegeman, EdD, RDH, RD, LD, CDE
Associate Professor
Dental Hygiene Department
University of Cincinnati Blue Ash
Blue Ash, Ohio

Amy Teague, RDH, MS
Senior Clinic Coordinator
Assistant Clinical Professor
Texas Woman's University
Dental Hygiene Program
Denton, Texas

Laura J. Webb, CDA, RDH, MS
Independent Consultant
Dental Hygiene and Dental Assisting
LJW Education Services
Fallon, Nevada

Reviewers

Lezlie M. Cantrell, RDH, PhD
Dental Hygiene Educational Consultant
Educator, Higher Education
Sheridan, Wyoming

Nicole Day, RDH
Dental Hygiene Educational Consultant
Los Angeles, California

Preface

The purpose of this book is to help prepare dental hygiene students by providing a thorough practice review of foundational dental hygiene knowledge. Dental hygiene students preparing to take the National Board Dental Hygiene Examination (NBDHE) are often so overwhelmed with the amount of information to be mastered that they don't know where to begin. It is important for candidates to remember that they have already successfully completed a demanding and competitive course of study and that they have the ability to successfully pass this high-stakes examination. In addition, it is important to remember that reviewing the material and practicing exam questions is much simpler than learning it for the first time.

Preparation is the key to success, and this book serves as a valuable resource in that preparation. Welcome to the rewarding career of dental hygiene patient care. We wish you every success!

The Editorial Team

The Learning Package

Mosby's Review Questions for the National Board Dental Hygiene Examination is a book and Evolve website package designed to provide the candidate preparing for the national board examination the most realistic and trustworthy practice testing available! Written by a variety of content experts who are familiar with the examination and who are also instructors in dental hygiene programs at accredited institutions, users can be assured that the practice questions and rationales will provide them realistic, meaningful test preparation. The number and quality of practice questions will also help the test candidates increase their readiness and go into the actual test with the experience and confidence necessary to improve their chances of passing.

BOOK

The chapters of *Mosby's Review Questions for the National Board Dental Hygiene Examination* follow the format and distribution of questions on the actual test. With more than 1200 unique questions, this product offers students more than six times the number of Component A test questions with which to practice. Each question includes an explanatory rationale to help exam candidates highlight the areas and topics with which they may need a more thorough content review. A listing of textbook resources is provided if more detailed information is needed (see Appendix A, Additional Resources).

EVOLVE WEBSITE

The companion Evolve website features all of the 1200+ questions found in the printed book in two formats—in *practice mode* by test category and in *exam-simulation mode* with a built-in test generator that allows the student to create a variety of unique practice tests, each of which matches the number and distribution of questions by category to ensure that the sample test provides the most realistic practice. In a practice mode, instant feedback is provided for users to view as they choose, and in exam-simulation mode, feedback is provided at the end of the exam.

Fifteen in-depth cases in the style of the National Board Dental Hygiene Examination (NBDHE) are also included on the Evolve website—each with detailed medical/dental histories, completed periodontal charts, radiographs, clinical photographs, and 15 to 30 multiple-choice questions to provide extensive Component B practice. Cases are categorized as they are on the exam—adult periodontal, pediatric, geriatric, medically compromised, and special needs—and again, users may practice them separately or randomly within the simulated exam.

The simulated exams also provide instant feedback upon completion and a timer function to simulate the test-taking environment and help with time management, which is one of the most common reasons students may fail the test.

Preparing for the National Board Dental Hygiene Examination

Preparation for the National Board Dental Hygiene Examination (NBDHE) is a critical component for success. It requires organization, planning, time management, discipline, and a positive attitude. Thorough preparation allows the dental hygienist to have confidence in his or her ability to satisfy board requirements using knowledge and skill and it helps reduce test anxiety. This book is designed to be systematically used to reinforce and refresh existing knowledge, identify areas where more study is needed, and apply concepts to patient care. Dental hygiene educators have shared their expertise and experience by integrating core concepts into the NBDHE question format, which allows the test-taker to become familiar and comfortable with the examination. Successful completion of the NBDHE is required for licensure in the United States, and this book can serve as a valuable resource in achieving that goal.

Success requires the dental hygienist to be not only physically, psychologically, and mentally prepared, but also to be thoroughly aware of the format, content, logistics, and test requirements of the NBDHE (see later for a discussion on candidate test preparation and the format of the NBDHE).

STRATEGIC PLANNING FOR SUCCESS

Dental hygiene curriculum is designed to be foundational with each new subject building on the existing knowledge base. The student should strive to master new information and integrate it into what has already been learned, not just memorize test material. Review of test content needs to begin 4 to 6 months in advance of the exam to allow the test candidate to be well prepared. Each individual should devise a study plan based on learning styles and strategies that have been successful in the past. Some additional success strategies are listed here:

- Obtain the *NBDHE Guide* and application materials from the Joint Commission on National Dental Examinations (JCNDE). Read the information thoroughly to become familiar with examination design, format, and administration.
- Obtain a copy of the most recently released NBDHE from the JCNDE, which is protected by copyright and available for a fee. This examination is a helpful practice tool. Other simulated exams, such as the questions

in this textbook and those on the Evolve website, are very useful for review.

- Analyze areas of strength and weakness and focus on mastering weaknesses first. Dental hygienists who have not been in educational programs or practice recently should focus on the basic sciences and changes in dental practice since graduation.
- Gather study resources (such as this textbook) for use during the review period. This book can be used as a primary study guide, which can be supplemented with textbooks, notes, websites, and review courses. Textbooks and reference material should be current. There is no specific textbook or review course that is recommended by the JCNDE, nor is there any textbook or review course affiliated with the JCNDE.
- If forming a study group, find study partners with similar habits, self-discipline, and efforts that will complement the group. Keep in mind that members of a study group are responsible for their own individual learning.
- Create an orderly schedule for review with goals and deadlines to ensure progress.
- Follow a schedule with a goal of finishing the review a few days before the exam.

SUGGESTIONS FOR STUDY SUCCESS

Learning as much as possible about the NBDHE—how the test is constructed, what type of questions are included, and how long the test is—is a critical first step toward success. NBDHE construction is discussed later. The suggestions found here are designed to help develop active study skills, not just reading and highlighting a textbook. Active learning skills increase the reader's chances of remembering important material. The NBDHE is constructed to test higher-level thinking skills (such as, analysis, synthesis, and application). Relating study material to information learned in the past is an important difference between critical thinking and simple memorization. Strategies to encourage active learning include:

- Ask yourself questions about material you have just studied. Predict how the material could be worded in the NBDHE.
- Form study groups to review, formulate, and ask questions to each other. Members should be willing to be actively

involved and devote sufficient time to the success of the group.
- Note key concepts and facts of importance. Note areas of weakness or uncertainty to emphasize study in these areas.
- Be interested and engaged in the material to improve learning.
- Use prepared test questions that are recent and relevant.
- Set a specific goal for each study period.
- Establish a schedule for each day and stick to the schedule.
- Schedule a 1- to 2-hour time period for studying with short 10-minute breaks every 20 minutes to increase retention of material.
- Write summaries of what you have studied, rephrasing the information so that you can better understand it.
- If information is confusing in one resource, check other textbooks or resources to see if there is a clearer explanation.
- Visualize or imagine how the information you have just read would look. How would a patient with those signs and symptoms look?
- Overlearn the material. Continuing to read and study even after the material is learned ensures less will be forgotten.
- Outline or map key material.

DEALING WITH TEST ANXIETY

Properly channeled, stress and anxiety can actually improve test-taking ability by increasing alertness and focus. Uncontrolled stress and anxiety can interfere with performance and negatively affect the performance of even the best candidate. Managing stress and anxiety effectively can be learned, although no one technique works for everyone. Taking specific steps to cope with and reduce anxiety-producing situations (such as studying and preparing for the board examinations) is the best way to reduce test anxiety. Other helpful hints for managing test anxiety include:

- Being well-prepared boosts confidence and test performance.
- Schedule study periods well in advance to avoid last minute panic.
- Maintain a positive attitude—94% of candidates are successful on the first attempt!
- Become familiar with the NBDHE by studying the contents of the *Candidate's Guide*.
- Regular exercise in the weeks before the examination reduces stress.
- Eat healthy foods and get plenty of rest in the time leading up to the exam.
- Accept the fact that you will not know everything.
- Replace negative thoughts with positive ones. Research has proven that positive imagery can be extremely helpful.

- The day and evening before the exam, plan a relaxing activity, such as seeing a movie with friends.

MASTERING THE MULTIPLE-CHOICE QUESTIONS

The components of multiple-choice questions include:
1. Stem: Poses a question or forms an incomplete statement. Usually you can determine what is being asked from the stem alone. Key words (such as best, most, first, or least) are usually emphasized in some way.
2. Distractors: The quality of the distractor determines the effectiveness of the question. Distractors often contain common misconceptions as well as responses that meet some but not all of the conditions posed in the stem.
3. Correct answer: Each test question will have only *one* option that is correct or clearly the *best* answer.

TEST-WISE STUDENTS

Being *test-wise* is the capacity to use the characteristics and formats of the test to achieve a higher score.

Test-taking is a skill that can be learned and improved like any other skill. A "test-wise" student is often able to find the correct response using context clues. Some principles that improve test-taking ability are:

- Use logic and common sense to determine the correct answer. Test items are usually based on typical situations that a dental hygienist would encounter, rather than rare or unusual findings. The most common response is usually the correct response.
- Uses cues in the stem and distractors to find the correct response.
- If a word is unfamiliar, try to find its meaning in the sentence context or divide the word into its prefix or suffix.
- Read each question thoroughly, but quickly. Do not read the question over and over. Select the response and move on. You can mark the question to come back to later.
- Read all options before deciding on the correct response. All responses will be plausible in a well-constructed test item, but it is important to choose the *best* response.
- Eliminate any distractors that are obviously incorrect.
- Do not make an item more difficult than it is or read anything into the meaning. Looking for tricks or hidden meaning is a waste of valuable test time.
- Relate each item to the stem to ensure that it fits the intent of the stem and is grammatically correct.
- Focus on key words in the stem.
- Select the most inclusive option. Between two similar options, choose the option with the most detail.

- In a long question, break the stem into smaller, manageable sections.
- Try answering the question before reading the distractors. This helps you find the correct response more quickly.
- Don't give up! If there are several questions in a row that are unfamiliar, move on to the items you know.
- Concentrate on one question at a time and do not worry about how many more questions remain.
- Focus on the intent of the question. Is it asking for a positive or negative response? Negative words (for example, *EXCEPT* or *NOT*) are usually emphasized in the stem to alert the reader to reverse the thought process.
- If there are calculations, work through each step of the process and then double-check the calculations.
- If a situation is unfamiliar, try to relate it to a situation that is familiar and determine which concepts would apply.
- Reword difficult questions to see if it helps with understanding.
- There is no penalty for guessing. Do not leave an item unanswered.

EXAMINATION DAY

A few tips to be prepared on the day of the examination include:

- Set multiple alarms to avoid oversleeping.
- Allow plenty of time for traffic, weather, and parking delays.
- Get up early enough to have a good breakfast with some protein.
- Dress comfortably in layers to adjust to temperature changes.
- Bring your admission card and valid photo identification card to the examination site.
- Leave all study materials and cell phones outside of the examination center.
- Arrive at least 15 minutes early. Most examination sites will not allow late arrivals.
- Anxiety is usually at its peak while waiting for the test to begin or in the first few minutes. To relax, take a few deep breaths and keep focused.
- Read the instructions slowly and carefully and follow all instructions exactly.

COMPONENTS OF THE NATIONAL BOARD DENTAL HYGIENE EXAMINATION

The purpose of the NBDHE is to "assess the ability to understand important information from basic biomedical, dental, and dental hygiene sciences, and the ability to apply such information in a problem-solving context." The NBDHE is designed to test the candidate's ability to apply the essential skills and knowledge as an entry-level safe practitioner regarding oral health care. The examination is based on the American Dental Education Association competencies for entry-level dental hygiene practice.

The NBDHE is computer-based and includes 350 multiple-choice questions in a variety of formats that are discussed later. Test items cover functions that a dental hygienist is expected to be able to perform, and only functions that may be legally delegated to a dental hygienist in a majority of states are included in the examination. The test is a comprehensive examination with two components.

Component A consists of 200 dental hygiene discipline-based questions offered in the first 3½-hour morning session. Component A covers three knowledge areas:

- Scientific basis for dental hygiene practice
- Provision of clinical dental hygiene services
- Community health/research principles

Component B is the second session that lasts 4 hours and presents 150 case-based items, which are related to no more than 15 dental hygiene patient cases. These cases contain information dealing with a variety of patients and include patient histories, dental charts, radiographs, and clinical photographs. Each examination contains at least one patient case of the following types: geriatric, adult-periodontal, pediatric, special needs, and medically compromised. The NBDHE defines a compromised patient as a patient whose health status requires modification of standard treatment or special treatment considerations. The purpose of these case-based items is to provide a simulation of actual clinical practice; these items are an application of the candidates' clinical experiences. Case-based items address the skills and knowledge required in each of the following areas:

- Assessing patient characteristics
- Obtaining and interpreting radiographs
- Planning and managing dental hygiene care
- Performing periodontal procedures
- Using preventive agents
- Providing supportive treatment service
- Professional responsibility

The patient history includes the following:

- Summary of the patient's history, sex, age, weight, and vitals
- Medical history with all pertinent information
- Dental history, including gingival condition, oral hygiene status, dental care, and concerns
  - Important information to know, such as tooth anatomy, Black's classifications of restoration and caries, and Angle's classification of malocclusion
  - Tooth numbers and letters for periodontics are on the chart
- Social history, tobacco and alcohol use, and occupational and social information
- Chief complaint: *Always address the chief complaint first!* (The only exception would be alleviation of pain.)

The clinical chart will represent the clinical findings. Carious lesions may be charted, but restorations usually are not. Periodontal probing depths, furcations, recession, attrition, plaque, and calculus may be included. Radiographs may be a complete series of periapical images, bitewing images, or panoramic images and will be labeled right or left. In addition, photos of study models and clinical photos may be included. Cases will include all relevant material, so *do not look for hidden information—it's in there!* There also may be extraneous information that has nothing to do with patient care, so disregard anything that is irrelevant to the case. Terminology is extremely important.

QUESTION FORMATS

This section gives examples of the two different question formats: traditional question formats and new question formats.*

Traditional Question Formats

Completion Format

In the completion format, the stem contains a statement that is completed by the addition of one of the options.

Question Format

In the question format, the stem contains a complete question. These are the most easily understood and most commonly used type of question.

Negative Format

The negative format is often used and contains a word (such as, EXCEPT, NOT, or LEAST), which is either capitalized or italicized in the stem. This type of question is useful for highlighting exemptions. *Helpful hint:* Underline the negative word.

Best Answer/Most Likely Answer Format

The best answer/most likely answer questions require careful attention and prioritizing. First, ask yourself, "What is the question asking?" Then answer it in your mind. Look for the responses and find the one that most closely matches your answer. Remember that there are often several responses that could work, but there is only one BEST answer.

Paired True/False Format

In this format, the stem is only part of the question that varies. The stem has two statements on the same topic, and the options have all of the possible variations. *Helpful hint:* Write T or F above each statement and then select the correct answer.

Cause-and-Effect Format

The cause-and-effect format is similar to the paired true/false format, because the only part of the question that changes is the stem. The stem contains a statement and a reason, and each is written as a separate statement and connected by "because."

Case Problems or "Testlets"

Case problems, or "testlets," are a variation of the old story problems we all loved so much in math!

A brief scenario, which is most commonly used in community health, is given, and the questions are based on the information presented. *Helpful hint:* All the information you need is within the scenario. Do not bring in extraneous factors.

New Question Formats

Three new question formats were introduced to the NBDHE in 2012. The new formats are ordering/sequence problems, extended matching, and multiple correct/multiple response. These formats are considered pretest questions and will not affect the candidate's results. However, these questions will be evaluated for statistical performance.

Ordering Format

These questions ask you to place the steps of a procedure in the correct order.

Matching Format

This is a variation of the multiple-choice question. A list of words or statements and a number of responses are listed with the correct word or statement to be matched with the correct response. This type of question works well with signs and symptoms that are linked to specific diseases or conditions.

Multiple Correct/Multiple Response Format

The multiple correct/multiple response format is used for determining what characteristics are associated with a specific disease, drug, treatment, or condition.

A FINAL TIP

Remember, you have spent the last several years preparing for this examination. Have confidence in yourself, prepare well, and you will succeed!

Barbara L. Bennett

*Consult the *NBDHE Guide* for examples of each question format.

Contents

PART 2   **COMPONENT B**

Component B practice is located on the companion Evolve website. See the inside front cover for details.

Scientific Basis for Dental Hygiene Practice

## CHAPTER 1

Anatomic Sciences

Vicki Gianopoulos, Ashley Martin Hale, Jodi L. Olmsted

QUESTIONS

1. Which paired muscle covers most of the lateral aspect
   of the ramus of the mandible?
   A. Temporalis
   B. Masseter
   C. Lateral pterygoid
   D. Medial pterygoid

2. During periodontal surgery, a fenestration is exposed
   on tooth #6. A fenestration is a defect of which type of
   bone?
   A. Compact
   B. Cancellous
   C. Interdental
   D. Interradicular

3. The fibrous connective tissue membrane covering the
   outside of bone is called the
   A. endosteum.
   B. periosteum.
   C. hyaline cartilage.
   D. articular cartilage.

4. What is the purpose of the synovial membrane in a
   synovial joint?
   A. Secrete fluid into the joint cavity
   B. Surround the joint like a fibrous sleeve
   C. Innervate the muscles that move the joint
   D. Convey a sense of position and movement

5. Which component of a nerve conducts impulses
   toward the cell body?
   A. Axon
   B. Soma
   C. Neuron
   D. Dendrite

6. Which spinal vertebrae fuse together to form a triangular mass?
   A. Sacral
   B. Lumbar
   C. Cervical
   D. Thoracic

7. The ophthalmic nerve is the first division of the fifth cranial nerve V, the trigeminal nerve. The maxillary nerve is the second division of the trigeminal nerve.
   A. Both statements are true.
   B. Both statements are false.
   C. The first statement is true, and the second statement is false.
   D. The first statement is false, and the second statement is true.

8. Which injections technique would be used to achieve anesthesia of teeth #15 and #16?
   A. Nasopalatine block
   B. Anterosuperior alveolar block
   C. Middle superior alveolar block
   D. Posterosuperior alveolar block

9. The infraorbital foramen is located in which bone?
   A. Frontal
   B. Maxilla
   C. Zygomatic
   D. Sphenoid

10. All of the following are foramina in the sphenoid bone EXCEPT the
    A. incisive foramen.
    B. superior orbital fissure.
    C. foramen ovale.
    D. foramen rotundum.

11. Which muscle retracts the tongue?
    A. Genioglossus
    B. Hyloglossus
    C. Styloglossus
    D. Palatoglossus

12. Which plane of dissection divides the body into anterior and posterior portions?
    A. Frontal
    B. Sagittal
    C. Horizontal
    D. Median

13. Teeth #3 and #14 are
    A. ipsilateral to each other.
    B. contralateral to each other.
    C. inferior to each other.
    D. superficial to each other.

14. The following characteristics describe muscle tissue EXCEPT one. Which one is the EXCEPTION?
    A. Each muscle has two ends.
    B. Muscle cells are called *sarcomeres*.
    C. Muscles are categorized according to their role in movement.
    D. The muscle origin is attached to the least movable part.
    E. The muscle insertion is attached to the most movable part.

15. Which lymph nodes drain both sides of the chin, the lower lip, the floor of mouth, the apex of tongue, and the mandibular incisors?
    A. Facial
    B. Submental
    C. Submandibular
    D. Retropharyngeal

16. Which endocrine gland matures T-lymphocytes for the immune system and undergoes involution (reduces in size) after puberty?
    A. Thyroid
    B. Thymus
    C. Pancreas
    D. Parathyroid

17. The corrugator supercilii is a muscle of facial expression in which region?
    A. Eye
    B. Nose
    C. Mouth
    D. Scalp

18. Which muscle elevates the mandible?
    A. Risorius
    B. Buccinator
    C. Medial pterygoid
    D. Lateral pterygoid

19. Which muscle originates from the alveolar process of the maxilla, the alveolar process of the mandible, and the pterygomandibular raphe?
    A. Masseter
    B. Risorius
    C. Buccinator
    D. Sternocleidomastoid

20. Which part of the brain regulates homeostasis?
    A. Medulla
    B. Thalamus
    C. Cerebellum
    D. Hypothalamus

21. Which branch of the trigeminal nerve contains both sensory and motor components?
    A. Ophthalmic V_1
    B. Maxillary V_2
    C. Mandibular V_3

22. Which of the following are the two main divisions or systems of the autonomic nervous system?
    A. Brain, spinal cord
    B. Afferent impulse, efferent impulse
    C. Sympathetic system, parasympathetic system

23. Which cranial nerve provides parasympathetic innervation to the cardiac muscles, thymus, and stomach?
    A. IV
    B. X
    C. XI
    D. XII

24. Which of the following is NOT innervated by the middle superior alveolar nerve?
    A. Tooth #4
    B. Tooth #12
    C. Distobuccal root of tooth #2
    D. Mesiobuccal root of tooth #14

25. The muscles of facial expression are innervated by which nerve?
    A. IV
    B. V
    C. VII
    D. VIII

26. Which vein receives blood flow from the superficial temporal vein and the facial vein and drains into the external jugular vein?
    A. Maxillary
    B. Ophthalmic
    C. Inferior alveolar
    D. Retromandibular

27. The articulation of the temporomandibular joint involves which two bones?
    A. Temporal bone, mental protuberance
    B. Sphenoid bone, coronoid process of the mandible
    C. Temporal bone, mandibular condyles

28. Which artery supplies the mandibular teeth and surrounding tissues with blood?
    A. Facial
    B. Lingual
    C. Inferior alveolar
    D. Pterygoid plexus

29. Which major artery supplies the brain with blood and is palpated during emergency situations?
    A. Aorta
    B. Subclavian
    C. Internal carotid
    D. Common carotid

30. Which artery is the source of the ophthalmic artery, has NO branches, and is located deep to the sternocleidomastoid muscle?
    A. Aorta
    B. Subclavian
    C. External carotid
    D. Internal carotid

31. The facial artery is a direct branch of which main artery?
    A. Subclavian
    B. Internal carotid
    C. External carotid
    D. Brachiocephalic

32. Which of the following arteries supplies maxillary anterior teeth with blood?
    A. Incisive
    B. Mylohyoid
    C. Greater palatine
    D. Anterior superior alveolar

33. The facial vein drains each region of the head and neck EXCEPT one. Which one is the EXCEPTION?
    A. Orbital region
    B. Upper lip area
    C. Lower lip area
    D. Submental region

34. Veins of teeth have alveolar branches and dental branches. Which branch type would drain the pulp tissue of teeth through the apical foramen?
    A. Alveolar branches
    B. Dental branches
    C. Both A and B
    D. Neither A nor B

35. Which vein has NO valves, drains most of the head and neck region, and does NOT drain any of the dentition?
    A. Internal jugular
    B. External jugular
    C. Internal maxillary
    D. Inferior alveolar

36. Many veins in the head and neck region lack valves. Valveless veins of the head and neck contribute to the severe and rapid spread of dental infections.
    A. Both statements are true.
    B. Both statements are false.
    C. The first statement is true, and the second statement is false.
    D. The first statement is false, and the second statement is true.

37. Each of the following is an afferent cranial nerve EXCEPT one. Which one is the EXCEPTION?
    A. Optic
    B. Vagus
    C. Olfactory
    D. Hypoglossal

38. Which muscle, upon contraction, protrudes the tongue?
    A. Genioglossus
    B. Hyloglossus
    C. Styloglossus

39. Each of the following is a suprahyoid muscle EXCEPT one. Which one is the EXCEPTION?
    A. Mylohyoid
    B. Geniohyoid
    C. Stylohyoid
    D. Sternohyoid

40. Cervical lymph nodes run along which muscle?
    A. Trapezius
    B. Buccinator
    C. Epicranial
    D. Sternocleidomastoid

41. For each numbered muscle, select the most closely linked facial expression from the list provided.

Muscles of Facial Expression	Facial Expression upon Contraction of Muscle
1. Mentalis	A. Frowning
2. Risorius	B. Raising chin and protruding lower lip
3. Corrugator supercilii	C. Chewing
4. Levator anguli oris	D. Stretching lips
5. Buccinator	E. Smiling

42. For each numbered structure, select the most closely linked primary nodes that drain those structures from the list provided.

Anatomic Structure	Lymph Node Drainage
1. Sublingual salivary gland	A. Deep parotid
2. Parotid salivary gland	B. Submandibular
3. Base of tongue	C. Superior deep cervical
4. Paranasal sinus	D. Submental
5. Lower lip	E. Retropharyngeal

43. For each numbered temporomandibular joint (TMJ) disk position, select the most closely linked description of the movement from the list provided.

TMJ Disk Positions	Movement
1. Elevation	A. Shifting the mandible to one side by unilateral contraction of the lateral pterygoid muscle
2. Lateral deviation	B. Opening the mouth by contraction of the inferior heads of the lateral pterygoid muscles and the suprahyoid muscles
3. Retraction	C. Moving the jaw forward by bilateral contraction of the lateral pterygoid muscles
4. Protrusion	D. Raising the lower jaw by contraction of all portions of the temporalis, masseter, and medial pterygoid muscles
5. Depression	E. Moving the jaw back by contraction of the posterior portions of both temporalis muscles

44. The first branchial arch is also called the *mandibular arch*. The cartilage forming within the mandibular arch is known as *Reichert cartilage.*
    A. Both statements are true.
    B. Both statements are false.
    C. The first statement is true, and the second statement is false.
    D. The first statement is false, and the second statement is true.

45. Each of the following is a period of prenatal development EXCEPT one. Which one is the EXCEPTION?
    A. Fetal
    B. Ovulation
    C. Embryonic
    D. Preimplantation

46. Which cells are responsible for producing dentin?
    A. Osteoblasts
    B. Ameloblasts
    C. Odontoblasts
    D. Cementoblasts

47. Each of the following is a component of the tooth germ EXCEPT one. Which one is the EXCEPTION?
    A. Enamel organ
    B. Dental sac
    C. Dental lamina
    D. Dental papilla
    E. Dental follicle

48. Order the stages of odontogenesis. Match each letter with its proper sequence number.
    ___ A. Cap stage
    ___ B. Bud stage
    ___ C. Bell stage
    ___ D. Maturation stage
    ___ E. Initiation stage

49. Division of a cell into two daughter cells occurs during which phase of mitosis?
    A. Prophase
    B. Anaphase
    C. Metaphase
    D. Telophase

50. The inner cells of the dental papilla will develop into which structure?
    A. Cementum
    B. Dentin
    C. Pulp
    D. Enamel

51. The earliest indication of a part or an organ during prenatal development is referred to as the
    A. primordium.
    B. stomodeum.
    C. zygote.
    D. nucleus.

52. Which primordial structure differentiates into the ameloblasts that produce enamel?
    A. Outer enamel epithelium
    B. Stellate reticulum
    C. Inner enamel epithelium
    D. Stratum intermedium

53. Which stage of tooth development occurs between the 11th and 12th weeks of prenatal development?
    A. Bud
    B. Cap
    C. Bell
    D. Initiation

54. Which of the following cells is/are DIRECTLY responsible for immunoglobulin production?
    A. Plasma
    B. Basophils
    C. Monocytes
    D. Neutrophils
    E. Eosinophils

55. Incremental lines that stain brown in preparations of mature enamel are
    A. neonatal lines.
    B. enamel tufts.
    C. lines of Retzius.
    D. enamel spindles.
    E. enamel lamellae.

56. Which period of prenatal development occurs during months 3 to 9?
    A. Fetal
    B. Embryonic
    C. Preimplantation
    D. A only
    E. Both A and B

57. From the following list, select the structures of the embryo that begin development in week 4 of prenatal development.
    A. Face
    B. Neck
    C. Palate
    D. Tongue
    E. Placenta

58. Each cell facilitates the exfoliation of a primary tooth EXCEPT one. Which one is the EXCEPTION?
    A. Ameloblast
    B. Osteoclast
    C. Odontoclast
    D. Cementoclast

59. The cervical loop is responsible for development of
    A. dentin.
    B. pulp.
    C. enamel.
    D. root.

60. Down syndrome is a developmental disturbance that occurs during which period of prenatal development?
    A. Fetal
    B. Embryonic
    C. Preimplantation

61. The incomplete developmental division of a tooth germ is called FUSION. Fusion takes place during the initiation stage of tooth development.
    A. Both statements are true.
    B. Both statements are false.
    C. The first statement is true, and the second statement is false.
    D. The first statement is false, and the second statement is true.

62. Which is the most common cell found in the lamina propria of the oral mucosa?
    A. Epiblast
    B. Odontoblast
    C. Osteoblast
    D. Osteoclast
    E. Fibroblast

63. The cells responsible for the development of the periodontal ligament come from the
    A. dental sac.
    B. dental papilla.
    C. enamel organ.
    D. successional lamellae.

64. The cusp of Carabelli is found on which permanent molars?
    A. #3, #14
    B. #2, #15
    C. #19, #30
    D. #18, #31

65. Eight bones compose the neurocranium, surrounding the brain. Fifteen bones compose the viscerocranium, or the bones of the face.
    A. Both statements are true.
    B. Both statements are false.
    C. The first statement is true, and the second statement is false.
    D. The first statement is false, and the second statement is true.

66. The sphenoid bone is composed of the
    A. palatine process.
    B. temporal fossa.
    C. superior orbital fissure of the orbit.
    D. base of skull anterior to occipital bone.
    E. B, C, and D.

67. Anatomically, the inferior alveolar artery supplies which structure?
    A. Soft floor of mouth
    B. Tongue muscles
    C. Sublingual gland
    D. Mandibular teeth

68. The functions of the lymphatic system include all EXCEPT one. Which one is the EXCEPTION?
    A. Filter fluids
    B. Fight infection
    C. Produce lymphocytes
    D. Produce thrombocytes
    E. Return plasma to venous bloodstream

69. For each division of the trigeminal nerve (V) listed, select its appropriate name from the list provided.

Trigeminal Nerve Division	Name
____ 1. Division I	A. Maxillary
____ 2. Division II	B. Mandibular
____ 3. Division III	C. Ophthalmic

70. The abducens (VI), trochlear (IV), and oculomotor (III) nerves all provide innervation to the muscles of the eye. These nerves provide sensory innervation.
    A. Both statements are true.
    B. Both statements are false.
    C. The first statement is true, and the second statement is false.
    D. The first statement is false, and the second statement is true.

71. Match each germ layer listed to the structure it forms in the developing embryo.

Germ Layer	Structure Formed in Embryo
____ 1. Endoderm	A. Gastrointestinal tract, epithelium, and associated glands
____ 2. Mesoderm	B. Nervous system, epidermis, sensory epithelium of the eye, ear, and nose; tooth enamel; and oral epithelium
____ 3. Ectoderm	C. Muscles, bone, cartilage, blood, dentin, pulp, cementum, and periodontal ligament

72. For each of the developing branchial arches listed, select the most appropriate anatomic structure that it gives rise to.

Developing Branchial Arch	Resulting Structure
____ 1. Mandibular arch (branchial I)	A. Muscles of facial expression, cranial nerve VII
____ 2. Hyoid arch (branchial II)	B. Tongue, cranial nerve IX
____ 3. Branchial arch III	C. Muscles of throat, inferior hyoid cartilage, cranial nerve X
____ 4. Branchial arch IV	D. Mandible, muscles of mastication, cranial nerve V

73. Match each cell type to the structure it forms.

Cell Type	Resulting Structure
____ 1. Ameloblasts	A. Cementum
____ 2. Cementoblasts	B. Dentin
____ 3. Odontoblasts	C. Alveolar bone
____ 4. Dental follicle	D. Enamel

74. The temporomandibular joint (TMJ) is capable of which two types of movement?
    A. Rotation, gliding
    B. Hinge, translation
    C. Pivot, ball and socket
    D. Ball and socket, saddle

75. Which arteries are the terminal branches of the external carotid artery?
    A. Superior thyroid, lingual
    B. Facial, ascending pharyngeal
    C. Posterior auricular and occipital
    D. Maxillary, superficial temporal

76. A hematoma that results from the administration of a posterior superior alveolar (PSA) nerve block is caused by bleeding from which arteries or veins?
    1. Posterior superior alveolar artery
    2. Pterygoid plexus of veins
    3. Temporal artery
    4. Facial artery
    5. Maxillary vein
    6. Posterior retromandibular vein
       A. 1, 2, 5
       B. 2, 3, 4
       C. 3, 4, 6
       D. 1, 2, 4

77. How many teeth are present in an individual with a full deciduous dentition?
    A. 20
    B. 24
    C. 28
    D. 32

78. Which is NOT a characteristic feature of the primary dentition?
    A. Thin enamel
    B. Thin dentin
    C. Large pulp cavity
    D. Whiter in color than permanent dentition

79. Which teeth have wider crowns mesiodistally than faciolingually?
    A. #5 and #12
    B. #7 and #10
    C. #24 and #25
    D. #23 and #26

80. Each is an important function of the cementoenamel junction (CEJ) EXCEPT one. Which one is the EXCEPTION?
    A. Prevention of caries
    B. Self-cleansing properties
    C. Food deflection resulting in gingival inflammation
    D. Health and maintenance of periodontal tissue in interproximal spaces

81. Match each dental anomaly listed with its description.

Dental Anomaly	Description
____ 1. Dwarf roots	A. Partial splitting of tooth germ
____ 2. Concrescence	B. Crown or root demonstrating sharp bends, curves
____ 3. Dilaceration	C. Fusion after root formation
____ 4. Mulberry molars	D. Extreme condition impacting crown-to-root ratio
____ 5. Gemination	E. Result of congenital syphilis
____ 6. Dens in dente	F. Tooth within a tooth

82. The clinical crown-to-root ratio is always the same. However, the anatomic crown–to-root ratio may change.
    A. Both statements are true.
    B. Both statements are false.
    C. The first statement is true, and the second statement is false.
    D. The first statement is false, and the second statement is true.

83. There is relatively constant mesial movement of the molars to compensate for proximal abrasion. Relatively consistent occlusal forces result in bone remodeling.
    A. Both statements are correct and related.
    B. Both statements are correct but NOT related.
    C. The first statement is correct, but the second is NOT.
    D. The first statement is NOT correct, but second is correct.
    E. Both statements are incorrect and unrelated.

84. Enamel is formed by ameloblasts, which are derived from the ectoderm. The ectoderm also signals the mesoderm to start the development of dentin and pulp.
    A. Both statements are true.
    B. Both statements are false.
    C. The first statement is true, and the second statement is false.
    D. The first statement is false, and the second statement is true.

85. Cellular metabolism occurs in the
    A. ribosomes.
    B. lysosome.
    C. mitochondria.
    D. Golgi apparatus.
    E. endoplasmic reticulum.

86. During facial development, the two structures forming the major facial structures are the frontonasal process and the pharyngeal (branchial) arch I. This process begins during week 6 in utero.
    A. Both statements are true.
    B. Both statements are false.
    C. The first statement is true, and the second statement is false.
    D. The first statement is false, and the second statement is true.

87. Each is a paranasal sinus EXCEPT one. Which one is the EXCEPTION?
    A. Frontal
    B. Mandibular
    C. Maxillary
    D. Sphenoidal
    E. Ethmoidal

88. Which muscle involved in facial expression does not have a bony attachment, shapes and controls the size of the mouth opening, and helps create lip positions and movements during speech?
    A. Risorius
    B. Zygomaticus major
    C. Orbicularis oris
    D. Levator anguli oris

89. Each is an anterior branch of the external carotid artery EXCEPT one. Which one is the EXCEPTION?
    A. Occipital
    B. Superior thyroid
    C. Facial
    D. Lingual

90. Which gland is associated with dry eye syndrome, (DES), also known as *keratoconjunctivitis sicca?* (KCS)?
    A. Thyroid
    B. Thymus
    C. Lacrimal
    D. Parathyroid

91. The face and its related tissues begin to form during week 6 of prenatal development, within the fetal period. Facial development is completed by week 12.
    A. Both statements are true.
    B. Both statements are false.
    C. The first statement is true and the second statement is false.
    D. The first statement is false, and the second statement is true.

92. Which developmental disturbance appears as a "tooth within a tooth" on radiologic examination?
    A. Fusion
    B. Tubercles
    C. Gemination
    D. Dens in dente

93. Each is a type of connective tissue EXCEPT one. Which one is the EXCEPTION?
    A. Bone
    B. Blood
    C. Muscle
    D. Cartilage

94. Enamel may be lost through attrition, abrasion, erosion, caries, or abfraction. Radiographically, enamel appears more radiolucent than dentin or pulp, both of which appear more radiopaque.
    A. Both statements are true.
    B. Both statements are false.
    C. The first statement is true, and the second statement is false.
    D. The first statement is false, and the second statement is true.

95. Which acronym defines the correct sequence of words used to describe a tooth?
    A. D-T-A-Q
    B. D-A-C-T
    C. C-A-D-Q
    D. D-A-Q-T

96. How many permanent anterior teeth are present in an adult mouth?
    A. 6
    B. 8
    C. 10
    D. 12

97. Which tooth numbers represent maxillary first premolars?
    A. #5 and #12
    B. #4 and #13
    C. #21 and #28
    D. #24 and #25

98. Which statement is correct? (Select all that apply.)
    A. Maxillary second premolars are bifurcated with a buccal and palatal root.
    B. Mandibular molars are bifurcated with a mesial and distal root.
    C. Maxillary molars are trifurcated with a mesiobuccal, distobuccal, and palatal root.
    D. Maxillary first premolars are bifurcated with a buccal and palatal root.

1. Which paired muscle covers most of the lateral aspect of the ramus of the mandible?

ANS: B
The masseter (B) muscle is located on the lateral aspect of the ramus of the mandible. The temporalis (A) muscle is a large, fan-shaped muscle attached to the coronoid process of the mandible. The lateral pterygoid (C) has two heads and lies superiorly to the medial pterygoid. The medial pterygoid (D) inserts on the medial surface of the mandibular ramus. All these muscles are muscles of mastication.

2. During periodontal surgery, a fenestration is exposed on tooth #6. A fenestration is a defect of which type of bone?

ANS: A
A fenestration is an opening or window in the solid plate of compact (A) cortical bone on the facial surface over the root of a tooth. Cancellous (B) bone is located between the alveolar bone proper and the plates of cortical bone. The interdental septum (C) is bone located between the roots of adjacent teeth. Interradicular (D) bone is located between the roots of the same tooth.

3. The fibrous connective tissue membrane covering the outside of bone is called the

ANS: B
Periosteum (B) is the fibrous connective tissue membrane covering the outside of bone except at the articular surfaces. Endosteum (A) is the connective tissue membrane lining the marrow cavity of the bone. Hyaline cartilage (C) is a flexible and slightly elastic cartilage found in joints, costal cartilages, the nasal septum, the larynx, and the trachea. Articular cartilage (D) is specialized, thin, smooth hyaline cartilage found on the joint surfaces of bones, for example, in a synovial joint.

4. What is the purpose of the synovial membrane in a synovial joint?

ANS: A
The synovial membrane secretes synovial fluid (A), which lubricates the synovial joint. The capsular ligament surrounds the joint like a fibrous sleeve (B). The sensory nerve endings innervate the muscles that move the joint (C). Proprioceptive nerve endings convey a sense of position and movement (D).

5. Which component of a nerve conducts impulses toward the cell body?

ANS: D
Dendrites (D) are branching cellular extensions of a nerve that conduct impulses toward the cell. An axon (A) is a cellular extension of a nerve that conducts impulses away from the cell. The soma (B) is the body of the cell containing the nucleus. A neuron (C) is the basic functional unit of the nervous system.

6. Which spinal vertebrae fuse together to form a triangular mass?

ANS: A
The sacral (A) vertebrae of the spinal cord fuse together to form a triangular mass, called the *sacrum*. The lumbar (B) region comprises the five large vertebrae located between the thoracic and sacral regions. The cervical (C) region comprises the seven vertebrae located between the base of the neck and the thoracic region. The thoracic (D) region comprises the 12 vertebrae between the cervical and lumbar regions.

7. The ophthalmic nerve is the first division of the fifth cranial nerve V, the trigeminal nerve. The maxillary nerve is the second division of the trigeminal nerve.

ANS: A
Both statements are true (A). Cranial nerve V is the trigeminal nerve, of which the ophthalmic nerve is the first division (V_1) and the maxillary nerve is the second division (V_2). The third division of the trigeminal nerve (V_3) is the mandibular nerve. Choices B, C, and D do not accurately reflect the statements.

8. Which injections technique would be used to achieve anesthesia of teeth #15 and #16?

ANS: D
The posterosuperior alveolar block (D) anesthetizes the mesiobuccal root of the first maxillary molar and the second and third maxillary molars. The nasopalatine block (A) anesthetizes the premaxillary area of the palate and the anterior maxillary teeth. The anterosuperior alveolar block (B) anesthetizes the gingiva and the anterior maxillary teeth. The middle superior alveolar block (C) anesthetizes the premolars and the mesiobuccal root of the first maxillary molar.

26. Which vein receives blood flow from the superficial temporal vein and the facial vein and drains into the external jugular vein?

    ANS: D
    The retromandibular (D) vein receives blood flow from the superficial temporal vein and the facial vein and drains into the external jugular vein. It is situated immediately posterior to the angle of the mandible. The maxillary vein (A) receives blood flow from the pterygoid plexus and drains into the retromandibular vein. The ophthalmic vein (B) drains the tissue of the orbit and proceeds into the facial vein. The inferior alveolar vein (C) forms from the merging of the dental, alveolar, and mental branches and drains into the pterygoid plexus.

27. The articulation of the temporomandibular joint involves which two bones?

    ANS: C
    Temporal bone and mandibular condyle (C) articulate to form part of the temporomandibular joint. Neither temporal bone and mental protuberance (A) nor sphenoid bone and the coronoid process of the mandible (B) articulate with each other.

28. Which artery supplies the mandibular teeth and surrounding tissues with blood?

    ANS: C
    The inferior alveolar artery (C) is a branch of the maxillary artery and supplies the mandibular teeth, the floor of the mouth, and the mental region with blood. The facial artery (A) is also known as the *external maxillary artery* and extends to the mid-face region to supply the oral, buccal, zygomatic, nasal, infraorbital, and orbital regions. The lingual artery (B) is an anterior branch from the external carotid artery and supplies the tissue superior to hyoid bone, including the suprahyoid muscles and the floor of the mouth. The pterygoid plexus (D) supplies the deep facial areas and the posterosuperior alveolar vein and the inferior alveolar vein.

29. Which major artery supplies the brain with blood and is palpated during emergency situations?

    ANS: D
    The common carotid artery (D) runs superiorly along the neck, lateral to the trachea and the larynx. When palpated against the larynx, the most reliable arterial pulse of the body can be monitored. The aorta (A) is a major artery, which gives rise to the common carotid artery and the subclavian artery (B) on the left side of the heart and the brachiocephalic artery on the right side of the heart. The internal carotid artery (C) supplies the anterior part of the brain and the eye and sends branches to the forehead and the nose. The aorta (A), the subclavian artery (B), and the internal carotid artery (C) cannot be reliably palpated in an emergency.

30. Which artery is the source of the ophthalmic artery, has NO branches, and is located deep to the sternocleidomastoid muscle?

    ANS: D
    The internal carotid artery (D) is a branchless division of the common carotid artery, which is covered by the sternocleidomastoid muscle, and supplies blood to the ophthalmic artery. The aorta (A), a major artery that is a portion of the heart itself gives rise to the common carotid artery and the subclavian artery (B) on the left side of the heart and the brachiocephalic artery on the right side of the heart. The external carotid artery (C) travels superiorly to the internal carotid artery and has four sets of branches.

31. The facial artery is a direct branch of which main artery?

    ANS: C
    The facial artery is the final anterior branch from the external carotid artery (C), not the subclavian artery (A), the internal carotid artery (B), or the brachiocephalic artery (D).

32. Which of the following arteries supplies maxillary anterior teeth with blood?

    ANS: D
    Maxillary anterior teeth are supplied by the anterosuperior alveolar artery (D). The incisive artery (A) supplies the periodontium of the mandibular anterior teeth, including the associated gingiva. The mylohyoid artery (B) supplies the floor of the mouth and the mylohyoid muscle. The greater palatine artery (C) supplies the hard and soft palates.

33. The facial vein drains each region of the head and neck EXCEPT one. Which one is the EXCEPTION?

    ANS: A
    The orbital region (A) is drained by the cavernous sinus and the pterygoid plexus, not the facial vein. The facial vein drains the upper lip (B), the lower lip (C), and the submental region (D).

34. Veins of teeth have alveolar branches and dental branches. Which branch type would drain the pulp tissue of teeth through the apical foramen?

    ANS: B
    The incisive artery branches off the inferior alveolar artery, remaining within the mandibular canal to divide

into dental and alveolar branches. The dental branches (B) of the pulp drain the mandibular anterior teeth by way of each tooth's apical foramen. The alveolar branches (A) of the periodontium drain the mandibular anterior teeth, including the gingiva. Choices C and D do not correctly address the statement.

35. Which vein has NO valves, drains most of the head and neck region, and does NOT drain any of the dentition?

ANS: A
The internal jugular vein (A) drains most of the head and the neck, except the dentition. The external jugular vein (B) is the only vein the head and neck with valves. The internal maxillary vein (C) drains the pterygoid plexus, whereas the inferior alveolar vein (D) drains the mandibular teeth and the periodontium.

36. Many veins in the head and neck region lack valves. Valveless veins of the head and neck contribute to the severe and rapid spread of dental infections.

ANS: A
The correct choice is A; both statements are true. Most veins in the head and neck lack valves, with the exception of the external jugular vein. The lack of valves in the veins of the head and neck may contribute to severe and rapid spread of dental infections. Choices B, C, and D do not correctly reflect the statements.

37. Each of the following is an afferent cranial nerve EXCEPT one. Which one is the EXCEPTION?

ANS: D
The hypoglossal nerve (D) is an efferent (motor) cranial nerve for both intrinsic and extrinsic muscles of the tongue. The optic nerve (A), the vagus nerve (B), and the olfactory nerve (C) are afferent, or sensory, nerves.

38. Which muscle, upon contraction, protrudes the tongue?

ANS: A
The genioglossus muscle (A) protrudes the tongue upon contraction. The hyloglossus muscle (B) depresses the tongue when it contracts. Upon contraction, the styloglossus muscle (C) retracts the tongue.

39. Each of the following is a suprahyoid muscle EXCEPT one. Which one is the EXCEPTION?

ANS: D
The sternohyoid muscle (D) is an infrahyoid muscle. The mylohyoid (A), geniohyoid muscle (B), and stylohyoid (C) muscles are all suprahyoid muscles.

40. Cervical lymph nodes run along which muscle?

ANS: D
The sternocleidomastoid muscle (D) is a landmark of the neck during the extraoral examination to define locations of superficial and deep cervical lymph nodes. Cervical lymph nodes do not lie adjacent to the trapezius (A), buccinator (B), or epicranial (C) muscles.

41. For each numbered muscle, select the most closely linked facial expression from the list provided.

ANS: 1B; 2D; 3A; 4E; 5C
When the mentalis muscle (1) contracts, the chin is raised and the lower lip protrudes (B). When the risorius muscle (2) contracts, the lips are stretched (D). When the corrugator supercilii (3) contracts, this action produces a frown (A). When the levator anguli oris (4) contracts, this action produces a smile (E). When the buccinator (5) contracts, food is pushed onto the occlusal plane, facilitating the chewing of food (C).

42. For each numbered structure, select the most closely linked primary nodes that drain those structures from the list provided.

ANS: 1B; 2C; 3E; 4A; 5D
The sublingual salivary gland (1) is drained by the submandibular lymph node (B). The parotid salivary gland (2) is drained by the superior deep cervical lymph node (C). The base of the tongue (3) is drained by the retropharyngeal lymph node (E). The paranasal sinus (4) is drained by the deep parotid lymph node (A). The lower lip (5) is drained by the submental lymph node (D).

43. For each numbered temporomandibular joint (TMJ) disk position, select the most closely linked description of the movement from the list provided.

ANS: 1D; 2A; 3E; 4C; 5B
Elevation of the TMJ disk (1) results in the raising of the lower jaw through contraction of all portions of the temporalis, masseter, and medial pterygoid muscles (D). Lateral deviation of the TMJ disk (2) results in shifting of the mandible to one side via unilateral contraction of the lateral pterygoid muscle (A). Retraction of the TMJ disk (3) results in backward jaw movement through contraction of posterior portions of both temporalis muscles (E). Protrusion of the TMJ disk (4) produces forward jaw movement through bilateral contraction of the lateral pterygoid muscles (C). Depression of the TMJ disk (5) produces opening of the mouth through contraction of the inferior heads of the lateral pterygoid and suprahyoid muscles (B).

44. The first branchial arch is also called the *mandibular arch*. The cartilage forming within the mandibular arch is known as *Reichert cartilage*.

   ANS: C
   Choice C is correct; the first statement is true, and the second statement is false. There are six branchial arches. The first branchial arch is considered the *mandibular arch*, and the second branchial arch is known as the *hyoid arch*. The cartilage that forms within the mandibular arch is Meckel cartilage, not Reichert cartilage, which forms in the second branchial arch. Choices A, B, and D do not correctly reflect the statements.

45. Each of the following is a period of prenatal development EXCEPT one. Which one is the EXCEPTION?

   ANS: B
   The ovulation period (B) occurs during a woman's menstrual cycle with the release of an ovum. The unfertilized egg is not part of prenatal development. The three distinct periods of prenatal development are the preimplantation period (D), occurring during the first week after fertilization; the embryonic period (C), occurring during the second to the eighth week; and the fetal period (A), which occurs from the third to the ninth month.

46. Which cells are responsible for producing dentin?

   ANS: C
   Odontoblasts (C) are responsible for producing dentin. Osteoblasts (A) are bone-producing cells. Ameloblasts (B) produce enamel and cementoblasts (D) produce cementum.

47. Each of the following is a component of the tooth germ EXCEPT one. Which one is the EXCEPTION?

   ANS: C
   The dental lamina (C) is not part of the tooth germ, although the proliferation of ectodermal cells into specific sites is the first stage of odontogenesis. This thickened sheet of epithelium will give way to become the enamel organ. The three components that make up the tooth germ are the enamel organ (A), the dental sac (B), and the dental papilla (D). DENTAL FOLLICLE (E) is another term for dental sac.

48. Order the stages of odontogenesis. Match each letter with its proper sequence number.

   ANS: 1E; 2B; 3A; 4C; 5D
   Odontogenesis begins with the initiation stage (1E) during the sixth to the seventh week. Next is the bud stage (2B), beginning in the eighth week, which is followed by the cap stage (3A) during weeks nine and ten. During the eleventh and twelfth weeks, the bell stage (4C) occurs, and the final stage of odontogenesis is the maturation stage (5D).

49. Division of a cell into two daughter cells occurs during which phase of mitosis?

   ANS: D
   Telophase (D) is the last phase in which the individual cell divides into two daughter cells. During prophase (A), the DNA (deoxyribonucleic acid) in the form of chromatin condenses into chromosomes. During metaphase (C), the chromosomes move and align themselves in the middle of the cell. Next is anaphase (B), during which the chromosomes separate and migrate to opposite poles of the cell.

50. The inner cells of the dental papilla will develop into which structure?

   ANS: C
   The inner cells of the dental papilla develop into dental pulp (C). Cementum (A) is produced by cementocytes that come from the dental sac. Dentin (B) is produced by the outer cells of the dental papilla. Enamel (D) is produced by ameloblast cells that come from the enamel organ.

51. The earliest indication of a part or an organ during prenatal development is referred to as the

   ANS: A
   The primordium (A) is the earliest indication of a part or an organ during prenatal development. The stomodeum (B) is also known as the *primitive mouth* and begins as just a slight depression but subsequently will give rise to the oral cavity. A zygote (C) is a fertilized egg, resulting from the union of a man's sperm and a woman's ovum. A nucleus (D) is a large organelle found in most cells, responsible for the regulation of all cellular function.

52. Which primordial structure differentiates into the ameloblasts that produce enamel?

   ANS: C
   Inner enamel epithelium (IEE) (C) comprises the columnar cells of the enamel organ that differentiate into ameloblasts. The outer enamel epithelium (OEE) (A) comprises cuboidal cells that protect the outer portion of the enamel organ. Between the IEE and OEE is the stellate reticulum (B), composed of star-shaped cells, and the stratum intermedium (D), composed of flat to cube-shaped cells; both support the production of enamel.

53. Which stage of tooth development occurs between the 11th and 12th weeks of prenatal development?

ANS: C
The bell stage (C) occurs between weeks 11 and 12 of prenatal development. The initiation stage (D) occurs between weeks 6 and 7 of tooth development. The bud stage (A) occurs during week 8, whereas the cap stage (B) happens between weeks 9 and 10.

54. Which of the following cells is/are DIRECTLY responsible for immunoglobulin production?

ANS: A
Activated B-cell lymphocytes form plasma cells (A), which are directly responsible for producing immunoglobulins (antibodies). Basophils (B), monocytes (C), neutrophils (D), and eosinophils (E) are all white blood cells, and all contribute to the immune response. A lymphocyte is a white blood cell that has three functional types, one of which is a B-cell lymphocyte.

55. Incremental lines that stain brown in preparations of mature enamel are

ANS: C
Incremental lines that stain brown in preparations of mature enamel are lines of Retzius (C). The neonatal line (A) is an incremental line of Retzius; however, it is more pronounced and marks trauma or stress placed on ameloblasts during birth. Enamel tufts (B) appear as small, dark hypocalcified, brushlike areas found near the dentinoenamel junction (DEJ). Enamel spindles (D) are actually short dentinal tubules that have been trapped in the enamel matrix. Enamel lamellae (E) extend from the DEJ all the way out to the occlusal surface and are partially calcified sheets of enamel matrix.

56. Which period of prenatal development occurs during months 3 to 9?

ANS: A
The final period of prenatal development is the fetal period (A), which spans months 3 to 9 or delivery. After fertilization, the zygote travels along until it implants itself into the uterus. This period is known as the PREIMPLANTATION PERIOD (C), which occurs during week 1. The embryonic period (B) follows during weeks 2 through 8. Choices D and E do not correctly address the statement.

57. From the following list, select the structures of the embryo that begin development in week 4 of prenatal development.

ANS: A, B, D
Facial development (A) begins during week 4 and continues into week 12. The neck (B) and the tongue (D) begin to develop in conjunction with the face. The placenta (E) begins development during week 2 from the interaction of the trophoblast layer and the endometrial tissues. The palate (C) begins formation during week 5 and also continues through week 12.

58. Each cell facilitates the exfoliation of a primary tooth EXCEPT one. Which one is the EXCEPTION?

ANS: A
The ameloblast (A) is the enamel-producing cell that does not facilitate exfoliation of teeth. The osteoclast (B) is necessary to resorb the alveolar bone anchoring the tooth. The odontoclast (C) is responsible for resorption of dentin. The cementoclast (D) is responsible for the resorption of cementum.

59. The cervical loop is responsible for development of

ANS: D
The cervical loop is responsible for root (D) development. Dentin (A) is developed from odontoblasts. Pulp (B) develops from the inner cells of the dental papilla. The enamel of the crown of the tooth (C) is formed from ameloblasts.

60. Down syndrome is a developmental disturbance that occurs during which period of prenatal development?

ANS: C
Down syndrome is a developmental disturbance that occurs during meiosis. The final stages of meiosis occur just after fertilization, which takes place during the preimplantation (C) period. The division of chromosomes occurs prior to the zygote being implanted and has already taken place by the embryonic (B) or fetal (A) periods.

61. The incomplete developmental division of a tooth germ is called FUSION. Fusion takes place during the initiation stage of tooth development.

ANS: B
Both statements are false (B). Fusion is the union of two tooth germs. Incomplete tooth germ division is referred to as GEMINATION. Fusion takes place during the cap stage of odontogenesis, not during the initiation stage. Choices A, C, and D do not accurately reflect the statements.

62. Which is the most common cell found in the lamina propria of the oral mucosa?

    ANS: E
    The fibroblast (E) is the most common cell found in the lamina propria of the oral mucosa. Epiblast (A) layers are high-columnar cells of the bilaminar embryonic disk. The odontoblast (B) is the cell that will produce dentin. The osteoblast (C) is a bone-forming cell, and the osteoclast (D) is a bone-resorbing cell.

63. The cells responsible for the development of the periodontal ligament come from the

    ANS: A
    The dental sac or follicle (A) consists of ectomesenchyme that surrounds the enamel organ and will produce not only the periodontal ligament but also cementum and alveolar bone. The dental papilla (B) has inner cells that will produce the pulp and outer cells that will produce dentin. The enamel organ (C) will produce enamel. The successional lamellae (D) comprise the epithelial tissue that will give rise to succedaneous teeth.

64. The cusp of Carabelli is found on which permanent molars?

    ANS: A
    The cusp of Carabelli is found on the lingual surface of maxillary first molars, which includes #3 and #14 (A). Teeth #2 and #15 (B) are maxillary second molars; #19 and #30 (C) are mandibular first molars; and #18 and #31 (D) are mandibular second molars.

65. Eight bones compose the neurocranium, surrounding the brain. Fifteen bones compose the viscerocranium, or the bones of the face.

    ANS: C
    The correct answer is (C); the first statement is true, and the second statement is false. Eight bones compose the neurocranium: the frontal, the sphenoid, the ethmoid, and the occipital bones, which are single bones. The paired temporal and parietal bones also are part of the neurocranium. The second statement is false. There are 14 bones, not 15, that make up the viscerocranium, including the single mandible and the vomer. The paired nasal, lacrimal, zygomatic, inferior nasal conchae, palatine, and maxillae are the remaining bones composing the face. Choices A, B, and D do not accurately reflect the statements.

66. The sphenoid bone is composed of the

    ANS: E
    The correct answer is (E). The complex, three-dimensional sphenoid bone contains the temporal fossa (B), the superior orbital fissure (C), the base of the skull anterior to occipital bone (D), and the pterygoid processes. The palatine process (A) is part of the maxillae.

67. Anatomically, the inferior alveolar artery supplies which structure?

    ANS: D
    The mandibular teeth (D) and the bone of the mandible are supplied by the inferior alveolar artery. The lingual artery supplies the floor of the mouth (A), and its branches supply the tongue (B). The sublingual gland (C) is supplied by the sublingual and submental arteries.

68. The functions of the lymphatic system include all EXCEPT one. Which one is the EXCEPTION?

    ANS: D
    The correct choice is D; thrombocytes are produced in bone marrow and not in the lymphatic system. The lymphatic system filters fluids (A), fights infection (B), produces lymphocytes (C), and returns plasma to the venous bloodstream (E).

69. For each division of the trigeminal nerve (V) listed, select its appropriate name from the list provided.

    ANS: 1C; 2A; 3B
    Division I (1) is known as the ophthalmic V_1 (C). Division II (2) is the maxillary V_2 (A). Division III (3) is the mandibular V_3 (B).

70. The abducens (VI), trochlear (IV), and oculomotor (III) nerves all provide innervation to the muscles of the eye. These nerves provide sensory innervation.

    ANS: C
    The correct choice is C. The first statement is true, and the second statement is false. The abducens, trochlear, and oculomotor nerves supply motor innervation to the muscle of the eye. Choices A, B, and D do not correctly reflect the statements.

71. Match each germ layer listed to the structure it forms in the developing embryo.

    ANS: 1A; 2C; 3B
    The endoderm (1) forms the gastrointestinal tract, epithelium, and associated glands (A). The mesoderm

(2) forms muscles, bone, cartilage, blood, dentin, pulp, cementum, and periodontal ligament (C). The ectoderm (3) forms the nervous system, epidermis, sensory epithelium of the eye, ear, and nose; the tooth enamel; and the oral epithelium (B).

72. For each of the developing branchial arches listed, select the most appropriate anatomic structure that it gives rise to.

ANS: 1D; 2A; 3B; 4C
The mandibular arch (1) gives rise to the mandible, muscles of mastication, and cranial nerve V (D). The hyoid arch (2) gives rise to the muscles of facial expression and cranial nerve VII (A). Branchial arch III (3) gives rise to the tongue and cranial nerve IX (B). Branchial arch IV (4) gives rise to the muscles of the throat, the inferior hyoid cartilage, and cranial nerve X (C).

73. Match each cell type to the structure it forms.

ANS: 1D; 2A; 3B; 4C
Ameloblasts (1) give rise to enamel (D). Cementoblasts (2) give rise to cementum (A). Odontoblasts (3) give rise to dentin (B). The dental follicle (4) gives rise to mesenchymal cells, which give rise to alveolar bone (C), the periodontal ligament, and cementum.

74. The temporomandibular joint is capable of which two types of movement?

ANS: A
The temporomandibular joint (TMJ) rotates and glides (A). Rotational movement occurs between the disk and the mandibular condyle in the lower synovial cavity. As the jaw opens further, an anterior gliding movement also occurs along the posterior slope of the articular eminence. Movements B, C, and D are not associated with the TMJ.

75. Which arteries are the terminal branches of the external carotid artery?

ANS: D
There are approximately eight main branches of the external carotid artery. The terminal branches are maxillary and superficial temporal branches (D) given off deep to the neck of the condyle. The superior thyroid and lingual (A) branches and the facial and ascending pharyngeal (B) branches are given off in the carotid triangle. The posterior auricular and occipital (C) arteries are posterior arteries given off below maxillary and superficial temporal arteries.

76. A hematoma that results from the administration of a posterior superior alveolar (PSA) nerve block is caused by bleeding from which arteries or veins?

ANS: D
The posterior superior alveolar artery (1), the pterygoid plexus of veins (2) and the facial artery (4) are located in the infratemporal fossa. This location may contain a high volume of blood if a hematoma occurs. The vessels listed in A, B, and C are not associated with the PSA nerve block.

77. How many teeth are present in an individual with a full deciduous dentition?

ANS: A
The full deciduous dentition contains 20 teeth (A). The full permanent dentition contains 32 teeth (D). Neither 24 (B) nor 28 (C) represents a full count of teeth at any stage.

78. Which is NOT a characteristic feature of the primary dentition?

ANS: B
Dentin in primary teeth is much thicker than dentin in permanent teeth (B). Primary teeth are characterized as having relatively thin enamel (A) and large pulp cavities (C) and are whiter in color than permanent teeth (D).

79. Which teeth have wider crowns mesiodistally than faciolingually?

ANS: B
Permanent maxillary incisors, teeth #7 and #10 (B), are wider mesiodistally than faciolingually. Maxillary premolars (A) and mandibular incisors (C and D) are wider faciolingually than mesiodistally.

80. Each is an important function of the cementoenamel junction (CEJ) EXCEPT one. Which one is the EXCEPTION?

ANS: A
Prevention of caries decay (A) is NOT a function of the cementoenamel junction (CEJ). The CEJ functions for self-cleansing by the natural spillways that are formed, lending to self-cleansing properties (B), food deflection (C), and both health and maintenance of periodontal tissues in the interproximal spaces (D).

81. Match each dental anomaly listed with its description.

ANS: 1D; 2C; 3B; 4E; 5A; 6 F
Dwarf roots (1) affect the crown-to-root ratio (D). Concrescence (2) involves fusion after roots are formed (C). In dilaceration (3), the crown or root

demonstrates sharp bends or curves (B). Mulberry molars (4) result from congenital syphilis (E). Gemination (5) involves the partial splitting of the root germ (A). Dens in dente (6) describes a tooth within a tooth (F).

82. The clinical crown-to-root ratio is always the same. However, the anatomic crown–to-root ratio may change.

    ANS: B
    Both statements are false (B). The clinical crown-to-root ratio may change, depending on the location of alveolar bone and the gingiva. The anatomic crown–to-root ratio (the crown and root are covered with enamel and cementum, respectively) always remains the same. Choices A, C, and D do not correctly reflect the statements.

83. There is relatively constant mesial movement of the molars to compensate for proximal abrasion. Relatively consistent occlusal forces result in bone remodeling.

    ANS: A
    Both statements are correct and related (A). Active eruption, mesial drift, and masticatory occlusal and orthodontic corrective forces are all examples of consistent forces in alveolar bone remodeling. Traumatic occlusal force is an example of a type of force that is NOT a consistent, constant force that results in bone remodeling. Choices B, C, D, and E do not correctly reflect the statements.

84. Enamel is formed by ameloblasts, which are derived from the ectoderm. The ectoderm also signals the mesoderm to start the development of dentin and pulp.

    ANS: A
    Both statements are true (A). Enamel develops from the enamel organ, which is derived from the ectoderm. The enamel organ will differentiate into the inner enamel epithelium, the stellate reticulum, the stratum intermedium, and the outer enamel epithelium. The inner enamel epithelium will give rise to ameloblasts. The ectoderm's production of ameloblasts is the signal to the mesodermal structure of the dental papilla to start the formation of dentin and pulp. Choices B, C, and D do not correctly reflect the statements.

85. Cellular metabolism occurs in the

    ANS: C
    Mitochondria (C) are the "power plants" of the cell and are responsible for the rate of energy production. Ribosomes (A) are the RNA (ribonucleic acid) of the cell and are also responsible for protein production. Lysosomes (B) act as "scavenger" cells, removing debris from within the cellular body. The Golgi apparatus (D) is involved in merocrine secretion. The endoplasmic reticulum (E) manufactures various products for use within and outside cells.

86. During facial development, the two structures forming the major facial structures are the frontonasal process and the pharyngeal (branchial) arch I. This process begins during week 6 in utero.

    ANS: C
    The correct choice is C. The first statement is true. The frontonasal process will form the forehead and the middle third of the face, including the nose, the philtrum, maxillary incisors, and the premaxillary area or the primary palate. The first pharyngeal (branchial) arch I forms the mandibular and maxillary processes, which will form the mandible, most of the maxillae, and palatine bones. The zygomatic bones of the cheek are also formed from these processes. The second statement is false. This process begins during week 3 in embryologic development. By week 6, the major facial structures have formed and are developing in complexity. Choices A, B, and D do not accurately reflect the statements.

87. Each is a paranasal sinus EXCEPT one. Which one is the EXCEPTION?

    ANS: B
    There is no structure called the mandibular sinus (B). Paranasal sinuses include the frontal (A), maxillary (C), sphenoidal (D), and ethmoidal (E) sinuses.

88. Which muscle involved in facial expression does not have a bony attachment, shapes and controls the size of the mouth opening, and helps create lip positions and movements during speech?

    ANS: C
    The orbicularis oris muscle (C) shapes and controls the size of the mouth opening and is important in the creation of lip positions and movements during speech. The risorius muscle (A) stretches the lips laterally, retracting the labial commissure and widening the mouth to produce a grimace. The zygomaticus major muscle (B) elevates the labial commissure of the upper lip and pulls it laterally, thus helping create to a smile. The levator anguli oris muscle (D) elevates the labial commissure, as when a person smiles.

89. Each is an anterior branch of the external carotid artery EXCEPT one. Which one is the EXCEPTION?

ANS: A
The occipital artery (A) is a posterior branch of the external carotid artery. The external carotid artery has four sets of branches, grouped according to location in relation to the main artery: (1) anterior, (2) medial, (3) posterior, and (4) terminal. The superior thyroid (B), facial (C), and lingual (D) arteries are all anterior branches of the external carotid artery.

90. Which gland is associated with dry eye syndrome (DES), also known as *keratoconjunctivitis sicca* (KCS)?

ANS: C
Lacrimal glands (C) are paired exocrine glands that secrete lacrimal fluid, or tears. With dry eye syndrome, the lacrimal glands produce less fluid, a condition often associated with aging or certain medications. The thyroid (A), thymus (B), and parathyroid (D) glands are all endocrine glands, not exocrine glands. The thyroid gland (A) is the largest endocrine gland and secretes thyroxine directly into the vascular system to stimulate the body's metabolic rate. The thymus gland (B) is part of the immune system and helps fight disease processes. The parathyroid gland (D) secretes parathyroid hormone directly into the vascular system to regulate phosphorus and calcium levels.

91. The face and its related tissues begin to form during week 6 of prenatal development, within the fetal period. Facial development is completed by week 12.

ANS: D
The correct choice is D. The first statement is false. The face and its related tissues begin to form at the beginning of week 4 in the embryonic period, not during week 6 in the fetal period. However, the second statement is true. Facial development starts during weeks 3 and 4 and is completed in the twelfth week. Choices A, B, and C do not correctly reflect the statements.

92. Which developmental disturbance appears as a "tooth within a tooth" on radiologic examination?

ANS: D
The abnormal invagination of the enamel organ into the dental papilla results in the developmental disturbance known as *dens in dente* (D) and appears as a "tooth within a tooth" on radiographic examination. In gemination (C), the single tooth germ tries unsuccessfully to divide into two tooth germs, resulting in a large single-rooted tooth with a common pulp cavity. With fusion (A), two adjacent tooth germs join together, leading to a large, falsely macrodontic tooth that can be verified with radiographic examination. Tubercles (B) are extra cusps that appear as small, round enamel extensions.

93. Each is a type of connective tissue EXCEPT one. Which one is the EXCEPTION?

ANS: C
Muscle tissue (C) is part of the muscular system and is a classification of basic tissue in the same way that connective tissue is also a classification of basic body tissue. Bone (A) is a rigid type of specialized connective tissue that makes up the majority of the body's mature skeleton. Blood (B) is a fluid specialized connective tissue that transports nutrients throughout the body. Cartilage (D) is a type of firm, noncalcified, specialized connective tissue that forms much of the temporary skeleton of the embryo and structurally supports certain soft tissues after birth.

94. Enamel may be lost through attrition, abrasion, erosion, caries, or abfraction. Radiographically, enamel appears more radiolucent than dentin or pulp, both of which appear more radiopaque.

ANS: C
Choice C is correct. The first statement is true. Enamel may be lost through attrition (wearing away from tooth-to-tooth contact), abrasion (loss through friction from toothbrushing or toothpaste), erosion (loss through chemical means that do not involve bacteria), caries (loss through chemical means from cariogenic bacteria), or abfraction (loss through tensile and compressive forces during tooth flexure). However, the second statement is false. On radiographs, enamel appears more radiopaque (lighter) than dentin or pulp, both of which appear more radiolucent (darker). Choices A, B, and D do not accurately reflect the statements.

95. Which acronym defines the correct sequence of words used to describe a tooth?

ANS: D
The correct sequence of words used to describe a tooth is based on the D-A-Q-T system (D), with *D* for dentition, *A* for arch, *Q* for quadrant, and *T* for tooth type. For example, a dental professional may refer to a permanent (D) mandibular (A) left (Q) premolar (T). Acronyms in choices A, B, and C are incorrectly sequenced.

96. How many permanent anterior teeth are present in an adult mouth?

    ANS: D
    An adult mouth has 12 total permanent anterior teeth (D): 8 incisors (4 each lateral and central incisors [two in each arch]) and 4 canines (two in each arch). Figures in choices A, B, and C are less than 12 (the normal number of permanent anterior teeth).

97. Which tooth numbers represent maxillary first premolars?

    ANS: A
    Teeth #5 and #12 (A) are maxillary first premolars.
    Teeth #4 and #13 (B) are maxillary second premolars.
    Teeth #21 and #28 (C) are mandibular first premolars.
    Teeth #24 and #25 (D) are mandibular central incisors.

98. Which statement is correct? (Select all that apply.)

    ANS: B, C, D
    The correct choices are B, C, and D. Mandibular molars have a bifurcated root: mesial and distal (B). Maxillary molars have trifurcated roots: mesiobuccal, distobuccal, and palatal (C). Maxillary first premolars may have a bifurcated root: buccal and palatal (D). Maxillary second premolars are rarely bifurcated (A).

## CHAPTER 2

Physiology

Gina Cano-Monreal, Ashley Martin Hale

QUESTIONS

1. Which definition BEST describes *diffusion*?
   A. Movement of molecules from a higher to lower concentration gradient
   B. Net movement of water down its concentration gradient
   C. Ability of a substance to move across a membrane
   D. Movement of substances across a plasma membrane

2. Neutrophils are known as which type of blood cell?
   A. Agranulocytes
   B. Platelets
   C. Granulocytes
   D. Erythrocytes

3. During gingivitis, which immune system cells are most likely to be the first to respond?
   A. Neutrophils
   B. Eosinophils
   C. Erythrocytes
   D. Agranulocytes

4. The merocrine glands are responsible for the secretion of which fluid?
   A. Testosterone
   B. Thyroxin
   C. Estrogen
   D. Sweat

5. Which type of tissue lines the surface of the lungs?
   A. Visceral pleura
   B. Peritoneal pleura
   C. Pericardial pleura
   D. Visceral peritoneum

6. Which BEST describes what happens to a nerve when there is an influx of sodium ions?
   A. Depolarization
   B. Myelination
   C. Polarization
   D. Excitation

7. The inferior alveolar nerve is difficult to anesthetize because it is has a thick myelin sheath. Myelin acts as an insulator that prevents the generation of electrical activity.
   A. Both statements are true.
   B. Both statements are false.
   C. The first statement is true, and the second statement is false.
   D. The first statement is false, and the second statement is true.

8. An elevated serum potassium level is known as
   A. hypernatremia.
   B. hyperkalemia.
   C. hypercarotenemia.
   D. hypokalemia.

9. A group of similar cells that perform a common function is called a/an
   A. tissue.
   B. cell.
   C. organ.
   D. ecosystem.

10. Negative feedback mechanisms oppose the direction of an initial stimulus. Defects in negative feedback mechanisms are the cause of most homeostatic imbalances.
    A. Both statements are true.
    B. Both statements are false.
    C. The first statement is true, and the second statement is false.
    D. The first statement is false, and the second statement is true.

11. Which cellular organelle is responsible for the detoxification of drugs, pesticides, and carcinogens?
    A. Golgi apparatus
    B. Mitochondria
    C. Cell membrane
    D. Ribosome
    E. Smooth endoplasmic reticulum

12. Which type of epithelium is multilayered to provide protection to underlying tissue and is found in areas subject to abrasion such as the mouth and the esophagus?
    A. Transitional
    B. Stratified squamous
    C. Simple squamous
    D. Pseudostratified columnar

13. A bone disease that results in fragile and thin bones when bone resorption is faster than bone deposit is called
    A. ostepenia.
    B. osteogenesis.
    C. osteoporosis.
    D. osteoarthritis.

14. Each is a property of muscle tissue EXCEPT one. Which one is the EXCEPTION?
    A. Contractility
    B. Excitability
    C. Conductivity
    D. Extensibility

15. At which sites are motor nerve impulses transmitted from nerve endings to skeletal muscle cells?
    A. Neuromuscular junctions
    B. Sarcomeres
    C. Z-disks
    D. Cross-bridges
    E. Myofilaments

16. The trigeminal nerve
    A. serves the sternocleidomastoid and trapezius muscles.
    B. provides the sensation of taste for the tongue.
    C. allows for chewing of food.
    D. helps to regulate heart activity.

17. Which of the following is NOT a characteristic of AB-positive blood?
    A. A and B antigens are present on the surface of red blood cells.
    B. No anti-A or anti-B antibodies are produced.
    C. Rh antigens are produced.
    D. Anti-A and anti-B antibodies are produced.

18. Which substance must be present for the thyroid gland to produce thyroxine?
    A. Iron
    B. Calcium
    C. Iodine
    D. Carbohydrates

19. Type 2 diabetes mellitus is best described by which statement?
    A. The pancreas produces insulin, but glucagon is not responsive to it.
    B. The pancreas produces insulin, but the insulin receptors on the body's cells are resistant.
    C. The thyroid gland produces insulin, but the insulin receptors on the body's cells are resistant.
    D. The pancreas produces insulin, and the insulin receptors on the body's cells allow too much of the insulin to enter the cell.
    E. The pancreas does not produce any insulin.

20. Which is the first step of blood clot formation (hemostasis)?
    A. Platelet plug formation
    B. Conversion of prothrombin to thrombin
    C. Vascular spasms
    D. Formation of prothrombin factor
    E. Thrombin conversion of fibrinogen to fibrin mesh

21. Which factor determines the movement of respiratory system gases?
    A. Water solubility
    B. Partial pressure gradients
    C. Temperature variations
    D. Molecular weight of respiratory system gases

22. Which of the following is NOT a functional activity of the digestive system?
    A. Mechanical digestion
    B. Chemical digestion
    C. Absorption
    D. Replication
    E. Propulsion

23. Cilia cannot be repaired or regenerated, even after quitting smoking. Emphysema is characterized by irreversible destruction of the walls of the alveoli and the production of abnormally large air spaces.
    A. Both statements are true.
    B. Both statements are false.
    C. The first statement is true, and the second statement is false.
    D. The first statement is false, and the second statement is true.

24. The pharynx is a passageway for air and food. But the larynx is a passageway only for air.
    A. Both statements are true.
    B. Both statements are false.
    C. The first statement is true, and the second statement is false.
    D. The first statement is false, and the second statement is true.

25. Chronic obstructive pulmonary disease (COPD) is a combination of chronic bronchitis and
    A. pneumonia.
    B. diabetes.
    C. emphysema.
    D. asthma.

26. Which is the most appropriate definition of the term *peristalsis*?
    A. Wavelike contraction of smooth muscle that moves food through the alimentary canal
    B. Movement across intestinal segments while digestive juices mix with foodstuffs
    C. Breakdown of fats upon interaction with bile
    D. The effect of gastric juices on the esophagus

27. Which nerve innervates the diaphragm?
    A. Saphenous
    B. Popliteal
    C. Brachial plexus
    D. Phrenic

28. These blood vessels permit nutrient and gas exchange between blood and tissue cells, while these blood vessels carry blood back to the heart under low-pressure conditions.
    A. Capillaries; veins
    B. Arteries; veins
    C. Arteries; capillaries
    D. Veins; capillaries

29. Which structure is the natural pacemaker of the heart?
    A. Purkinje fiber
    B. Atrioventricular (AV) node
    C. Sinoatrial (SA) node

30. Select the correct sequence of steps in the acute inflammatory process:
    A. (1) Vasodilation, (2) vascular permeability, (3) exudation, (4) vascular stasis
    B. (1) Vascular permeability, (2) vasodilation, (3) exudation, (4) vascular stasis
    C. (1) Vascular stasis, (2) vasodilation, (3) vascular permeability, (4) exudation
    D. (1) Vasodilation, (2) exudation, (3) vascular stasis, (4) vascular permeability

Answers and Rationales

1. Which definition BEST describes *diffusion*?

   ANS: A
   Diffusion is the movement of molecules from a higher concentration gradient to a lower concentration gradient (A). Osmosis is the net movement of water down its concentration gradient (B). Permeability is the ability of substances to move across a membrane (C). Carrier-mediated transport is the movement of substances across plasma membrane (D).

2. Neutrophils are known as which type of blood cell?

   ANS: C
   Neutrophils are a type of white blood cells (leukocytes) and are further classified as granulocytes (C) for the granules in the cytoplasm. Agranulocytes (A) are a type of white blood cells that do not contain granules in the cytoplasm. Platelets (B) are cell fragments involved in blood clotting. Erythrocytes (D) are red blood cells.

3. During gingivitis, which immune system cells are most likely to be the first to respond?

   ANS: A
   Neutrophils (A) are a type of white blood cells that are usually the first to appear to fight infections. Eosinophils (B) increase during allergic reactions. Erythrocytes (C) are red blood cells and are not directly involved in the immune response. Agranulocytes (D) are also a type of white blood cells that respond later in the inflammatory response.

4. The merocrine glands are responsible for the secretion of which fluid?

   ANS: D
   The merocrine gland is responsible for the secretion of sweat (D). Testosterone (A) is secreted by the testes. Thyroxin (B) is secreted by the thyroid gland. Estrogen (C) is secreted by the follicular cells of the ovaries.

5. Which type of tissue lines the surface of the lungs?

   ANS: A
   The visceral pleura (A) lines the surface of the lungs; the viscera lines organs, and the pleura associates that lining with the thoracic cavity. Peritoneal pleura (B) lines the abdominal cavity. Pericardial pleura (C) lines the cardiac tissues. The visceral peritoneum (D) is associated with the surface lining of an organ in the abdominal cavity.

6. Which BEST describes what happens to a nerve when there is an influx of sodium ions?

   ANS: A
   Depolarization (A) occurs when there is an influx of sodium, causing the nerve to send an impulse. Myelination (B) is the covering of a nerve axon with myelin, a type of protective sheath. Polarization (C) occurs when there is an influx of potassium back into the cell, stopping the nerve impulse. Excitation (D) describes what happens when a gate channel of a cell is opened, allowing for an influx of sodium or potassium.

7. The inferior alveolar nerve is difficult to anesthetize because it is has a thick myelin sheath. Myelin acts as an insulator that prevents the generation of electrical activity.

   ANS: A
   Both statements are true (A). The thick myelin sheath covering the inferior alveolar nerve acts as an insulator that prevents the generation of electrical activity. Choices B, C, and D do not accurately reflect the statements.

8. An elevated serum potassium level is known as

   ANS: B
   Hyperkalemia (B) is defined as elevated potassium concentrations in blood. Hypernatremia (A) is an elevated serum sodium level. Hypercarotenemia (C) is excessive levels of carotene in blood. Hypokalemia (D) is low potassium concentrations in blood.

9. A group of similar cells that perform a common function is called a/an

   ANS: A
   A tissue (A) is a group of cells that performs a common function. One cell (B) cannot perform a function. A group of tissues with a similar function makes up an organ (C). An ecosystem (D) is a community of living organisms working together.

10. Negative feedback mechanisms oppose the direction of an initial stimulus. Defects in negative feedback mechanisms are the cause of most homeostatic imbalances.

    ANS: A
    Both statements are true (A). Negative feedback mechanisms or loops reverse the direction of an initial stimulus to keep the body in a state of homeostasis.

If negative feedback mechanisms that oppose stimuli to return the body to homeostasis are not working properly, the body strays from homeostasis and is in a state of homeostatic imbalance. Choices B, C, and D do not accurately reflect the statements.

11. Which cellular organelle is responsible for the detoxification of drugs, pesticides, and carcinogens?

ANS: E
The smooth endoplasmic reticulum (E) functions in the detoxification of toxins such as drugs, pesticides, and carcinogens. The Golgi apparatus (A) is responsible for the proper modification and packaging of proteins. Mitochondria (B) are responsible for the production of adenosine triphosphate (ATP) in a cell. The cell membrane (C) is responsible for regulating what enters and exits a cell. A ribosome (D) is the site of protein synthesis.

12. Which type of epithelium is multilayered to provide protection to underlying tissue and is found in areas subject to abrasion such as the mouth and the esophagus?

ANS: B
Stratified squamous epithelium (B) is multilayered, functions to protect underlying tissues, and is found in the mouth and the esophagus. Transitional epithelium (A) is single layered and is found in organs such as the bladder, where expansion is important. Simple squamous epithelium (C) is also single layered and is found in organs in which diffusion across the tissue is allowed. Pseudostratified columnar epithelium (D) is single layered, even though it gives the illusion of containing multiple layers.

13. A bone disease that results in fragile and thin bones when bone resorption is faster than bone deposit is called

ANS: C
Osteoporosis (C) is a bone disease in which bone resorption outpaces bone deposition, which results in thin and fragile bones. Osteopenia (A) is a significant reduction in bone mineral density. Osteogenesis (B) is the process by which the osteoblasts lay down new bone material. Osteoarthritis (D) is a joint disorder rather than a bone disorder.

14. Each is a property of muscle tissue EXCEPT one. Which one is the EXCEPTION?

ANS: C
Conductivity (C) is a property of nerve tissue and is not associated with muscle tissue. Muscle tissue has the ability to contract (A), become excited (B), and extend (D).

15. At which sites are motor nerve impulses transmitted from nerve endings to skeletal muscle cells?

ANS: A
The neuromuscular junction (A) is the space in between a nerve ending and a skeletal muscle cell, across which neurotransmitters cross. Sarcomeres (B), Z-disks (C), and myofilaments (E) all refer to muscle structure. Sarcomeres are functional units of myofibrils (muscle cells); myofilaments make up the myofibrils, and Z-disks are the areas between repetitive sarcomeres. The term *cross-bridges* (D) refers to the sliding of thick and thin filaments across one another to allow for muscle contraction.

16. The trigeminal nerve

ANS: C
The trigeminal nerve innervates the muscles involved in mastication and is responsible for functions such as biting, swallowing, and chewing (C). The sternocleidomastoid and trapezius muscles are innervated by cranial nerve XI, or the accessory nerve (A). Taste to the anterior two thirds of the tongue comes from the chorda tympani branch of cranial nerve VII (the facial nerve), and taste and sensation to the posterior third of the tongue is provided by cranial nerve IX, the glossopharyngeal nerve (B). Heart activity is regulated by the autonomic nervous system, with cranial nerve X or the vagus nerve (D).

17. Which of the following is NOT a characteristic of AB-positive blood?

ANS: D
AB-positive blood type cannot produce anti-A or anti-B antibodies (D); if it did, the antibodies would bind to the A and B antigens on the surface of the red blood cells, causing them to lyse. In the AB-positive blood group, red blood cells have A and B antigens (proteins) on their surfaces (A). The red blood cells in this blood group do not produce anti-A or anti-B antibodies (B). The word *positive* in the name of this blood group refers to the production of the Rh antigens (C).

18. Which substance must be present for the thyroid gland to produce thyroxine?

ANS: C
Iodine (C) is necessary for the production of thyroid hormones, including thyroxine. Iron (A) is a major component of hemoglobin, which transports oxygen from the lungs to tissues. Calcium (B) is critical for skeletal function. Carbohydrates (D) are the major source of energy for humans.

19. Type 2 diabetes mellitus is best described by which statement?

    ANS: B
    In type 2 diabetes, the pancreas produces insulin, but the insulin receptors on the body's cells are resistant (B). Receptors on cells of the body must be responsive to insulin, not to glucagon, so that insulin can guide glucose into the cells that need it (A). Insulin is produced by the beta-cells of the pancreas, not the thyroid (C). In type 2 diabetes, even though insulin is produced by the beta-cells of the pancreas, the insulin receptors on the body's cells do not respond to it; glucose cannot enter into the cells that need it (D). Type 2 diabetes is also referred to as *non–insulin-dependent diabetes* because the pancreas does produce insulin, which differentiates it from type 1, or insulin-dependent, diabetes (E).

20. Which is the first step of blood clot formation (hemostasis)?

    ANS: C
    Vascular spasms (C) are the first step of blood clot formation. The steps of hemostasis fall under the general categories of vasoconstriction, which involves vascular spasms; followed by platelet plug formation (A); and finally blood clotting, which involves the formation of prothrombin (D), subsequent conversion to thrombin (B), and formation of the fibrin mesh (E).

21. Which factor determines the movement of respiratory system gases?

    ANS: B
    Respiratory system gases move down the partial pressure gradients (B) from an area in which the partial pressure is higher to an area in which the partial pressure is lower. Water solubility (A), temperature variations (C), and molecular weight (D) do not determine movement of gases in the respiratory system.

22. Which of the following is NOT a functional activity of the digestive system?

    ANS: D
    Replication is NOT a function of the digestive system (D); replication occurs when a strand of DNA produces a copy of itself. Mechanical (A) and chemical (B) digestion are both functions of the digestive system; mechanical digestion primarily functions in the mouth, in contrast to chemical digestion, which mainly functions in digestion at the stomach and intestines (and to a lesser extent, the mouth). Absorption (C) is a

vital function of the digestive system that occurs in the intestine. Propulsion (E) is necessary to propel food through the digestive or alimentary canal.

23. Cilia cannot be repaired or regenerated, even after quitting smoking. Emphysema is characterized by irreversible destruction of the walls of the alveoli and the production of abnormally large air spaces.

    ANS: D
    The first statement is false, and the second statement is true (D). Damage to the respiratory cilia can be reversed if a person quits smoking; the cilia begin to quickly repair themselves and regenerate after cessation of smoking. However, the alveoli of those with emphysema are irreversibly destroyed by smoking, resulting in the formation of large air spaces that can trap air and reduce breathing efficiency. Choices A, B, and C do not accurately reflect the statements.

24. The pharynx is a passageway for air and food. But the larynx is a passageway only for air.

    ANS: A
    Both statements are true (A). The pharynx is a part of two systems: (1) the respiratory system and (2) the digestive system. As such, it can function in the passage of both air and food. The larynx is the voicebox and functions in the respiratory system by providing a passageway for air to the lungs. Choices B, C, and D do not accurately reflect the statements.

25. Chronic obstructive pulmonary disease (COPD) is a combination of chronic bronchitis and

    ANS: C
    Chronic obstructive pulmonary disease (COPD) is a combination of chronic bronchitis and emphysema (C). Pneumonia (A), diabetes (B), and asthma (D) are not components of COPD.

26. Which is the most appropriate definition of the term *peristalsis*?

    ANS: A
    Peristalsis refers to characteristic wavelike movements of the smooth muscle in the alimentary canal to move food along (A). Movement across intestinal segments describes the process of segmentation rather than peristalsis (B). The breakdown of fats is not a movement but a process (C). The effect of gastric juices on the esophagus refers to the condition known as *heartburn* (D).

27. Which nerve innervates the diaphragm?

ANS: D
The phrenic nerve (D) innervates the diaphragm, where it plays a role in breathing and diaphragmatic movement. The saphenous nerve (A) innervates the medial aspect of the leg. The popliteal nerve (B) innervates the lower extremities. The brachial plexus (C) innervates the upper appendages.

28. These blood vessels permit nutrient and gas exchange between blood and tissue cells, while these blood vessels carry blood back to the heart under low-pressure conditions.

ANS: A
Capillaries and veins (A) are described in the statements. The thin walls of the capillaries (A, C, D) allow for nutrient and gas exchange across them. Veins (A, B, D) are low-pressure blood vessels that return blood to the heart. Arteries (B, C) are thick-walled blood vessels that permit the flow of blood under high pressure. Choice D is a reverse of the correct answer.

29. Which structure is the natural pacemaker of the heart?

ANS: C
The sinoatrial (SA) node (C) is the natural pacemaker of the heart. However, if the SA node fails, then the atrioventricular (AV) node (B) may take over this role. Purkinje fibers (A) are not a component of the intrinsic cardiac conduction system.

30. Select the correct sequence of steps in the acute inflammatory process:

ANS: A
The correct sequence of steps (A) in acute inflammation is as follows:
1. Vasodilation increases blood, resulting in redness and heat.
2. Vascular permeability: Endothelial cells become "leaky" from either direct endothelial cell injury or via chemical mediators.
3. Exudation: Fluid, proteins, red blood cells, and white blood cells escape from the intravascular space as a result of increased osmotic pressure extravascularly and increased hydrostatic pressure intravascularly.
4. Vascular stasis: Slowing of the blood in the bloodstream allows chemical mediators and inflammatory cells to collect and respond to the stimulus.

Choices B, C, and D are incorrectly sequenced.

5. For each of the numbered vitamins, select the most closely associated deficiency or excess.

Vitamin	Deficiency or Excess
_____ 1. Vitamin A	A. Deficiency results in beriberi.
_____ 2. Vitamin D	B. Deficiency during pregnancy results in neural tube defects.
_____ 3. Thiamin	C. Deficiency results in weakened collagen, excessive bleeding, and poor wound healing.
_____ 4. Niacin	D. Excess may cause increased activity of osteoclasts.
_____ 5. Folic acid	E. Deficiency results in rickets.
_____ 6. Vitamin B$_{12}$	F. Deficiency results in pellagra.
_____ 7. Vitamin C	G. Deficiency results in pernicious anemia.

6. Protein energy malnutrition is known as
   A. marasmus.
   B. atherosclerosis.
   C. Crohn disease.
   D. scurvy.
   E. Cushing syndrome.

7. Intrinsic factor in the stomach is needed for the absorption of
   A. vitamin A.
   B. thiamin.
   C. vitamin B$_{12.}$
   D. vitamin C.
   E. calcium.

8. Chronic iron deficiency anemia is known as
   A. megaloblastic anemia.
   B. pica.
   C. hyperosmolar hyperglycemic state.
   D. Sjögren syndrome.
   E. Plummer-Vinson syndrome.

9. Which fatty acid has the first double bond at the third carbon atom from the omega end?
   A. Trans
   B. Stearic acid
   C. Alpha-linolenic acid
   D. Triglyceride
   E. Cholesterol

10. Which snack creates the most cariogenic environment in the oral cavity?
    A. Almonds
    B. Raisins
    C. Cheddar cheese
    D. Grapefruit
    E. Fried eggs

11. How many minutes of acid exposure in the oral cavity will one peppermint candy disk provide?
    A. 0
    B. 4
    C. 20
    D. 40
    E. 60

12. Chewing gum used to reduce the risk of dental caries should contain which of the following cariostatic sugar alcohols?
    A. Erythritol
    B. Lactitol
    C. Mannitol
    D. Sorbitol
    E. Xylitol

13. Protein, casein, phosphorus, and calcium have anticariogenic properties. Milk is always a good beverage to recommend for patients with a high caries risk because of its anticariogenic properties.
    A. Both statements are true.
    B. Both statements are false.
    C. The first statement is true, and the second statement is false.
    D. The first statement is false, and the second statement is true.

14. Each is a source of cholesterol EXCEPT one. Which one is the EXCEPTION?
    A. Skim milk
    B. Low-fat fruit yogurt
    C. Lean hamburger
    D. Butter
    E. Margarine

15. Which foods constitute a complete protein? (Select all that apply.)
    A. Beans and rice
    B. Whole-wheat bagel
    C. Eggs
    D. Peanut butter
    E. Macaroni and cheese

16. The basic unit of a protein is a glycerol. The distinguishing feature of a protein, compared with a carbohydrate or a fat, is the source of oxygen.
    A. Both statements are true.
    B. Both statements are false.
    C. The first statement is true, and the second statement is false.
    D. The first statement is false, and the second statement is true.

17. Which food exemplifies a vegan (strict vegetarian) diet? (Select all that apply.)
    A. Maple syrup
    B. Corn oil
    C. Cream cheese
    D. Soy milk
    E. Grilled cheese sandwich

18. Each factor inhibits the absorption of calcium EXCEPT one. Which one is the EXCEPTION?
    A. Excessive caffeine intake
    B. Pregnancy
    C. Smoking
    D. Excessive alcohol intake
    E. Use of antacids

19. The animal form of vitamin A is
    A. tocopherol.
    B. carotene.
    C. retinol.
    D. calciferol.
    E. renin.

20. Each vitamin can be synthesized by the body EXCEPT one. Which one is the EXCEPTION?
    A. B_6
    B. B_{12}
    C. C
    D. D
    E. K

21. Ham and roast beef are excellent sources of
    A. calcium.
    B. folate.
    C. vitamin B_{12}.
    D. vitamin C.
    E. vitamin K.

22. Which vitamin aids the body in converting tryptophan to niacin?
    A. Folic acid
    B. Pantothenic acid
    C. Vitamin B_6
    D. Vitamin B_{12}
    E. Vitamin E

23. Which vitamin is NOT a fat-soluble vitamin?
    A. D
    B. E
    C. K
    D. A
    E. C

24. Which phrase BEST describes the process of anabolism?
    A. Splitting complex substances into simpler substances
    B. Depositing inorganic elements onto an organic matrix

C. Dividing insoluble molecules (fats) into smaller particles
    D. Using absorbed nutrients to build or synthesize more complex compounds
    E. Hydrolyzing triglycerides for use in the Krebs cycle

25. For a manufacturer to label a food as containing "zero" trans fats, the maximum number of grams that the U.S. Food and Drug Administration (FDA) allows the product to contain is
    A. 0.2.
    B. 0.5.
    C. 0.75.
    D. 1.2.
    E. 2.0.

26. Energy intake is balanced by appetite (the desire to eat) and hunger (the physiologic desire to eat). The pituitary gland regulates hunger.
    A. Both statements are true.
    B. Both statements are false.
    C. The first statement is true, and the second statement is false.
    D. The first statement is false, and the second statement is true.

27. Linoleic acid is an essential fatty acid that cannot be synthesized by the body. Good sources of linoleic acid include meat, fish, poultry, and eggs.
    A. Both statements are true.
    B. Both statements are false.
    C. The first statement is true, and the second statement is false.
    D. The first statement is false, and the second statement is true.

28. Order the steps of iron deficiency development, from first to last. Match each letter with its proper sequence number.

    1. _____   A. Hemoglobin production falls.
    2. _____   B. Iron stores diminish.
    3. _____   C. Transport of iron decreases.

29. Serum ferritin test measures the first stage of iron deficiency. For this first stage, accurate measures may be made in infants, children, and adults with this diagnostic test.
    A. Both statements are true.
    B. Both statements are false.
    C. The first statement is true, and the second statement is false.
    D. The first statement is false, and the second statement is true.

ANS: 1B; 2C; 3A
In the development of iron deficiency, iron stores in the body first diminish (B), followed by a decrease in the transport of iron (C). Subsequently, a decrease occurs in hemoglobin production (A).

29. Serum ferritin test measures the first stage of iron deficiency. For this first stage, accurate measures may be made in infants, children, and adults with this diagnostic test.

ANS: C
The first statement is true, and the second statement is false (C). Serum ferritin testing is used to measure the initial stage of iron deficiency. Accurate measures can be made for children and adults, as serum ferritin cut-off values can be determined. However, serum ferritin is not a reliable diagnostic tool for infants, as normal serum ferritin values are often present in conjunction with iron-responsive anemia. Choices A, B, and D do not correctly reflect the statements.

30. Which laboratory finding reflects the most cardioprotective lipoprotein profile?

ANS: B
The presence of low very-low-density lipoproteins (VLDLs) and high high-density lipoproteins (HDLs) (B) is the most cardioprotective lipoprotein profile. Lipoproteins are water-soluble compounds that carry lipids throughout the body. The best lipid profile is a high HDL to low low-density lipoproteins (LDL) and VLDL level. VLDLs transport cholesterol and triglycerides in the body, and high levels (A, D) may lead to the development of atherosclerosis. LDLs primarily carry cholesterol from the liver to other peripheral sites, and high levels of LDLs (C, D) are also associated with the development of atherosclerosis. HDLs are often termed "good cholesterol" because they carry cholesterol away from the arteries and back to the liver.

31. Protein energy malnutrition (PEM) is commonly measured by using serum albumin and total lymphocyte counts. Albumin synthesis depends on functioning liver cells and an appropriate supply of amino acids.

ANS: A
Both statements are true (A). PEM is commonly measured by using serum albumin and total lymphocyte counts. Serum albumin accounts for more than 50% of total serum proteins. Albumin synthesis depends on functioning liver cells and an appropriate supply of amino acids. Choices B, C, and D do not correctly reflect the statements.

32. Conditions other than malnutrition may depress albumin concentration. Advanced kidney disease, liver disease, infection, cancer, and burns may all depress albumin concentration.

ANS: A
Both statements are true (A). In addition to malnutrition, advanced kidney disease, liver disease, infection, cancer, and burns may all depress albumin concentration. Choices B, C, and D do not correctly reflect the statements.

33. Measuring prothrombin time (PT) provides an important indication of which nutrient level?

ANS: D
Measuring prothrombin time (PT) is an important indicator for vitamin K (D) levels in those individuals taking warfarin (Coumadin). Blood clotting is affected in patients taking anticoagulants such as warfarin. Vitamin K levels affect PT and may result in increased or excessive bleeding during clinical treatment if not closely monitored. Measuring PT would not reliably indicate levels of vitamin A (A), vitamin C (B), niacin (C), or potassium (E).

34. Each factor contributes to vitamin D deficiency EXCEPT one. Which one is the EXCEPTION?

ANS: D
Skin diseases (D) do not contribute to vitamin D deficiency. Vitamin D deficiency may be caused by dietary insufficiency (A), malabsorption (B), kidney disease (C), and sunscreen (E), all of which may prevent the conversion of vitamin D precursors to active vitamin D.

35. Brittle, ridged, or spoon-shaped nails; scaly, flaky, off-colored or cracked facial skin; and pale epithelial lining of the eyes and gingiva are signs of which nutritional deficiency?

ANS: D
Iron deficiencies (D) may be characterized by brittle, ridged, or spoon-shaped nails; scaly, flaky, off-colored or cracked facial skin; and pale epithelial lining of the eyes and gingiva. Deficiency of vitamin A (A) is associated with loss of night vision, keratomalacia, corneal ulceration, or Bitot spots. Angular cheilitis or cheilosis (cracks around the corners of the mouth) and glossitis (inflammation of the tongue) are associated with deficiencies of several B-complex vitamins (B). Zinc deficiency (C) is associated with changes in the epithelium of the tongue, flattened filiform papillae, increased susceptibility to periodontal disease, and loss of taste

and smell acuity. Vitamin K deficiencies (E) are associated with bleeding problems, including gingival hemorrhaging.

36. For each numbered nutritional element, select its most closely linked deficiency symptom.

ANS: 1A; 2E; 3C; 4B; 5D
Zinc deficiency (1) is associated with thickened oral epithelium and tongue and impaired taste (A). Vitamin A deficiency (2) is associated with ameloblast atrophy and accelerated periodontal destruction (E). Riboflavin deficiency (3) is associated with angular cheilosis, burning tongue, and blue-to-purple–colored mucosa (C). Vitamin K deficiency (4) is linked to gingival hemorrhaging (B). Vitamin C deficiency (5) is associated with odontoblast atrophy and slow wound healing (D).

37. Which are the physiologic roles of potassium? (Select all that apply.)

ANS: A, B, C
Muscle contraction (A), facilitation of nerve impulses (B), and maintenance of the electrical conductivity of the heart (C) are all the physiologic roles of potassium. Osmotic equilibrium (D) and electrolyte balance (E) are the physiologic roles of chloride, not potassium.

38. Which electrolytes are cations? (Select all that apply.)

ANS: A, B, C, E
Cations (electrolytes that have a positive charge) include sodium (A), potassium (B), magnesium (C), and calcium (E). Phosphate (D) is an anion, or an electrolyte that has a negative charge.

39. Which factors impact the basal metabolic rate (BMR)? (Select all that apply.)

ANS: A, B, D, E
Factors affecting the basal metabolic rate (BMR) include age (A), starvation or fasting (B), body composition and gender (D), and state of health (E). Other factors affecting BMR include sleep, exercise, and endocrine function. Kilocalories measure metabolic energy (C), not BMR.

40. All are plasma components of hyperlipidemia EXCEPT one. Which one is the EXCEPTION?

ANS: B
Hyperlipidemia describes an elevation of lipids or fats in the blood. Lipids include triglycerides (A), cholesterol esters, phospholipids (C), high-density lipoproteins (D), and low-density lipoproteins (E). Trans fats (B) are artificially manufactured lipids created by saturating carbon bonds.

6. Which cellular characteristic describes why gram-positive bacteria stain differently from how gram-negative bacteria stain?
   A. Thinner peptidoglycan
   B. Thicker peptidoglycan
   C. Less cytoplasm
   D. More cytoplasm

7. An ideal antibiotic has the ability to inhibit a wide range of microorganisms, including normal flora. It will only act on the pathogen, with no harmful effect to the human host.
   A. Both statements are true.
   B. Both statements are false.
   C. The first statement is true, and the second statement is false.
   D. The first statement is false, and the second statement is true.

8. Which term BEST describes the ability of a microorganism to cause disease?
   A. Stability
   B. Virulence
   C. Productivity
   D. Transmissibility

9. The cellular structure that is used to classify a bacterial species as gram-positive or gram-negative is the
   A. flagellum.
   B. cell wall.
   C. cell membrane.
   D. pilus.
   E. glycocalyx.

10. All are typical bacterial cell shapes EXCEPT one. Which one is the EXCEPTION?
    A. Spirochete
    B. Coccus
    C. Bacillus
    D. Disk

11. The prefix *strepto-* designates bacteria that take on which type of arrangement?
    A. Chain
    B. Tetrad
    C. Cluster
    D. Sarcina
    E. Diploid

12. Which is the MOST appropriate definition of a microorganism?
    A. An organism with individual cells that can be seen with the unaided eye
    B. An organism that does not contain a nucleus
    C. An organism with individual cells that are too small to be seen with the unaided eye
    D. An organism that does not contain a cell membrane

13. The key to Alexander Fleming's recognition of penicillin as a tool for fighting bacterial infections was his observation that
    A. bacteria inhibited the growth of nearby bacteria.
    B. mold inhibited the growth of nearby bacteria.
    C. mold inhibited the growth of nearby yeast.
    D. viruses could produce penicillin.

14. The best definition of a virus is
    A. a eukaryotic microorganism with branching hyphae.
    B. an acellular microorganism that requires a host for replication.
    C. a eukaryotic microorganism with the ability for locomotion.
    D. a prokaryotic microorganism that may exist singly, in pairs, chains, or clusters.
    E. a photosynthetic cell classified by differences in pigmentation.

15. You are observing a cell through a microscope and note that it does not have a nucleus. From this observation, you can also conclude that it most likely
    A. has a cell wall containing peptidoglycan.
    B. is a fungi.
    C. moves with the aid of cilia.
    D. does not have a cell membrane.

16. Structures that enable the transfer of genetic material between bacterial cells are
    A. fimbriae.
    B. capsules.
    C. cilia.
    D. pili.

17. Observation of microbial cell arrangement can be used to differentiate between streptococci and staphylococci. Observation of microbial cell shape can be used to differentiate between streptococci and staphylococci.
    A. Both statements are true.
    B. Both statements are false.
    C. The first statement is true, and the second statement is false.
    D. The first statement is false, and the second statement is true.

18. A patient is believed to be infected by *Mycobacterium tuberculosis,* the causative agent of tuberculosis. These microorganisms have a waxy cell wall. Which of the following staining methods can verify this assumption?
    A. Gram
    B. Flagellar
    C. Acid-fast
    D. Endospore

19. Which type of microorganism is most likely to be found in the large intestine, where there is no exposure to oxygen?
    A. Obligate aerobe
    B. Obligate anaerobe
    C. Facultative anaerobe
    D. Airborne bacteria

20. Which type of microorganism generally uses aerobic metabolism when oxygen is available but can carry on fermentation in an anaerobic environment when necessary?
    A. Aerotolerant anaerobes
    B. Facultative anaerobes
    C. Obligate anaerobes
    D. Obligate aerobes

21. All increase the virulence of bacteria EXCEPT one. Which one is the EXCEPTION?
    A. Exotoxins
    B. Bacterial glycocalyx
    C. Lipopolysaccharides
    D. Glycosaminoglycans

22. Most human pathogens are classified as
    A. mesophiles.
    B. thermophiles.
    C. psychrophiles.
    D. hyperthermophiles.

23. Microbes that are classified as beta-hemolytic have the ability to
    A. lyse white blood cells.
    B. produce endotoxins.
    C. lyse red blood cells.
    D. ferment glucose.

24. Which kind of relationship is exhibited by bacterial normal flora in a host's large intestine?
    A. Commensal
    B. Parasitic
    C. Symbiotic
    D. Competitive

25. Antibiotics may lead to septic shock if used to treat
    A. viral infections.
    B. gram-positive bacteria that produce exotoxins.
    C. protozoan infections.
    D. helminth infestations.
    E. gram-negative bacteria that produce endotoxins.

26. A change in the location of normal flora may result in an opportunistic infection. Opportunistic infections contribute to nosocomial infections.
    A. Both statements are true.
    B. Both statements are false.
    C. The first statement is true, and the second statement is false.
    D. The first statement is false, and the second statement is true.

27. New viruses rarely cause disease, but if disease is produced, it is very severe. On the basis of this characteristic, the pathogenicity and virulence of a particular virus would be considered
    A. low, high.
    B. low, low.
    C. high, low.
    D. high, high.

28. Convalescence is the disease stage in which the number of microorganisms causing the disease and the intensity of signs and symptoms decrease. During convalescence, the host is beginning to feel better, but the pathogen causing the disease may still be spread to others.
    A. Both statements are true.
    B. Both statements are false.
    C. The first statement is true, and the second statement is false.
    D. The first statement is false, and the second statement is true.

29. Which condition is a symptom of a disease?
    A. Fever
    B. Sore throat
    C. Vomiting
    D. High blood pressure

30. The virus that causes influenza is often transmitted over a distance less than 1 meter (m) by an unprotected sneeze. This is an example of what type of transmission?
    A. Vector
    B. Droplet
    C. Fomite
    D. Vehicle

31. The mucous membranes of the body are portals of entry for pathogens. Which mucous membranes are the MOST common site of entry for infectious agents?
    A. Oral cavity
    B. Genitourinary tract
    C. Gastrointestinal tract
    D. Respiratory tract

32. Bacterial endospores or spores are a problem in sterilizing instruments and equipment because
    A. endospores can transform into a vegetative state.
    B. most pathogenic bacteria are spore-formers.
    C. spores are resistant to physical and chemical agents.
    D. spores are protected by a waxy coating.

33. Which object is a fomite?
    A. Water
    B. Droplets from a sneeze
    C. Body fluids
    D. Insects
    E. Hypodermic needle

34. Interferons nonspecifically inhibit the spread of which type of infections?
    A. Viral
    B. Bacterial
    C. Protozoan
    D. Parasitic worm

35. All are considered nonspecific body immune defenses EXCEPT one. Which one is the EXCEPTION?
    A. Antibodies
    B. Mucous membranes
    C. Intact skin
    D. Phagocytic cells
    E. Lysozyme in tears

36. T-helper cells produce
    A. antibodies.
    B. cytolytic enzymes.
    C. plasma cells.
    D. cytokines.

37. Which is NOT a characteristic of adaptive immunity?
    A. Nonspecific
    B. Possesses memory
    C. Requires activation
    D. Represents third line of defense

38. Antigens are
    A. cells that protect the body against invaders.
    B. enzymes secreted by white blood cells.
    C. molecules that the body specifically recognizes as foreign.
    D. proteins the body produces against invading substances.
    E. proteins on the surface of the cell which determine tissue type.

39. An antibiotic binds to the 30S ribosomal subunit. On the basis of this information, this antibiotic inhibits which of the following processes?
    A. Transcription in eukaryotes
    B. Transcription in prokaryotes
    C. Translation in eukaryotes
    D. Translation in prokaryotes

40. A viral infection may be treated with an antibiotic. Antivirals are difficult to develop because viruses use host cell machinery for their replication.
    A. Both statements are true.
    B. Both statements are false.

C. The first statement is true, and the second statement is false.
D. The first statement is false, and the second statement is true.

41. The BEST definition of *sterilization* is
    A. disinfection of living tissue.
    B. use of a chemical agent to destroy pathogens.
    C. killing or removal of all microorganisms in a material or an object.
    D. reduction in the number of pathogenic microorganisms in a material or an object.

42. Standard methods of sterilization are NOT effective in destruction of
    A. viruses.
    B. bacteria.
    C. prions.
    D. protozoa.
    E. fungi.

43. A chemical agent that kills pathogenic microbes in general is a(n)
    A. sanitizer.
    B. germicide.
    C. disinfectant.
    D. fungicide.
    E. antiseptic.

44. Proper filtration of air and liquids relies on which property?
    A. Addition of pressure
    B. Sterile liquids
    C. Filter size
    D. Filter pore size

45. Which BEST describes the selective toxicity characteristic of antimicrobials?
    A. The ability to harm microbes without significantly harming host cells
    B. The ability to cause host cell damage without significantly damaging microbes
    C. The ability to harm the host cell and leave viruses alone
    D. The ability to titrate dosage that can be selectively and safely administered to a host

46. The mechanism of action for naturally occurring penicillin and its synthetic derivatives such as methicillin and ampicillin is the inhibition of cell wall synthesis. The spectrum of action for beta-lactam antibiotics equally includes gram-negative and gram-positive bacteria.
    A. Both statements are true.
    B. Both statements are false.
    C. The first statement is true, and the second statement is false.
    D. The first statement is false, and the second statement is true.

47. Erythromycin and tetracycline both act by
    A. disrupting cell membranes.
    B. disrupting cell wall synthesis.
    C. disrupting nucleic acid synthesis.
    D. inhibiting viral attachment.
    E. inhibiting protein synthesis.

48. The total number of existing cases of a particular disease in a particular population within a given period is referred to as the
    A. rate.
    B. prevalence.
    C. incidence.
    D. proportion.

49. All are thought to be beneficial aspects of fever EXCEPT one. Which one is the EXCEPTION?
    A. Stimulating interferon responses
    B. Inhibiting microbial growth
    C. Stimulating the action of phagocytes
    D. Stimulating tissue repair

50. Which reaction is characterized by degranulation of mast cells as a result of antigen–antibody complexes affixed to cell surfaces?
    A. Immune complex
    B. Cytotoxic
    C. Anaphylactic
    D. Delayed hypersensitivity

51. What is the etiologic agent of syphilis?
    A. *Borrelia vincentii*
    B. *Actinomyces israelii*
    C. *Treponema pallidum*
    D. *Treponema denticola*
    E. *Histoplasma capsulatum*

52. All are cardinal signs of inflammation EXCEPT one. Which one is the EXCEPTION?
    A. Pain
    B. Redness
    C. Swelling
    D. Localized heat
    E. Pale color
    F. Loss of function

53. All of these cellular components increase disease virulence EXCEPT one. Which one is the EXCEPTION?
    A. Flagellae
    B. Glycocalyx
    C. Fimbriae
    D. Pili
    E. Lipopolysaccharides

54. A memory or secondary immune response will generate a more rapid antibody response. It is more powerful than a primary immune response.
    A. Both statements are true.
    B. Both statements are false.
    C. The first statement is true, and the second statement is false.
    D. The first statement is false, and the second statement is true.

55. Which condition describes the body's immune system reacting to its own tissues as if they were foreign?
    A. Hyperimmune reaction
    B. Autoimmune reaction
    C. Allergic reaction
    D. Immunodeficiency reaction

56. The relationship between herpes simplex 1 and herpes simplex 2 MOST closely matches the relationship between
    A. measles and mumps.
    B. chickenpox and shingles.
    C. smallpox and chickenpox.

57. Which virus enters the respiratory system and spreads via blood to the parotid glands to present as a characteristic disease sign?
    A. Severe acute respiratory syndrome (SARS) virus
    B. H1N1 influenza virus
    C. Mumps virus
    D. Rhinovirus

58. Which disease is characterized by the production of toxins that cause respiratory tract inflammation, paralysis of cilia, and a characteristic cough?
    A. Pertussis
    B. H1N1 influenza
    C. Tuberculosis
    D. Respiratory syncytial virus infection
    E. Chickenpox

59. Which oral pathogen can cause an infection that may lead to cardiovascular disease?
    A. *Mycobacterium tuberculosis*
    B. *Fusobacterium nucleatum*
    C. *Borrelia burgdorferi*
    D. *Streptococcus mutans*

60. Koplik spots are a distinctive oral manifestation of which diseases?
    A. Measles
    B. Mumps
    C. Rubella
    D. Meningitis
    E. Pneumonia

Answers and Rationales

1. Which inflammatory mediator is produced by B-cells and T-cells?

   ANS: A
   Cytokines (A) are inflammatory mediators produced by B-cells and T-cells. Immunoglobulins (B) are produced by plasma cells, which are produced by B-lymphocytes. Interleukin-4 (C) and interleukin-6 (D) are found in T-cells and stimulate the B-lymphocyte response.

2. Which is the predominant antibody in saliva?

   ANS: A
   Immunoglobulin A (A) is the predominant antibody found in saliva and is termed the *secretory antibody*. The other antibodies—immunoglobulin E (B), immunoglobulin D (C), and immunoglobulin G (D)—may be found in saliva but not in amounts as large as that of immunoglobulin A.

3. Which cells are most involved in cell-mediated immunity?

   ANS: D
   T-lymphocytes (D) are responsible for cell-mediated immunity. Mast cells (A) release histamine and other vasoreactive mediators in allergic reactions, and plasma cells (B) produce immunoglobulin G. Neutrophils (C) are a type of white blood cells.

4. Contact dermatitis is considered which type of hypersensitivity reaction?

   ANS: D
   Contact dermatitis is considered a type IV hypersensitivity reaction (D), involving a T-cell–mediated response, not an antibody. Types I (A), II (B), and III (C) are associated with the formation of antibodies.

5. Saliva has each of these protective mechanisms EXCEPT one. Which one is the EXCEPTION?

   ANS: A
   Saliva does not increase (A) because of an increase in inflammation. Buffering the acids created by oral bacteria (B), containing secretory antibodies (C), and lubricating mucosal tissues (D) are the protective mechanisms of saliva.

6. Which cellular characteristic describes why gram-positive bacteria stain differently from how gram-negative bacteria stain?

   ANS: B
   The cell walls of gram-positive bacteria contain a thicker layer of peptidoglycan (B) than those of gram-negative bacteria, absorbing more stain and thus staining darker. Gram-negative bacterial cell walls contain less peptidoglycan than those of gram-positive bacteria (A), staining lighter. Cytoplasm amounts (C, D) do not directly affect the staining capabilities of bacteria.

7. An ideal antibiotic has the ability to inhibit a wide range of microorganisms, including normal flora. It will only act on the pathogen, with no harmful effect to the human host.

   ANS: D
   The correct choice is (D). The first statement is false as an ideal antibiotic should have the ability to inhibit a wide range of microorganisms but NOT the normal flora. The second statement is true. Choices A, B, and C do not accurately reflect the statements.

8. Which term BEST describes the ability of a microorganism to cause disease?

   ANS: B
   A microorganism's virulence (B) best describes its ability to cause disease. Stability (A), productivity (C), and transmissibility (D) do not directly influence the ability of a microorganism to cause disease.

9. The cellular structure that is used to classify a bacterial species as gram-positive or gram-negative is the

   ANS: B
   Differences between cell wall structure (B) and composition classify bacterial species as gram-positive or gram-negative. Gram-positive bacteria contain a large amount of peptidoglycan in a single, thick layer, whereas gram-negative bacteria contain a thin layer of peptidoglycan sandwiched between the cell membrane and an outer membrane containing lipopolysaccharides. A flagellum (A) is a hairlike structure that projects from the cell body and aids in movement. A cell membrane (C) is the outer covering of a cell. The pilus (D) is a hairlike projection found on the surface of many bacteria. Glycocalyx (E) is a glycoprotein–polysaccharide covering that surrounds many cells. None of these structures differentiates between gram-positive and gram-negative cells.

10. All are typical bacterial cell shapes EXCEPT one. Which one is the EXCEPTION?

    ANS: D
    A disk (D) is not a shape typical of bacterial cells viewed under the microscope. A spirochete (A) is

a corkscrew-shaped bacterium. A coccus (B) is a round-shaped bacterium. A bacillus (C) is a rod-shaped bacterium.

11. The prefix *strepto-* designates bacteria that take on which type of arrangement?

ANS: A
The prefix *strepto-* is the designation for bacterial cells arranged in a chainlike fashion (A). Two common examples are streptococci and streptobacilli. Tetrad (B) describes an arrangement of four cocci in a square shape. The cluster arrangement (C) contains cocci that are divided in numerous random planes. Sarcina (D) designates a cubelike arrangement. The diploid (E) arrangement consists of two joined bacterial cells.

12. Which is the MOST appropriate definition of a microorganism?

ANS: C
A microorganism is an organism in which the individual cells cannot be seen with the unaided eye (C). A microscope must be used to view individual microbial cells (A). Eukaryotic microorganisms do contain a nucleus in their cells (B). All microbial cells contain cell membranes (D).

13. The key to Alexander Fleming's recognition of penicillin as a tool for fighting bacterial infections was his observation that

ANS: B
Alexander Fleming observed that the growth of *Staphylococcus aureus* bacterial colonies were inhibited on plates contaminated with the mold *Penicillium notatum* (B), leading to the identification of the antibacterial agent penicillin. Bacteria are not inhibited by growth of nearby bacteria (A). Mold does not inhibit the growth of nearby yeast (C). Viruses do not produce penicillin (D).

14. The best definition of a virus is

ANS: B
A virus is an acellular microorganism that requires the nuclear materials of the host to replicate. Because viruses are not composed of cells, they are referred to as *acellular*; in addition, they do not contain the resources needed for replication and so must use host cell resources to complete their replication (B). A eukaryote is a cell that contains complex structures, including a nucleus bound within a membrane (A, C). Prokaryotic cells do not have a nucleus, a nuclear membrane, or any other membrane-bound organelles (D). A virus is not a cell (E) and cannot be classified as either prokaryotic or eukaryotic.

15. You are observing a cell through a microscope and note that it does not have a nucleus. From this observation, you can also conclude that it most likely

ANS: A
Prokaryotic cells (bacteria) have cell walls containing peptidoglycan, and only prokaryotic cells do not have a nucleus (A). Fungi are made up of eukaryotic cells, which do contain a nucleus (B). Cilia are only found on the surface of eukaryotic cells, which have a nucleus (C). All cells, prokaryotic and eukaryotic, have a cell membrane (D).

16. Structures that enable the transfer of genetic material between bacterial cells are

ANS: D
The only structures in this list of choices that can transfer genetic material are pili (D). Fimbriae (A) allow for attachment to host cells. Capsules (B) are protective structures around bacterial cells. Cilia (C) allow for movement of protozoan cells.

17. Observation of microbial cell arrangement can be used to differentiate between streptococci and staphylococci. Observation of microbial cell shape can be used to differentiate between streptococci and staphylococci.

ANS: C
The first statement is true, and the second is false (C). The arrangements of streptococci and staphylococci are different; streptococci are arranged in a chainlike fashion, whereas staphylococci are arranged in clusters. Both streptococci and staphylococci have the same coccal, or round, shape. Choices A, B and D do not correctly reflect the statements.

18. A patient is believed to be infected by *Mycobacterium tuberculosis,* the causative agent of tuberculosis. These microorganisms have a waxy cell wall. Which of the following staining methods can verify this assumption?

ANS: C
The standard stain for identifying bacteria from the *Mycobacterium* genus, including *Mycobacterium tuberculosis,* is the acid-fast stain (C). The components of this stain allow for penetration of the characteristic waxy cell walls of cells in this genus. Gram stain (A) is used for staining of bacterial cell walls and differentiation between gram-positive and gram-negative bacteria. The flagellar stain (B) is used to identify bacteria containing a flagella. The endospore (D) is used to differentiate between bacteria that form endospores.

The ability to produce endospores is restricted to the bacterial genera *Bacillus* and *Clostridium* (B). *Mycobacterium* species have a waxy, protective coating, not endospores (D).

33. Which object is a fomite?

ANS: E
A *fomite* is an inanimate object such a hypodermic needle (E) used in indirect-contact transmission to spread a pathogen from one reservoir to the next susceptible host. Water (A) is used in vehicle transmission. Droplets from a sneeze (B) are involved in droplet transmission. Bodily fluids (C) would be involved in direct-contact spread if the next susceptible host came into direct contact with this secretion from the pathogen's reservoir. Insects (D) are involved in vector transmission.

34. Interferons nonspecifically inhibit the spread of which type of infections?

ANS: A
Interferons are a part of the nonspecific, or first-line bodily defense. Their release inhibits viral infection (A) by activating the production of antiviral proteins in cells, which will stop the spread of viral infection to other host cells. Bacterial (B) and protozoal infections (C) are primarily controlled through stimulation of humoral immunity. Parasitic worm infestations (D) are primarily controlled through stimulation of cell-mediated immunity.

35. All are considered nonspecific body immune defenses EXCEPT one. Which one is the EXCEPTION?

ANS: A
Antibodies (A) are components of the body's specific immune system. They are produced by B-cells, which must be stimulated or called into action to produce plasma cells that produce antibodies. The antibodies will then specifically target the pathogens that caused their production in response. Mucous membranes (B), intact skin (C), phagocytic cells such as neutrophils and macrophages (D), and lysozyme in tears (E) are components of the body's nonspecific defenses that are always present and ready to defend the body against pathogens.

36. T-helper cells produce

ANS: D
T-helper cells produce cytokines (D), which are chemical messengers that activate other components of the immune system. Antibodies (A) are produced by

plasma cells, which are a product of B-lymphocytes. Cytolytic enzymes (B) are produced by killer T-cells and serve to lyse infected cells. Plasma cells (C) are a product of B-lymphocytes and cannot be produced by T-cells, although T-helper cells can send signals to them to produce antibodies.

37. Which is NOT a characteristic of adaptive immunity?

ANS: A
"Nonspecific" is incorrect because adaptive immune response is a *specific* immune response that specifically targets the pathogen that stimulated it (A). The remaining choices all define adaptive immunity. Memory cells are generated so that the immune system will remember a pathogen if it enters the body again (B) and generate a quick response. This arm of the immune system must be activated (C), usually by components of the nonspecific or innate immune system. Adaptive immunity is considered the third line of the body's defense (D).

38. Antigens are

ANS: C
Antigens are specific modules of a pathogen or substances secreted by the pathogen that the body recognizes as foreign (C). Cells that protect the body against invaders include white blood cells and antibodies (A). Enzymes secreted by white blood cells include collagenase, lysozyme, and matrix metalloproteinases (B). Complement proteins are produced to protect the body against foreign invaders (D). Proteins on the surface of cells that code for tissue type and transplant compatibility are called the major histocompatibility complex (MHC) (E).

39. An antibiotic binds to the 30S ribosomal subunit. On the basis of this information, this antibiotic inhibits which of the following processes?

ANS: D
Ribosomes are responsible for translation or protein synthesis. Ribosomes in eukaryotes are composed of a large 60S subunit and a small 40S subunit in comparison with ribosomes in prokaryotes that are composed of a large 50S subunit and a small 30S subunit. Some antibiotics prevent protein synthesis in bacteria, which are prokaryotes (D). Transcription is the process by which messenger ribonucleic acid (mRNA) is synthesized from a deoxyribonucleic acid (DNA) template and is not part of the mechanism of action for antibiotics (A, B). Protein synthesis in eukaryotes (C) is not affected by antibiotics.

40. A viral infection may be treated with an antibiotic. Antivirals are difficult to develop because viruses use host cell machinery for their replication.

ANS: D
The first statement is false, and the second statement is true (D). Antibiotics are specific for treating bacterial infections, whereas antivirals are used for the treatment of viral infections. Viruses do not contain the resources needed for replication, so they use host cell nucleic acids to complete their replication. This makes the development of antivirals difficult because there are significantly fewer antiviral targets. In addition, the necessity of replication inside a host cell makes it difficult to develop an antiviral that can target and destroy the virus while leaving the host cell unaffected. Choices A, B, and C do not accurately reflect the statements.

41. The BEST definition of *sterilization* is

ANS: C
Sterilization is the removal or destruction of all microorganisms, including endospores (C). Disinfection of living tissue (A) describes the term *antisepsis*. The use of a chemical agent to destroy pathogens is termed *disinfection* (B). Not all microorganisms are pathogens (D).

42. Standard methods of sterilization are NOT effective in destruction of

ANS: C
Prions (C), or proteinaceous infectious particles, are not destroyed by standard sterilization techniques. Additional measures such as incineration are needed to destroy prions. Standard sterilization methods can destroy viruses (A), bacteria (B), protozoa (D), and fungi (E).

43. A chemical agent that kills pathogenic microbes in general is a(n)

ANS: B
A germicide (B) is capable of killing pathogenic microbes in general. The suffix *-cide* indicates that a particular agent has killing capability. A sanitizer (A) does not kill all pathogenic microbes but simply reduces them to a safe level. Disinfectants (C) are applied to nonliving objects to destroy microorganisms on surfaces. Fungicide (D) is a chemical that specifically kills fungi. Antiseptics (E) are substances that inhibit the growth and development of microorganisms and are applied to living tissues.

44. Proper filtration of air and liquids relies on which property?

ANS: D
A filter used for the elimination of microbes in the air or in liquid relies on the presence of pores of a particular size to keep out, or filter out, microbes (D). The application of pressure (A) would not properly filter out air and liquids. Sterile liquids (B) are produced following the filtration process. Filter size (C) is irrelevant; it is the size of the pores in the filters that determine what microbes can or cannot pass through them.

45. Which BEST describes the selective toxicity characteristic of antimicrobials?

ANS: A
Selective toxicity is especially important in the design of an antimicrobial, ensuring that the antimicrobial is selectively toxic for the pathogen that is causing an infection and disease while leaving the host unharmed (A). Harming the host cell (B, C) is an unacceptable choice. Titration (D) is not related to the selective toxicity of an antimicrobial.

46. The mechanism of action for naturally occurring penicillin and its synthetic derivatives such as methicillin and ampicillin is the inhibition of cell wall synthesis. The spectrum of action for beta-lactam antibiotics equally includes gram-negative and gram-positive bacteria.

ANS: C
The first statement is true, and the second statement is false (C). Penicillin and its synthetic derivatives such as methicillin and ampicillin are beta-lactam drugs that target the assembly of peptidoglycan in bacterial cell walls. The second statement is false. Gram-positive bacteria are targeted more efficiently by this group of antibiotics because their cell walls contain a higher amount of peptidoglycan and do not contain an outer lipid membrane external to the peptidoglycan layer such as the one found in gram-negative bacterial cells. Choices A, B, and D do not accurately reflect the statements.

47. Erythromycin and tetracycline both act by

ANS: E
The mechanism of action for erythromycin and tetracycline is to inhibit protein synthesis (E). Erythromycin is a macrolide that binds to the 50S large ribosomal subunit in prokaryotic cells. Upon binding, it prevents messenger ribonucleic acid movement through the ribosome, thereby halting protein synthesis.

Tetracycline blocks the docking site of transfer ribonucleic acid so that an amino acid chain cannot be elongated to make a protein. These two antibiotics do not target the cell membrane (A), cell wall (B), or nucleic acids (C) of bacteria. In addition, antibiotics do not target viruses (D).

48. The total number of existing cases of a particular disease in a particular population within a given period is referred to as the

    ANS: B
    The definition of *prevalence* (B) is total number of already existing cases of a particular disease in a particular population within a given period. Rate (A) is the number of cases in a population expressed as a percentage. Incidence (C) only concerns the number of new cases in a given area or population during a period. It does not include the number of already existing cases that contribute to the total number of cases of a particular disease. Proportion (D) compares one population with the larger one to which it belongs.

49. All are thought to be beneficial aspects of fever EXCEPT one. Which one is the EXCEPTION?

    ANS: D
    Fever usually occurs in the acute inflammatory phase, which is not the period when tissue repair occurs (D). Fever is a nonspecific immune response that stimulates the actions of interferons (A) and phagocytes (C). The higher body temperature inhibits the growth of microorganisms (B) that may need the body to be at normal temperature for maximal replication efficiency.

50. Which reaction is characterized by degranulation of mast cells as a result of antigen–antibody complexes affixed to cell surfaces?

    ANS: C
    An anaphylactic reaction (C) is the most severe example of a type I, immediate hypersensitivity reaction. Within minutes after exposure to a previously encountered allergen, preformed immunoglobulin E (IgE) antibodies cause mast cells to be produced in the tissue and basophils in the circulating bloodstream to release histamine and other vasoreactive granules. Massive vasodilation results in a drop in blood pressure, and bronchoconstriction and edema of the airways may cause a life-threatening reaction. Immune complex (A), or type III, hypersensitivity reactions occur when antigen–antibody complexes leave the circulation and are deposited in body tissues or in a localized area, resulting in an acute inflammatory response. Lysosomal enzymes released from neutrophils cause the type of tissue destruction

seen in autoimmune diseases such as systemic lupus erythematosus. Cytotoxic (B), or type II, hypersensitivity occurs when the antibody attaches to the surface of a tissue cell, usually a red blood cell. Antibodies activate other complement antibodies such as immunoglobulin G and immunoglobulin M in blood, destroying the targeted red blood cells. Reactions to blood transfusions of incompatible blood types and fetal Rh incompatibility are examples of this type of hypersensitivity reaction. The delayed hypersensitivity (D), or type IV, cell-mediated immune response involves production of lymphokines from sensitized T-lymphocytes, causing conditions such as contact dermatitis and the skin reaction seen in the tuberculin skin test.

51. What is the etiologic agent of syphilis?

    ANS: C
    Syphilis is caused by the bacterial spirochete *Treponema pallidum* (C). *Borrelia vincentii* (A) and fusiform bacilli are the microorganisms associated with necrotizing ulcerative gingivitis (NUG). *Actinomyces israelii* (B) is the infectious agent in actinomycosis, a disease with abscesses draining from the bacteria into tissue. *Treponema denticola* (D) is one of the red complex of microorganisms that are associated with periodontitis. *Histoplasma capsulatum* (E) is one of the causative pathogens associated with histoplasmosis, a fungal infection of the lung.

52. All are cardinal signs of inflammation EXCEPT one. Which one is the EXCEPTION?

    ANS: E
    Pale color (E), or *pallor,* is not a cardinal sign of inflammation. The typical signs and symptoms of inflammation are pain (A), or *dolor*; redness (B), or *rubor*; swelling (C), or *tumor*; localized heat (D), or *calor*; and loss of function (F), or *laso functio*. These changes are primarily caused by increased vasodilation and increased capillary permeability, which bring additional blood flow to the area.

53. All of these cellular components increase disease virulence EXCEPT one. Which one is the EXCEPTION?

    ANS: A
    Flagellae (A) are long, threadlike appendages with a whiplike motion that allows the bacteria to move through fluids and are not linked to virulence. Glycocalyx (B), which is a capsule found on some bacteria, aids in adherence and resistance to phagocytosis, greatly enhancing bacterial virulence. Fimbriae (C) are cellular projections that promote

bacterial adherence and virulence. Pili (D) are tubelike structures that allow transfer of genetic material between bacteria, increasing drug resistance and virulence. Lipopolysaccharides (E) are a component of the cell wall of gram-negative bacteria.

54. A memory or secondary immune response will generate a more rapid antibody response. It is more powerful than a primary immune response.

ANS: A
Both statements are true (A). Memory or secondary immune responses are much quicker and more intense or powerful compared with primary immune responses. The memory cells produced during the primary immune response allow for a much quicker response to a pathogen that has been previously encountered by the host immune system. Primary immune responses are slower and less powerful because they must be activated on their first exposure to the pathogen and are producing memory cells for the first time. Choices B, C, and D do not accurately reflect the statements.

55. Which condition describes the body's immune system reacting to its own tissues as if they were foreign?

ANS: B
An autoimmune reaction (B) is the condition in which the body's immune system treats its own tissues as if they were foreign. A hyperimmune reaction (A) refers to an overproduction of antibodies but not necessarily against the body's own tissues. An allergic reaction (C) is also an overreaction of the body's immune system but not to the body's own tissues. An immunodeficiency (D) is caused when the body's immune system is deficient.

56. The relationship between herpes simplex 1 and herpes simplex 2 MOST closely matches the relationship between

ANS: B
The varicella-zoster virus causes both chickenpox and shingles (B), which are different clinical manifestations of the same virus. This is similar to the relationship between herpes simplex 1 (oral herpes) and herpes simplex 2 (genital herpes). Measles is caused by a virus that is entirely different from the mumps virus. Measles may include a rash that appears as flat, discolored areas (macules) and solid, red, raised areas (papules), whereas mumps causes enlargement of the parotid glands (A). Smallpox has been eradicated, and its pustules are firm and more embedded in skin compared with those of chickenpox (C).

57. Which virus enters the respiratory system and spreads via blood to the parotid glands to present as a characteristic disease sign?

ANS: C
The mumps virus (C) originates in the respiratory system and travels in the bloodstream to the salivary glands to cause the characteristic sign of enlarged parotid glands. The SARS virus (A), H1N1 influenza virus (B), and rhinovirus (which causes common cold) (D) infections are diseases of the respiratory system but manifest primarily with respiratory symptoms.

58. Which disease is characterized by the production of toxins that cause respiratory tract inflammation, paralysis of cilia, and a characteristic cough?

ANS: A
Bordetella pertussis, the causative agent of pertussis (A), or "whooping cough," produces a tracheal cytotoxin and results in a characteristic "whoop" cough. H1N1 influenza (B), known as the "swine flu," may produce severe respiratory symptoms but does not produce toxins. Tuberculosis (C) causes respiratory tract inflammation and causes a cough but does not produce toxins. Respiratory syncytial virus infection (D) causes a mild respiratory disease in adults but may cause severe respiratory problems in infants and young children. Respiratory syncytial virus does not produce toxins. Chickenpox (E) is transmitted by respiratory droplets but does not fit the description above.

59. Which oral pathogen can cause an infection that may lead to cardiovascular disease?

ANS: B
The only pathogen on the list that can cause an infection leading to a cardiovascular disease and is only found in the oral cavity is *Fusobacterium nucleatum* (B). *Mycobacterium tuberculosis* (A) causes tuberculosis. *Borrelia burgdorferi* (C) is the bacterium that causes Lyme disease. *Streptococcus mutans* (D) is the bacterium that causes dental caries.

60. Koplik spots are a distinctive oral manifestation of which diseases?

ANS: A
Koplik spots, which are small erythematous macules with white necrotic centers, are a distinctive oral manifestation of measles (A). Mumps (B) presents as swelling of the parotid glands. Rubella (C) is similar to measles but does not present with Koplik spots. Meningitis (D) presents with neurologic signs and symptoms such as numbness and stiff neck. *Pneumonia* (E) is the general term for respiratory infections of the lungs.

6. There are several types of candidiasis, including erythematous candidiasis and denture candidiasis. Regardless of the type, all forms must be treated with antibiotics.
   A. Both statements are true.
   B. Both statements are false.
   C. The first statement is true, and the second statement is false.
   D. The first statement is false, and the second statement is true.

7. Enamel hypoplasia is caused by ameloblast formation of too much enamel. Enamel hypocalcification occurs when there is too little enamel formation.
   A. Both statements are true.
   B. Both statements are false.
   C. The first statement is true, and the second statement is false.
   D. The first statement is false, and the second statement is true.

8. Which lesion may be associated with hormonal changes?
   A. Thyroid nodule
   B. Pyogenic granuloma
   C. Fordyce granules
   D. Hemangioma

9. Which response is NOT a sign or implication of a local inflammation?
   A. Redness
   B. Swelling
   C. Heat
   D. Lymphadenopathy

10. Cross-reactive (C-reactive) protein is produced in the
    A. liver.
    B. thyroid.
    C. spleen.
    D. stomach.

11. Bulimia is often associated with which oral condition?
    A. Attrition
    B. Abrasion
    C. Erosion
    D. Abfraction

12. Aspirin burn will appear
    A. as a nonpainful, chronic lesion on the hard palate.
    B. as an acute, painful, white lesion on the buccal mucosa.
    C. as an acute, nonpainful, red lesion the floor of the mouth.
    D. as a red-and-white, chronic, painless lesion requiring biopsy.

13. The dental hygienist has just done an in-service presentation to the nurses' aides at the nursing home, and one of the nurses' aides calls and states to the office that she just noticed a hard lump on the roof of the mouth of one of the residents, and although it does not hurt, she is worried that it might be cancer, since the resident is a smoker. What is the MOST likely clinical diagnosis?
    A. Torus palatinus
    B. Paget disease of the bone
    C. Compound odontoma
    D. Osteosarcoma

14. Crack cocaine use may exhibit all clinical findings EXCEPT one. Which one is the EXCEPTION?
    A. Parched lips
    B. Xerostomia
    C. Irritation of the palate
    D. Irritation of the floor of the mouth
    E. Increased heart rate and blood pressure

15. Traumatic ulcers are usually diagnosed through which diagnostic procedure?
    A. History of lesion
    B. Clinical appearance only
    C. Microscopic diagnosis
    D. Therapeutic diagnosis

16. What is the BEST method of diagnosis of linea alba?
    A. Clinical appearance
    B. Biopsy
    C. VELscope™
    D. Brush test

17. Nicotine stomatitis first appears clinically as a/an
    A. overall erythroplakia.
    B. white lesion.
    C. ulcerated area.
    D. brown stain.

18. Actinic cheilitis is only caused by
    A. smoking.
    B. use of lip gloss.
    C. sun.
    D. consistent trauma from a pipe stem.

19. Necrotizing sialometaplasia is clinically characterized by
    A. ulceration in the affected area.
    B. fever.
    C. lymphadenopathy.
    D. lack of saliva.

20. Pyogenic granuloma is associated with
    A. acute infection.
    B. older age.

C. chronic inflammation.
D. a genetic condition.

21. Which drug does NOT cause gingival enlargement?
    A. Phenytoin (Dilantin)
    B. Nifedipine (Procardia)
    C. Penicillin
    D. Amlodipine (Norvasc)

22. Chronic hyperplastic pulpitis is seen clinically
    A. within an open carious crown of a tooth.
    B. at the apex of the root.
    C. between roots.
    D. at the gingival margin.

23. Which does NOT describe the characteristics of a radicular cyst?
    A. Is a true cyst
    B. Is caused by caries
    C. Is a pseudocyst
    D. Occurs in nonvital tooth

24. The radicular cyst will have a similar radiographic appearance to all of these pathologies EXCEPT one. Which one is the EXCEPTION?
    A. Periapical granuloma
    B. Abscess
    C. Dentigerous or follicular cyst
    D. Periapical cyst

25. Which recurrent aphthous ulcer occurs most commonly?
    A. Major aphthous ulcer
    B. Minor aphthous ulcer
    C. Herpetiform ulcer
    D. Sutton disease ulcer

26. What is another term for hives?
    A. Urticaria
    B. Sutton disease
    C. Pruritus
    D. Contact dermatitis

27. All are characteristics of lichen planus EXCEPT one. Which one is the EXCEPTION?
    A. Benign, chronic condition
    B. Wickham striae
    C. Desquamative gingivitis
    D. Bull's-eye skin lesions

28. A triad of symptoms—joint pain, urethritis, and conjunctivitis—are associated with which condition?
    A. Behçet syndrome
    B. Hand-Schüller-Christian disease
    C. Reactive arthritis
    D. Lichen planus

29. Patients with systemic lupus erythematosus (SLE) may require modifications to dental hygiene treatment EXCEPT one. Which one is the EXCEPTION?
    A. Treatment of erosive oral lesions
    B. Delay of treatment because of immunosuppression
    C. Increased use of fluorides
    D. Use of adaptive oral hygiene aids

30. Acantholysis occurs in:
    A. lichen planus.
    B. normal mucosa.
    C. pemphigus vulgaris.
    D. mucosal membrane pemphigoid.

31. Oral and genital ulcers and ocular inflammation are characteristics of which condition?
    A. Erythema multiforme
    B. Behçet syndrome
    C. Hand-Schüller-Christian disease
    D. Reactive arthritis

32. Which condition is a bacterial skin infection?
    A. Impetigo
    B. Erythema multiforme
    C. Lichen planus
    D. Systemic lupus erythematosus (SLE)

33. Strawberry tongue is associated with which condition?
    A. Rheumatic fever
    B. Scarlet fever
    C. Tuberculosis
    D. Chickenpox

34. Which is the MOST characteristic clinical feature of herpes zoster?
    A. Fever
    B. Unilateral lesions
    C. Patient's age
    D. Ulcers throughout the oral mucosa

35. Which condition is NOT associated with tuberculosis?
    A. Positive protein derivative (PPD)
    B. Granulomatous disease
    C. Primary infection in oral tissues
    D. Kidney and liver involvement

36. Actinomycosis is caused by a/an
    A. fungus.
    B. filamentous bacterium.
    C. abscess.
    D. spirochete.

37. Syphilis is caused by
    A. *Actinomyces israelii.*
    B. *Treponema pallidum.*
    C. *Mycobacterium tuberculosis.*
    D. *Borrelia vincentii.*

38. An operculum contributes to which condition?
    A. Necrotizing ulcerative gingivitis (NUG)
    B. Syphilis
    C. Tuberculosis (TB)
    D. Pericoronitis

39. Which condition is MOST often associated with loss of vascularity in bone?
    A. Paget disease
    B. Sickle cell disease
    C. Radiation to bone
    D. Periapical cemento-osseous dysplasia

40. Candidiasis is an overgrowth of a
    A. yeastlike fungus.
    B. spirochete.
    C. filamentous bacterium.
    D. fusiform bacillus.

41. Clinically, pseudomembranous candidiasis is described as
    A. a white, curdlike material that cannot be rubbed off.
    B. denture stomatitis.
    C. a white, curdlike material that can be wiped off.
    D. red and painful mucosa.

42. The MOST common type of candidiasis affecting the oral mucosa is
    A. pseudomembranous candidiasis.
    B. hypertrophic candidiasis.
    C. candidal leukoplakia.
    D. chronic atrophic candidiasis.

43. Types 16 and 18 of human papillomavirus (HPV) have been specifically linked to anal, cervical, vulvar, and oropharyngeal cancers. HPV types 6 and 11, which cause condyloma acuminatum, are also considered oncogenic viruses.
    A. Both statements are true.
    B. Both statements are false.
    C. The first statement is true, and the second statement is false.
    D. The first statement is false, and the second statement is true.

44. What is the primary feature that distinguishes herpes simplex 1 from herpes zoster?
    A. Painful, burning gingiva
    B. Vesicles in oral cavity

C. Depressed immunologic function
D. Unilateral distribution of vesicles

45. Varicella-zoster-virus (VZV) causes chickenpox and what other disease?
    A. Measles
    B. Mumps
    C. Shingles
    D. Mononucleosis

46. A negative test for human immunodeficiency virus (HIV) indicates that a person is free of HIV. This is because antibodies are produced within days of exposure to HIV.
    A. Both statements are true.
    B. Both statements are false.
    C. The first statement is true, and the second statement is false.
    D. The first statement is false, and the second statement is true.

47. Hairy leukoplakia is caused by which virus?
    A. Epstein-Barr virus (EBV)
    B. Human-immunodeficiency virus (HIV)
    C. Human papilloma virus (HPV)
    D. Herpes simplex virus (HSV)

48. Characteristics of ankyloglossia include all EXCEPT one. Which one is the EXCEPTION?
    A. The cause is a short lingual frenum.
    B. The patient may experience speech problems.
    C. Corrective treatment is frenectomy.
    D. Ankyloglossia is associated with other congenital syndromes.

49. All are examples of hypersensitivity reactions involving antibodies EXCEPT one. Which one is the EXCEPTION?
    A. Asthma
    B. Hay fever
    C. Contact dermatitis
    D. Anaphylaxis
    E. Angioedema

50. Which type of cyst develops in place of a tooth?
    A. Dentigerous
    B. Primordial
    C. Botryoid
    D. Lateral periodontal

51. The type of immunity received after the full series of immunizations against hepatitis B is called
    A. natural passive immunity.
    B. acquired or artificial passive immunity.

C. natural active immunity.

D. acquired or artificial active immunity.

52. Which cyst often appears as a heart-shaped radiolucency?
   A. Radicular
   B. Nasopalatine canal
   C. Globulomaxillary
   D. Lateral periodontal

53. Which cyst does NOT have alveolar bone involvement?
   A. Nasopalatine canal
   B. Nasolabial
   C. Residual
   D. Radicular

54. Which cyst is filled with salivary gland tissue?
   A. Simple bone
   B. Traumatic bone
   C. Static bone
   D. Dermoid

55. The most common supernumerary tooth is the
   A. mesiodens.
   B. distomolar.
   C. maxillary permanent lateral.
   D. third molar.

56. The enamel pearl is
   A. seen as a radiopaque sphere on the root.
   B. an extra cusp seen on the crown of permanent incisors.
   C. the same as a taurodont.
   D. the same as a talon cusp.

57. Enamel hypoplasia may result from all conditions EXCEPT one. Which one is the EXCEPTION?
   A. Trauma
   B. Local infection
   C. Fluoride
   D. Tetracycline

58. Autosomes are
   A. nonsex-linked chromosomes.
   B. located at the periphery of the nucleus of cells in women.
   C. codons.
   D. centromeres.

59. The difference between primitive germ cells and mature germ cells is
   A. 23 chromosomes.
   B. 46 chromosomes.
   C. trisomy.
   D. phenotype.

60. Which is NOT associated with trisomy 21?
   A. Failure of chromosome pairs to separate or nondisjunction
   B. Down syndrome
   C. Three identical chromosomes at the same allele
   D. Increased intelligence

61. Most cases of Turner syndrome result from
   A. nondisjunction of dividing chromosome pair.
   B. trisomy.
   C. XXY chromosomes.
   D. deletion.

62. Which is the MOST important consideration in the treatment of a dental hygiene patient with cyclic neutropenia?
   A. High neutrophil count
   B. Patient malaise
   C. Low neutrophil count
   D. Frequency of recall appointments

63. All conditions have an autosomal–dominant trait EXCEPT one. Which one is the EXCEPTION?
   A. Cyclic neutropenia
   B. Focal palmoplantar and gingival hyperkeratosis
   C. Papillon-Lefèvre syndrome
   D. Laband syndrome

64. Progressive bilateral facial swelling is the first clinical manifestation in which autosomal–dominant condition?
   A. Cherubism
   B. Papillon-Lefèvre syndrome
   C. Kostmann syndrome
   D. Mandibulofacial dysostosis

65. Which characteristic is NOT a major feature in osteogenesis imperfecta?
   A. Abnormally formed bones that fracture
   B. Blue sclerae
   C. Dentinogenesis imperfecta
   D. Severe deafness

66. Multiple cysts of the jaws are associated with which condition?
   A. Dentinogenesis imperfecta
   B. Cherubism
   C. Nevoid basal cell carcinoma syndrome
   D. Mandibulofacial dysostosis

67. For which component of Gardner syndrome would a medical referral be recommended?
   A. Odontomas
   B. Supernumerary teeth
   C. Cottonwool appearance of alveolar bone
   D. Intestinal polyps

68. Multiple capillary dilations of skin and the mucous membrane are seen in which genetic condition?
    A. Hematoma
    B. White sponge nevus
    C. Gorlin syndrome
    D. Hereditary hemorrhagic telangiectasia

69. In which condition do intestinal polyps most frequently undergo malignant transformation?
    A. Gardner syndrome
    B. Peutz-Jeghers syndrome
    C. White sponge nevus
    D. Ellis-van Creveld syndrome

70. The autosomal–dominant, "pitted variety" of amelogenesis imperfecta is called
    A. hypoplastic.
    B. enamel agenesis.
    C. hypocalcified.
    D. hypomaturation.

71. All are characteristics of hypohidrotic ectodermal dysplasia EXCEPT one. Which one is the EXCEPTION?
    A. Hypotrichosis
    B. Hypodontia
    C. Reduced ability to sweat
    D. X-linked–recessive only

72. A lesion that has a stemlike base is described as being
    A. pedunculated.
    B. lobulated.
    C. sessile.
    D. bullous.

73. The clinical term used to describe a red lesion with unknown cause is a(an)
    A. hematoma.
    B. leukoplakia.
    C. erythroplakia.
    D. squamous cell carcinoma.

74. Which condition is frequently observed radiographically as a radiolucent scalloping around the roots of teeth?
    A. Traumatic bone cyst
    B. Static bone cyst
    C. Stage II periapical cemento-osseous dysplasia
    D. Radicular cyst

75. The dental hygienist typically uses the following types of diagnostic tools when collecting clinical data EXCEPT one. Which one is the EXCEPTION?
    A. Clinical
    B. Radiographic
    C. Historical
    D. Histologic

76. Which condition is NOT diagnosed by clinical diagnosis alone?
    A. Tori
    B. Black hairy tongue
    C. Fistula
    D. Lingual varicosities

77. All conditions are thought to be immunologically related EXCEPT one. Which one is the EXCEPTION?
    A. Erythema multiforme
    B. Pemphigus vulgaris
    C. Geographic tongue
    D. Aphthous ulcers

78. Pituitary adenoma may cause
    A. hyperpituitarism.
    B. hypothyroidism.
    C. hyperthyroidism.
    D. hypodontia.

79. A significant clinical finding in Addison disease is
    A. exophthalmos.
    B. bronzing of skin.
    C. gigantism.
    D. renal failure.

80. Which is NOT an etiologic factor in iron deficiency anemia?
    A. Chronic blood loss
    B. Nutritional deficiency
    C. Pregnancy
    D. Genetics

81. Pernicious anemia is a deficiency in vitamin
    A. B_{12}.
    B. D.
    C. B_6.
    D. C.

82. Which condition results from a chronic decrease in neutrophils?
    A. Leukemia
    B. Polycythemia
    C. Plummer-Vinson syndrome
    D. Agranulocytosis

83. A decrease in neutrophils is termed
    A. leukopenia.
    B. sickle cell anemia.
    C. thrombocytopenic purpura.
    D. leukemia.

84. Which drug is associated with osteonecrosis of the jaws?
   A. Phenytoin (Dilantin)
   B. Tetracycline
   C. Alendronate (Fosamax)
   D. Nifedipine (Procardia)

85. Which drug is NOT a calcium channel blocker?
   A. Diltiazem (Cardizem)
   B. Nifedipine (Procardia)
   C. Isradipine (DynaCirc)
   D. Cyclosporine (Sandimmune)

86. Sickle cell anemia occurs MOST commonly in which ethnic group?
   A. African Americans
   B. Caucasians
   C. Native Americans
   D. Asians

87. Which skin condition may be associated with type 2 diabetes mellitus?
   A. Bull's-eye lesion
   B. Acanthosis nigricans
   C. Butterfly rash
   D. Iris-eye lesion

88. Which severe, progressive autoimmune disease affecting skin and mucous membranes is characterized by a positive Nikolsky sign?
   A. Erythema multiforme
   B. Behçet syndrome
   C. Lichen planus
   D. Systemic lupus erythematosus (SLE)
   E. Pemphigus vulgaris

89. Bence-Jones proteins are found in the urine of patients with
   A. thalassemia.
   B. leukemia.
   C. multiple myeloma.
   D. carcinoma in situ.

90. *Neoplasia* is defined as an abnormal, uncontrolled proliferation of cells. Neoplasms may be either benign or malignant.
   A. Both statements are true.
   B. Both statements are false.
   C. The first statement is true, and the second statement is false.
   D. The first statement is false, and the second statement is true.

91. Raynaud phenomenon is characterized by all EXCEPT one. Which one is the EXCEPTION?
   A. Causes vasospasm of fingers and toes
   B. Causes tissue ischemia

C. Is triggered by medications and hot temperatures
D. May occur with rheumatoid arthritis or systemic lupus erythematosus

92. Which malignant skin tumor has the BEST prognosis?
   A. Basal cell carcinoma
   B. Squamous cell carcinoma
   C. Melanoma
   D. Epidermoid carcinoma

93. Which is NOT a characteristic feature of ameloblastoma?
   A. Benign
   B. Locally aggressive
   C. Unencapsulated
   D. Frequently fatal

94. An adenomatoid odontogenic tumor (AOT) often simulates which cyst?
   A. Lateral periodontal
   B. Dentigerous
   C. Nasopalatine
   D. Globulomaxillary

95. Pain is a frequent symptom of which lesion?
   A. Periapical cemento-osseous dysplasia
   B. Central ossifying fibroma
   C. Benign cementoblastoma
   D. Odontoma

96. All conditions may be found on the tongue EXCEPT one. Which one is the EXCEPTION?
   A. Neurofibroma
   B. Schwannoma
   C. Granular cell tumor
   D. Congenital epulis

97. The MOST common location of intraoral Kaposi sarcoma is the
   A. floor of the mouth.
   B. tongue.
   C. gingiva.
   D. buccal mucosa.

98. Which neoplasm is a malignant tumor of bone-forming tissue?
   A. Torus
   B. Rhabdomyosarcoma
   C. Osteosarcoma
   D. Osteoma

99. Inability to fully open the mouth is called
   A. trismus.
   B. crepitus.
   C. articulation.
   D. apertognathia.

100. In iron-deficiency anemia, the loss of which type of papillae of the tongue accounts for the red, beefy appearance?
    A. Fungiform
    B. Filiform
    C. Foliate
    D. Circumvallate

101. Which laboratory result provides the BEST information for diagnosing iron-deficiency anemia?
    A. Elevated hemoglobin
    B. B_{12} deficiency
    C. Deficiency of intrinsic factor
    D. Reduced hematocrit

102. All are clinical signs of pernicious anemia EXCEPT one. Which one is the EXCEPTION?
    A. Weakness
    B. Fatigue
    C. Burning tongue
    D. Tooth erosion

103. Which test is used to diagnose pernicious anemia?
    A. Western blot
    B. Pels-Macht
    C. Venereal Disease Research Laboratories (VDRL)
    D. Schilling

104. Which term refers to enamel hypoplasia of a permanent tooth resulting from infection of a deciduous tooth?
    A. Turner tooth
    B. Ghost tooth
    C. Hutchinson incisor
    D. Talon cusp

105. The MOST common odontogenic tumor is
    A. central ossifying fibroma.
    B. peripheral ossifying fibroma.
    C. osteoma.
    D. odontoma.

106. Which two nutrients are necessary for DNA synthesis?
    A. Folic acid
    B. Vitamin B_{12}
    C. Vitamin D
    D. All of the above
    E. A and B only

107. Which condition is present in polycythemia vera?
    A. Excessive number of platelets
    B. Insufficient number of white blood cells (WBCs)
    C. Excessive number of red blood cells (RBCs)
    D. Insufficient number of RBCs
    E. Excessive number of WBCs

108. The MOST common malignant soft tissue tumor of the head and neck in children is
    A. squamous cell carcinoma.
    B. chondrosarcoma.
    C. rhabdomyosarcoma.
    D. osteosarcoma.

109. The normal prothrombin time (PT) is
    A. 1 to 6 minutes.
    B. 10 minutes.
    C. 11 to 16 seconds.
    D. 30 minutes.

110. Thrombocytopenic purpura results from a severe reduction in
    A. red blood cells.
    B. platelets.
    C. international normalized ratio (INR).
    D. white blood cells.

111. Which are the MOST common sites for squamous cell carcinoma?
    A. Labial mucosa, buccal mucosa, and hard palate
    B. Labial mucosa, maxillary gingiva, and buccal mucosa
    C. Floor of the mouth, ventrolateral tongue, and soft palate
    D. Anterior tongue, gingiva, and retromolar area

1. Which intraosseous cyst occurs around the crown of an unerupted tooth?

   ANS: C
   A dentigerous cyst (C) occurs around the crown of an unerupted or developing tooth. An eruption cyst (A), which is similar to a dentigerous cyst, is found in the soft tissue around the crown of an erupting tooth. A primordial cyst (B) develops in the place of a tooth because of a disturbance in the tooth germ. A globulomaxillary cyst (D) is a well-defined, pear-shaped radiolucency found between the roots of the maxillary lateral incisor and the canine.

2. Which condition occurs when the cementum or dentin of a tooth fuses with the surrounding alveolar bone?

   ANS: B
   Ankylosis (B) is the condition in which the cementum or dentin of a tooth fuses with the surrounding alveolar bone. A primary or permanent tooth fuses with the surrounding alveolar bone, with no intervening periodontal ligament. Concrescence (A) is fusion of the cementum of two adjacent teeth only. With impaction (C), or when a tooth is said to be impacted, the tooth cannot erupt because of a physical obstruction. Gemination (D) is a developmental anomaly that occurs when a single tooth germ attempts to divide and results in the incomplete formation of two teeth.

3. Aphthous ulcers typically occur in all of these sites EXCEPT one. Which one is the EXCEPTION?

   ANS: B
   Aphthous ulcers typically do not occur in the keratinized attached gingiva (B). Aphthous ulcers typically occur on nonkeratinized mucosa such as the labial commissure (A), the buccal mucosa (C), and the soft palate (D).

4. Which bluish-gray lesion may appear as a radiopaque area on a dental image?

   ANS: B
   An amalgam tattoo (B) may appear intraorally as a flat, bluish-gray lesion of the oral mucosa. If any amalgam particles are dispersed in tissue, the tattoo may appear radiopaque on a dental image and appear bluish-gray intraorally. A hematoma (A) is a collection of blood within tissue as a result of trauma. An epulis fissuratum (C) is a soft tissue lesion associated with ill-fitting dentures and is not likely

to be seen radiographically. A traumatic neuroma (D) is a benign neoplasm of nerve cells. Soft tissue lesions such as a hematoma, an epulis fissuratum, or a traumatic neuroma are not visible on dental images.

5. Pericoronitis occurs most commonly in which location?

   ANS: C
   Mandibular third molars (C) are the most common locations for the occurrence of pericoronitis, an inflammation of the tissue around a partially erupted tooth. Pericoronitis occasionally occurs during the eruption of mandibular second molars (D), but much less frequently than with mandibular third molars. Pericoronitis does not commonly occur around maxillary first premolars (A) or maxillary central incisors (B).

6. There are several types of candidiasis, including erythematous candidiasis and denture candidiasis. Regardless of the type, all forms must be treated with antibiotics.

   ANS: C
   The first statement is true, and the second statement is false (C). Several different types of candidiasis exist, including erythematous candidiasis and denture candidiasis. Candidiasis is a fungal infection, so antibiotics are ineffective in treating this condition. The treatment of choice is an antifungal medication. Choices A, B, and D do not accurately reflect the statement.

7. Enamel hypoplasia is caused by ameloblast formation of too much enamel. Enamel hypocalcification occurs when there is too little enamel formation.

   ANS: B
   Both statements are false (B). Enamel hypoplasia occurs when there is too *little* enamel formation (not too much), and enamel hypocalcification is caused by a defect in mineralization of enamel, not the amount of enamel formed. Both enamel hypoplasia and enamel hypocalcification have many causes, including damage to the ameloblast by infectious agents, excess fluoride ingestion during enamel formation, and inherited conditions such as amelogenesis imperfecta. Choices A, C, and D do not accurately reflect the statements.

8. Which lesion may be associated with hormonal changes?

   ANS: B
   A pyogenic granuloma (B), sometimes called a *pregnancy tumor*, may be associated with hormonal

89. Bence-Jones proteins are found in the urine of patients with

ANS: C
Bence-Jones proteins (BJPs) are fragments of immunoglobulins found in the urine of patients with multiple myeloma (C), a cancer caused by systemic proliferation of plasma cells. BJPs are not specific to thalassemia (A), leukemia (B), or carcinoma in situ (D).

90. *Neoplasia* is defined as an abnormal, uncontrolled proliferation of cells. Neoplasms may be either benign or malignant.

ANS: A
Both statements are true (A). Neoplasms, or tumors, are caused by abnormal, uncontrolled proliferation of cells. Benign neoplasms remain localized and may be encapsulated or walled off. Benign neoplasms resemble normal cells and are described as well differentiated. Benign tumors are rarely fatal unless they are adjacent to vital structures but cannot spread to distant sites. Malignant neoplasms may invade and destroy surrounding tissue and have the ability to spread or metastasize. *Cancer* is another term for malignancy. Malignant tumors may be well differentiated to undifferentiated, or anaplastic, with little resemblance to normal cells. The nuclei of malignant tumors are darker (hyperchromatic) compared with normal nuclei, with increased and abnormal mitotic figures. Choices B, C, and D are not consistent with the statements.

91. Raynaud phenomenon is characterized by all EXCEPT one. Which one is the EXCEPTION?

ANS: C
Raynaud phenomenon is triggered by stress or cold temperatures, not medications or hot temperatures (C). It is a disorder that causes vasospasm of fingers and toes (A), which can lead to reduced blood flow and tissue ischemia (B). It often accompanies other autoimmune diseases such as rheumatoid arthritis, systemic lupus erythematosus, and Sjögren syndrome (D).

92. Which malignant skin tumor has the BEST prognosis?

ANS: A
Basal cell carcinoma (A) occurs only on skin and has a very good prognosis if diagnosed in its early stages. Squamous cell carcinoma (B) is the most common primary malignancy found in the oral cavity. It is also found on skin and is more aggressive than basal cell carcinoma, so early detection and treatment are important for a good prognosis. Melanoma (C) is a

malignant skin tumor that may occur intraorally in rare cases. It is the most aggressive of skin cancers, so early detection and treatment are critical. *Epidermoid carcinoma* (D) is another name for squamous cell carcinoma.

93. Which is NOT a characteristic feature of ameloblastoma?

ANS: D
Ameloblastoma, when diagnosed in the maxilla, is fatal if it extends into the brain (D); however, this is a rare occurrence. In general, ameloblastoma is benign (A), locally aggressive (B), and unencapsulated (C). Approximately 80% of ameloblastomas occur in the posterior mandible.

94. An adenomatoid odontogenic tumor (AOT) often simulates which cyst?

ANS: B
An adenomatoid odontogenic tumor (AOT) simulates a dentigerous cyst (B) because it is frequently associated with an impacted tooth. Radiographically, it appears as a radiolucency that extends beyond the cementoenamel junction (CEJ), as in a dentigerous cyst. The AOT may encompass 50% to 60% of the root. The lateral periodontal cyst (A) is found between the roots of the mandibular cuspid and the premolar. The nasopalatine cyst (C) often appears as a heart-shaped radiolucency in the anterior maxilla. The globulomaxillary cyst (D) is usually pear shaped and appears between the maxillary lateral and the cuspid.

95. Pain is a frequent symptom of which lesion?

ANS: C
Pain is associated with benign cementoblastoma (C), a cementum-producing tumor that is fused with the root or roots of vital teeth; this tumor typically occurs in young adults. Periapical cemento-osseous dysplasia (A) is a fairly common disease that affects periapical bone in the anterior mandible. It is asymptomatic, and the etiology is unknown. Central ossifying fibroma (B) is an asymptomatic tumor with mixed globular calcifications resembling cementum and bone, originating from the periodontal ligament cells' potential to produce both types of tissue. Odontomas (D) are odontogenic tumors derived from tooth-forming tissues and do not have pain as an associated feature.

96. All conditions may be found on the tongue EXCEPT one. Which one is the EXCEPTION?

ANS: D
Congenital epulis (D) is a benign tumor of female newborns and occurs on the gingiva, not on the

tongue. Neurofibroma (A) is a benign tumor derived from Schwann cells and perineural fibroblasts, and the tongue is the most common intraoral location. Schwannoma (B) is a benign tumor derived from Schwann cells, the connective tissue component surrounding nerves, and the tongue is the most common intraoral location. Granular cell tumors (C) often occur on the tongue and the buccal mucosa and are benign tumors composed of large cells with a granular cytoplasm.

97. The MOST common location of intraoral Kaposi sarcoma is the

ANS: C
The gingiva (C) and palatal tissue are the most common intraoral sites of Kaposi sarcoma. The floor of the mouth (A), tongue (B), and buccal mucosa (D) are not the most common sites for this condition. Squamous cell carcinoma is commonly found on the floor of the mouth and tongue. Verrucous carcinoma is commonly found on the buccal (and vestibule) mucosa.

98. Which neoplasm is a malignant tumor of bone-forming tissue?

ANS: C
Osteosarcoma (C) is a malignant tumor of bone. Torus (A) is a benign tumor of bone. Rhabdomyosarcoma (B) is a malignant tumor of striated muscle. Osteoma (D) is a benign tumor of normal, compact bone.

99. Inability to fully open the mouth is called

ANS: A
Trismus (A) refers to the inability to fully open the mouth. Crepitus (B) is a dry, crackling sound at the temporomandibular joint (TMJ). Articulation (C) is the term for the joining of bones at a location. Apertognathia (D) is an anterior open bite.

100. In iron-deficiency anemia, the loss of which type of papillae of the tongue accounts for the red, beefy appearance?

ANS: B
Filiform (B) papillae are the most numerous and have the highest metabolic requirements and disappear early in iron-deficiency anemia, causing the red, beefy appearance of the tongue. Fungiform (A) papillae are affected in severe cases of iron-deficiency anemia. Foliate (C) and circumvallate (D) papillae are not usually affected by the condition.

101. Which laboratory result provides the BEST information for diagnosing iron-deficiency anemia?

ANS: D
A reduced hematocrit (D) in laboratory results is the best information for the diagnosis of iron-deficiency anemia. Hematocrit is the volume percentage of red blood in whole blood cells, and hemoglobin is the iron-containing oxygen-transport protein in red blood cells (RBCs). A reduction in hematocrit indicates a decrease in RBCs and the resulting iron levels. A finding of reduced hemoglobin, not elevated hemoglobin (A), helps in the diagnosis of iron-deficiency anemia. Vitamin B_{12} (B) or pernicious anemia is caused by a deficiency in intrinsic factor (C), and this finding does not help diagnose iron-deficiency anemia.

102. All are clinical signs of pernicious anemia EXCEPT one. Which one is the EXCEPTION?

ANS: D
Tooth erosion (D) is not a clinical sign of pernicious anemia, which is a vitamin B_{12} deficiency caused by lack of intrinsic factor secreted by the parietal cells of the stomach required for absorption of vitamin B_{12}. Weakness (A), fatigue (B), and burning tongue (C) are all clinical signs of pernicious anemia.

103. Which test is used to diagnose pernicious anemia?

ANS: D
The Schilling (D) test, which determines the body's inability to absorb an oral dose of vitamin B_{12}, is used in the diagnosis of pernicious anemia. The Western blot (A) test is used in detecting human immunodeficiency virus. The Pels-Macht (B) test is used to identify pemphigus. The Venereal Disease Research Laboratories (C) test is used to diagnose syphilis.

104. Which term refers to enamel hypoplasia of a permanent tooth resulting from infection of a deciduous tooth?

ANS: A
Turner tooth (A) is a condition in which a permanent tooth displays enamel hypoplasia from exposure to infection or trauma in the preceding primary tooth. Ghost tooth (B) is a developmental problem in which one or several teeth in the same quadrant exhibit significant reduction in radiodensity radiographically. This condition is also termed *regional odontodysplasia*, and teeth have a ghostlike appearance and display very thin enamel and dentin. A Hutchinson incisor (C) is a malformed incisor formed as a result of exposure to congenital syphilis during tooth development. The tooth is shaped like a

41. The U.S. Food and Drug Administration (FDA) has indicated that the maximum daily dose of acetaminophen (Tylenol) should be 3000 mg. Which is the major toxicity concern for acetaminophen that prompted this reduced dose?

ANS: B
In high doses, acetaminophen may be converted to toxic radicals, which damage the liver (B). Patients with preexisting liver disease, those with alcoholism, and others are more susceptible. Acetaminophen poisoning accounts for a large number of emergency visits to the hospital, as well as many deaths as a result of liver damage. Although kidney damage (A) has been associated with the use of nonnarcotic analgesics, these disorders have usually occurred after long-term chronic use and when combinations of these types of drugs have been used. Acetaminophen does not have noticeable sedative (C) properties. It does not worsen asthma (D) unless an allergic reaction to acetaminophen occurs, which is rare. There is no known link between acetaminophen and bladder infections (E), since the drug has no major effect on structures in the urinary tract.

42. Which analgesic drug reduces blood clotting for the longest period?

ANS: E
Only aspirin (E) irreversibly inhibits cyclooxygenase, which inhibits the synthesis of thromboxane A_2, and inhibits platelet aggregation for the life of the platelet (7–10 days). Nonsteroidal antiinflammatory drugs (NSAIDs) such as ibuprofen (A) and naproxen (B) may also affect blood clotting but do so only for a short time because they reversibly inhibit cyclooxygenase and inhibit the synthesis of thromboxane A_2. Acetaminophen (C) has a minor effect on blood clotting in most cases. Codeine (D) has no major effect on blood clotting mechanisms, including platelet aggregation.

43. Which drug's antimicrobial action is based on its ability to inhibit cross-linking of the peptidoglycan chains in bacterial cell walls?

ANS: A
Amoxicillin (Amoxil) (A), like other penicillins, inhibits the enzyme transpeptidase, which catalyzes cross-linking in bacterial cell walls. Clindamycin (Cleocin) (B), clarithromycin (Biaxin) (C), and gentamicin (Garamycin) (E) all inhibit ribosomal protein synthesis in bacteria. Ciprofloxacin (Cipro) (D) inhibits deoxyribonucleic acid (DNA) function by inhibiting DNA enzymes.

44. Drugs that inhibit hydroxymethylglutaryl coenzyme A (HMG CoA) reductase are often used to treat which type of disorder?

ANS: C
HMG CoA reductase is an important enzyme in the synthesis of cholesterol in the liver (C). Drugs such as Lovastatin (Mevacor) and other "statins" reduce plasma cholesterol by this mechanism. Statins have a less direct effect on cardiac arrhythmias (A) and hypertension (B), although lowering plasma cholesterol often has a beneficial effect in patients receiving these agents. Statins have little if any effect on fungal organisms (D). Statins do not treat the inflammation or the pain of osteoarthritis (E).

45. Which drug has the MOST potent antiinflammatory effect?

ANS: B
Prednisone (Deltasone) (B), a glucocorticoid, has several mechanisms that make it a potent antiinflammatory drug used in a variety of settings. Inhibition of phospholipase A_2, a key enzyme in the inflammatory prostanoid and leukotriene pathway is a primary antiinflammatory action. Alendronate (Fosamax) (A) is a bisphosphonate that is used to reduce bone turnover. Atenolol (Tenormin) (C) is a beta-adrenergic receptor blocker that has a number of cardiovascular effects but not an antiinflammatory effect. Raloxifene (Evista) (D) is an estrogen receptor agonist–antagonist, more commonly known as a selective estrogen receptor modulator (SERM), with a beneficial effect in the treatment of postmenopausal osteoporosis, but no antiinflammatory action. Fluoxetine (Prozac) (E) is a selective serotonin reuptake inhibitor (SSRI), whose action in the brain mediates its antidepressant effect.

46. The patient has recently been prescribed a drug by a neurologist to treat a painful jaw. The pain was sharp and intermittent and seemed to be triggered by the slightest touch. The patient could not remember the name of the disorder, but it was explained to the patient that the prescribed "pain killer" was an antiepileptic drug used for this type of pain. Which would be the most likely drug prescribed?

ANS: D
The pain described is consistent with trigeminal neuralgia (tic douloureux) because of the type of pain, the location of the pain involving cranial nerve V, and the fact that a neurologist made the diagnosis. Carbamazepine (Tegretol) (D) is a drug commonly used to treat trigeminal neuralgia. It is effective in inhibiting nerve conduction by blocking neuronal sodium channels, and this also makes it useful to

treat certain types of seizure disorders. Oxycodone (Percodan, Percocet) (A) and dihydrocodeine (Synalgos DC) (B) are both opioids and are useful in treating pain but are less effective in treating the neuropathic type pain described here. Celecoxib (Celebrex) (C) is a cyclooxygenase-2 (COX-2) inhibitor and is used as an antiinflammatory and analgesic agent. Acetaminophen (Tylenol) (E) is not particularly effective in treating neuropathic pain.

47. A patient being treated for xerostomia with pilocarpine (Salagen) is most likely to experience which side effect?

ANS: A
Sweating (A) is the most common complaint of patients taking muscarinic cholinergic receptor agonists such as pilocarpine (Salagen) for the treatment of xerostomia. Although innervated by the sympathetic nervous system, sweat glands have muscarinic receptors that respond to postganglionic cholinergic nerves, resulting in increased secretion and these receptors also respond to pilocarpine. Cholinergic postganglionic nerves are otherwise rare in the sympathetic nervous system. Although tachycardia (B) is a possibility because of vasodilation, the vasodilation is usually mild or nonexistent with the oral doses used in this situation. Muscarinic receptor stimulation would tend to have very mild effects opposite to urinary retention (C) and constipation (E). Hypertension (D) is not likely to occur with the effect of pilocarpine, since cholinergic agonists usually decrease blood pressure and slow heart rate.

48. Which drug most effectively blocks the itching, pain, and swelling from histamine released in the skin?

ANS: D
Diphenhydramine (Benadryl) (D) is an antihistamine that blocks histamine H_1 receptors and inhibits the above effects of histamine on nerves and blood vessels. Chlorthalidone (Hygroton) (A) is a thiazide-type diuretic. Doxazosin (Cardura) (B) is an alpha 1-adrenergic receptor blocker. Candesartan (Atacand) (C) is an angiotensin II receptor blocker. Isoproterenol (Isuprel) (E) is a nonselective beta-adrenergic receptor agonist. These drugs are typically used in the treatment of hypertension but have no or minimal effects on acute responses to histamine because they do not block histamine receptors or alleviate acute inflammation.

49. Each of these drugs is used to treat asthma EXCEPT one. Which one is the EXCEPTION?

ANS: B
Metoprolol (Lopressor) (B) is a selective beta 1-adrenergic receptor blocker. Beta-blockers are

contraindicated in asthma because by blocking the beta 2-adrenergic receptors in the lung, bronchoconstriction may occur. Selective beta 1-adrenergic receptor blockers have primarily cardiac effects and are less likely to cause bronchoconstriction than nonselective beta-adrenergic receptor blockers. These drugs should still be used with caution in patients with asthma, since these drugs have no direct benefit in the relief of asthma symptoms. Fluticasone (Flonase) (A) is a glucocorticoid, with an antiinflammatory effect in the lung, reducing the inflammatory component of asthma. Salmeterol (Serevent) (C) is a long-acting beta 2-adrenergic receptor agonist, which causes bronchodilation. Ipratropium (Atrovent) (D) is an antimuscarinic, anticholinergic drug that blocks the bronchoconstricting effect of acetylcholine that is released in the lung. Montelukast (Singulair) (E) is a cysteinyl leukotriene 1 receptor blocker. Cysteinyl leukotrienes are inflammatory mediators that contribute to bronchoconstriction.

50. The antipsychotic effect of thioridazine (Mellaril) is largely caused by which mechanism in the brain?

ANS: E
Potencies of traditional antipsychotic drugs such as thioridazine are correlated with their affinities for D_2 dopamine receptors (E). Blocking the reuptake of norepinephrine and serotonin (A) is the mechanism of action of several antidepressants. Blocking sodium channels in the central nervous system (CNS) (B) is a mechanism of action of several antiepileptic drugs such as phenytoin. Blocking calcium channels in the CNS (C) is a characteristic of several antiepileptic drugs used in the treatment of absence (petit mal) seizures. Most sedatives act by enhancing the effect of GABA (D), an inhibitory neurotransmitter, on chloride channels.

51. A patient who has asthma and has been taking oral theophylline (Theolair) for several months develops an acute infection in the oral cavity. Since the patient reports an allergy to penicillin, oral erythromycin ethylsuccinate (E.E.S.), at a dose of 400 mg four times a day, is prescribed. Two days later, the patient begins to feel ill, reporting dizziness, nervousness, confusion, nausea and vomiting, and rapid heart rate. Which is the most likely explanation for the patient's symptoms?

ANS: E
Erythromycin inhibits the liver enzymes (the cytochromes) needed to metabolize many drugs, including theophylline (E). The symptoms described are consistent with theophylline toxicity, which

occurred when failure to metabolize theophylline caused the plasma levels to rise to harmful levels. Erythromycin does not affect renal excretion of other drugs (A). Erythromycin may cause severe gastrointestinal distress but does not enhance absorption of other drugs (B). Theophylline does not affect cell affinity for erythromycin (C), or decrease its excretion (D). Because of the low therapeutic index of theophylline, another choice of antibiotic would be better.

52. Which major neurotransmitter in autonomic ganglia leads to a rapid excitatory postsynaptic potential?

ANS: D
Acetylcholine (D) is the major neurotransmitter in ganglia and carries the stimulatory message from the preganglionic neuron to the postganglionic neuron. Acting on nicotinic cholinergic receptors linked to sodium channels, acetylcholine causes a rapid excitatory postsynaptic potential. Dopamine (A), norepinephrine (C), or both are released from interneurons in sympathetic ganglia, but they cause an inhibitory postsynaptic potential. Epinephrine (B) plays no major role in preganglionic transmission. Serotonin (E) may have a minor role in neurotransmission in some ganglia, but only in a delayed response in the postganglionic neurons.

53. Sumatriptan (Imitrex, Alsuma) is a drug that is commonly used to treat which disorder?

ANS: B
Sumatriptan (Imitrex, Alsuma) is an agonist at serotonin $5HT_{1B/1D}$ receptors. Sumatriptan and other triptans cause constriction of intracranial blood vessels, reduce pain fiber activity, and reduce inflammation associated with migraine headaches (B). The triptans have little effect at other receptors and the mechanism of action of sumatriptan has little benefit in the treatment of other disorders. Sumatriptan does little to change cholesterol metabolism (A) or to reduce bronchoconstriction in asthma attacks (C). Sumatriptan has no obvious benefit on ion channel activity in the heart (D) and may even be associated with certain arrhythmias. Sumatriptan has no activity on opioid receptors (E).

54. Which of the following BEST describes the mechanism of action of phentolamine?

ANS: C
Phentolamine is a drug that causes reversal of sodium channel blockage (C), shortening the time of soft tissue anesthesia following a dental procedure. The mechanism is related to its ability to block the vasoconstriction resulting from alpha-adrenergic receptor stimulation caused by epinephrine and norepinephrine. The resulting vasodilation leads to more rapid removal of the local anesthetic from the area of injection after the phentolamine is injected. Reversal of calcium channel blockage (A) is not an action of phentolamine (OraVerse). Calcium channel blockage (B) is the action of hypertensive medications such as verapamil (Calan, Isoptin). Blockage of sodium channels (D) is the action of the local anesthetic agent, not phentolamine.

55. Which drug has the broadest antibacterial spectrum?

ANS: A
Amoxicillin (Amoxil) (A) is the penicillin with a broadest spectrum of action and is called an "extended-spectrum" penicillin because it has greater activity compared with the other penicillins listed against gram-negative bacilli. Clavulanic acid (in Augmentin) (B) is not a penicillin, although its structure resembles penicillin with a beta-lactam ring, it has little antibacterial effect by itself. It is a beta-lactamase inhibitor and is added to amoxicillin to prevent amoxicillin's destruction by bacterial penicillinases. Dicloxacillin (Dynapen) (C) is a narrow-spectrum penicillin but is resistant to some penicillinases. Penicillin G (Pfizerpen) (D) and penicillin V (Penicillin VK) (E) have both have essentially the same narrow spectrum of action against many gram-positive bacteria and some gram-negative cocci. Although less active than penicillin G and penicillin V, dicloxacillin's resistance to penicillinase makes it useful in the treatment of infections caused by penicillinase-producing *Staphylococcus aureus*.

56. Which drug reduces coagulation by inhibiting the activation (carboxylation) of certain clotting factors in the liver?

ANS: E
Warfarin (Coumadin) (E) competitively inhibits vitamin K epoxide reductase, acting as a vitamin K antagonist. This action leads to inhibition of carboxylation of prothrombin factors VII, IX, and X, as well as other factors leading to reduced coagulation capacity. The other drugs listed act on elements in blood. Aspirin (A) and clopidogrel (Plavix) (C) are inhibitors of platelet aggregation; aspirin, due to its effect on cyclooxygenase, inhibits the production of thromboxane A_2, and clopidogrel inhibits the effect of adenosine diphosphate on platelets. Alteplase (t-PA, Activase) (B) binds to fibrin and leads to the hydrolysis and breakup of fibrin. Heparin (D) reduces blood clotting by accelerating the activity of antithrombin III and by other mechanisms.

57. Which is NOT a characteristic associated with nitrous oxide (NO) used for conscious sedation?

ANS: C
NO is not an effective skeletal muscle relaxant (C) even at higher anesthetic doses. NO has significant analgesic effects (A). It is noted for rapid induction (B) because of its low blood-to-gas solubility coefficient. NO is heavier than air (D) and may accumulate at floor level under conditions of poor ventilation or conditions of poor scavenging. It is odorless (E) and tasteless to the patient.

58. Which drug is used as an antidepressant and is considered an SSRI?

ANS: E
Paroxetine (Paxil) (E) is an antidepressant that primarily blocks the reuptake of serotonin in the brain. Amitriptyline (Elavil) (A), also an antidepressant, blocks both serotonin and norephinephrine reuptake mechanisms nonselectively. The mechanism of bupropion (Wellbutrin) (B) is not as well understood, although reuptake of dopamine may play a role. Haloperidol (Haldol) (C) is an antipsychotic drug that blocks the dopamine receptors. Lithium (Eskalith) (D) is used in treatment of the manic phase of bipolar disease or manic-depressive illness.

59. Which drug would be indicated in the treatment of methicillin-resistant *Staphylococcus aureus* (MRSA)?

ANS: E
Vancomycin (Vancocin) (E) is the antibiotic indicated for the treatment of *S. Aureus*. It is active in the presence of penicillinases produced by *S. aureus* and other mechanisms of resistance to beta-lactams. MRSA is largely resistant to clarithromycin (Biaxin) (B). Dicloxacillin (Dynapen) (C) is very similar to methicillin and is ineffective against this infection. Resistance by MRSA also extends to other beta-lactam antibiotics such as cephalexin (Keflex) (A) and penicillin V (Pen-Vee-k) (D).

60. Curare-type drugs such as vecuronium (Norcuron) cause muscle relaxation by which mechanism?

ANS: B
Curare-type drugs are competitive blockers of the nicotinic type of cholinergic receptors in the skeletal neuromuscular junction (B). Activation of chloride channels (A), either through GABA or independently of GABA, is the mechanism that applies to many sedative hypnotics that have some ability to relax skeletal muscle. Reducing blood flow (C) is not relevant to the action of any muscle relaxer. Reducing calcium release

from intracellular stores (D) is the mechanism of action of dantrolene (Dantrium), which is not a curare-type drug. Blocking ganglionic transmission (E) would be ineffective in causing skeletal muscle relaxation because skeletal muscles are innervated by somatic nerves, which do not have ganglia.

61. A drug that has an effect on the fetal development is said to have a/an

ANS: D
A drug that causes an adverse reaction in the developing fetus is termed *teratogenic effect* (D). The FDA has ranked drugs into five pregnancy categories: A, B, C, D, and X, ranked from least risky to most risky. A side effect (A) is a dose-related reaction that is not part of the desired therapeutic effect. A toxic effect (B) is an extension of the pharmacologic effect resulting from the drug's excessive and harmful effect on the target organ. The therapeutic effect (C) is the desired drug effect on target organs. An idiosyncratic effect or reaction (E) is a genetically related abnormal drug response that is atypical compared with that in the general population.

62. Which drug or drug class is most likely to result in bone loss when administered chronically in typical clinical doses?

ANS: E
Prednisone (Deltasone) (E), as well as other glucocorticosteroids, promotes a negative calcium balance by decreasing calcium absorption from the gastrointestinal (GI) tract. They also increase osteoclast activity and decrease osteoblast activity in bone and have other mechanisms as well. These effects may, and often do, lead to osteoporosis. Alendronate (Fosamax) (A) is a bisphosphonate, and bisphosphonates bind to bone remodeling surfaces, reducing the number and activity of osteoclasts. This is useful in treating certain bone loss disorders such as osteoporosis and Paget disease. Estrogens, including ethinyl estradiol (Estinyl) (B) and conjugated estrogens (Premarin) (C), increase osteoblast activity, which then suppresses the action of osteoclasts. Raloxifene (Evista) (D) is a selective estrogen receptor modulator (SERM), which has a similar beneficial effect on bone. It is more selective than ethinyl estradiol or conjugated estrogens in its ability to stimulate estrogen receptors.

63. Which anesthetic has the longest duration of action?

ANS: B
Bupivacaine (Marcaine) (B) is chemically similar to mepivacaine but with an additional substitution that is highly lipid soluble. This change increases the

potency and duration of the action of bupivacaine for up to 8 hours of analgesia, making it the longest-acting local anesthetic that is commonly used in dentistry. Articaine (Septocaine) (A) has a duration of action of 3 to 4 hours, making it an intermediate-acting local anesthetic. Lidocaine (Xylocaine) without epinephrine (C) and mepivacaine (Carbocaine) (D) have a short duration of 30 to 90 minutes of analgesia. Prilocaine (Citanest) (E) without epinephrine has an intermediate duration of 2 to 4 hours of analgesia.

64. Which drug inhibits renin release from the kidneys?

ANS: D
Metoprolol (Lopressor) (D), blocks beta 1-adrenergic receptors in the juxtaglomerular cells of the kidney's afferent arterioles, inhibiting the release of renin. Renin catalyzes the conversion of angiotensinogen to angiotensin I, which causes vasoconstriction, and stimulates aldosterone release. Aldosterone promotes sodium retention in the kidney, further raising blood pressure by vasoconstriction. Blocking the renin–angiotensin pathway reduces blood pressure and the demand on the heart, making this class of drugs important in the treatment of hypertension and heart failure. Candesartan (Atacand) (A) and enalapril (Vasotec) (C) also inhibit this pathway but do so "downstream" from renin release: Enalapril inhibits angiotensin-receptor-enzyme (ACE); and candesartan blocks the angiotensin II receptor. Digoxin (Lanoxin) (B) stimulates the heart directly, increasing its force of contraction. It does so by inhibiting the sodium–potassium pump (Na^+,K^+–adenosine triphosphatase [ATPase]) in the plasma membranes of cardiac cells. Nifedipine (Procardia) (E) is a calcium channel blocker, which reduces the contraction of cardiac muscle and increases vasodilation of the arteries—two methods of reducing blood pressure. This action is not linked to renin release.

65. While obtaining a patient's medical history, the dental hygienist learns that the patient takes cimetidine (Tagamet) prescribed for peptic ulcer. Which is the MOST likely scenario if local anesthesia (LA) is administered?

ANS: B
Cimitidine (Tagamet) is a prototype of the H_2-receptor antagonists which inhibit secretion of gastric acid by competitive inhibition of the H_2-receptors of the parietal cells of the stomach. One of the most serious adverse effects of cimitidine is its ability to inhibit liver microsomal enzymes via the cytochrome P-450 enzymes, slowing the elimination of some drugs in blood plasma. This may lead to increased drug levels and toxicity (B), even when drugs such as lidocaine are given in therapeutic doses. The clinician should exercise caution and use the lowest possible dose of local anesthetic in patients on cimetidine. Concurrent administration of cimitidine (Tagamet) would not negate lidocaine's local anesthetic properties (A). The efficacy of lidocaine would be increased with administration of cimitidine (Tagamet) (C). Allergic reactions to lidocaine are rare, and cimitidine (Tagamet) does not increase these types of reactions (D).

Provision of Clinical Dental Hygiene Services

## CHAPTER 7

Assessing Patient Characteristics

Frieda Atherton Pickett

QUESTIONS

1. Body temperature exceeding 37.5 °C (99.1 °F) but less than 41.0 °C (105.8 °F) is termed
   A. anoxia.
   B. pyrexia.
   C. hyperthermia.
   D. hypothermia.

2. The first stage of physical assessment begins before the patient is seated. At this time, it can be determined that the patient does not have a communicable disease.
   A. Both statements are true.
   B. Both statements are false.
   C. The first statement is true, and the second statement is false.
   D. The first statement is false, and the second statement is true.

3. The technique of using the sense of touch to obtain information is termed
   A. palpation.
   B. percussion.
   C. auscultation.
   D. observation.

4. When the medical history includes a history of myocardial infarction, which assessment is used to determine when it is safe to provide oral care?
   A. Six months have passed since the event.
   B. Three months have passed since the event.
   C. The patient has functional capacity to run a short distance and climb a flight of stairs.
   D. The patient has the functional capacity to run a long distance and climb two flights of stairs.

5. Which of the following categories in the American Society of Anesthesiologists (ASA) risk classification describes a healthy client with no systemic disease?
   A. ASA I
   B. ASA II
   C. ASA III
   D. ASA IV
   E. ASA V

6. Which ASA risk classification is appropriate for the patient who has a history of myocardial infarction but can perform vigorous, intense activity (10 metabolic equivalent [MET] functional capacity)?
   A. ASA I
   B. ASA II
   C. ASA III
   D. ASA IV
   E. ASA V

7. When the health history reveals that the patient has had a prior unpleasant dental experience that has led to dental phobia, which of the following is the MOST likely potential emergency situation?
   A. Exercise-induced asthma
   B. Tonic-clonic seizure
   C. Vasovagal syncope

8. According to the *Fourth Report on the Diagnosis, Evaluation, and Treatment of High Blood Pressure in Children and Adolescents*, at which age should a child's blood pressure be measured at health care appointments?
   A. >3 years
   B. >6 years
   C. >10 years
   D. >12 years

9. All of the following medical conditions are associated with hypertension EXCEPT one. Which one is the EXCEPTION?
   A. Heart failure
   B. Hyperthyroidism
   C. Diabetes mellitus
   D. Type I hypersensitivity reaction

10. Under which category does a blood pressure reading of 126/86 mm Hg fall?
    A. Prehypertension
    B. Normal blood pressure
    C. Stage 1 hypertension
    D. Stage 2 hypertension

11. When evaluating respiration, the clinician should observe all of the following factors EXCEPT one. Which one is the EXCEPTION?
    A. Rate of respiration
    B. Depth of respiration
    C. Quality of respiration
    D. Patient position during respiration
    E. Patient pulse rate during respiration

12. When nasal congestion is present, which oral procedure would MOST compromise the airway?
    A. Ultrasonic scaling
    B. Periodontal probing
    C. Taking dental images
    D. Periodontal scaling
    E. Intraoral or extraoral examination

13. The patient is a 10-year-old who presents with a body temperature of 100.5°F. Treatment considerations for this patient include
    A. having the patient rinse with mouthwash before providing treatment.
    B. questioning the parent about recent exposure to others with infectious conditions.
    C. immediately referring the patient to a physician to minimize exposure to other patients.

14. During a medical emergency, the pulse should be taken from which artery?
    A. Radial
    B. Carotid
    C. Brachial
    D. Femoral

15. All of the following are risk factors in the development of type II diabetes mellitus (T2DM) EXCEPT one. Which one is the EXCEPTION?
    A. Obesity
    B. Smoking
    C. Genetics
    D. Middle age
    E. Sedentary lifestyle

16. Your client presents with a blood pressure (BP) of 165/102 mm Hg, right arm, sitting. Treatment considerations include all of the following EXCEPT one. Which one is the EXCEPTION?
    A. Provide routine oral services
    B. Delay treatment until BP is controlled
    C. Keep appointment duration short
    D. Provide referral for medical evaluation of BP within 1 month
    E. Use a stress-reduction protocol and good pain control

17. Blood pressure (BP) classifications in pediatric individuals are based on all of these factors EXCEPT one. Which one is the EXCEPTION?
    A. Age
    B. Gender
    C. Height
    D. Weight

18. Indurated, movable retroauricular lymph nodes suggest examination of which area for etiology?
    A. Scalp behind ear
    B. Auricular tragus
    C. Zygomatic region
    D. Maxillary posterior teeth

19. Submandibular lymph nodes are best examined by
    A. rolling the node over the inferior border of the mandible.
    B. pushing the node superiorly to contact the mylohyoid muscle.
    C. asking the patient to swallow as the nodes are palpated bilaterally.

20. All of the following techniques will detect the presence of cysts or lymphadenopathy during the extraoral examination of the neck EXCEPT one. Which one is the EXCEPTION?
    A. Taking medical history
    B. Rolling the nodes over a hard surface
    C. Visual observation as the head is turned to the side
    D. Palpation of areas where the lymphatic system is present

21. The presence of cystic acne indicates the probable finding of which microorganism?
    A. *Staphylococcus aureus*
    B. *Neisseria gonorrhoeae*
    C. *Treponema pallidum*
    D. *Streptococcus sanguis*

22. A periodontal infection surrounding tooth #24 would be related to which condition?
    A. Enlargement of submental nodes
    B. Induration of submandibular nodes
    C. Formation of a mucocele in the lower lip
    D. Prominent sublingual ductal mucosa

23. An objective abnormal finding during the head and neck examination that can be identified by a health care professional is called a *symptom*. A patient report of pain is a good example of a symptom.
    A. Both statements are true.
    B. Both statements are false.
    C. The first statement is true, and the second statement is false.
    D. The first statement is false, and the second statement is true.

24. During examination of the temporomandibular joint (TMJ), all of the following are issues to be considered EXCEPT one. Which one is the EXCEPTION?
    A. Noises
    B. Tenderness
    C. Deviations of movement
    D. Crowding of mandibular incisors

25. When the oral cavity exhibits a reduction of saliva, all of the following are potential findings EXCEPT one. Which one is the EXCEPTION?
    A. Caries
    B. Candidiasis
    C. Coated tongue
    D. Periodontal disease

26. Examination of breath odors is a component of all of the following conditions EXCEPT one. Which one is the EXCEPTION?
    A. Alcoholism
    B. Carcinoma
    C. Tobacco use
    D. Diabetes mellitus

27. Which area of the tongue has the greatest predisposition to development of carcinoma?
    A. Dorsal surface
    B. Lateral borders
    C. Ventral surface
    D. Area of foramen cecum

28. Palpation of the lymph nodes during the head and neck examination reveals all of the following conditions EXCEPT one. Which one is the EXCEPTION?
    A. Metastatic lesions
    B. Fibrous hyperplasia
    C. Acute inflammation
    D. Latent tuberculosis (TB) infection

29. During oral examination, the patient is asked to occlude the teeth and swallow. What is the reason for this?
    A. Assessment for tremitus
    B. Assessment for centric occlusion
    C. Assessment for mouth breathing
    D. Assessment for reverse swallowing

30. A lesion that is attached by a stemlike or stalklike base is described as
    A. sessile.
    B. diffuse.
    C. papillary.
    D. corrugated.
    E. pedunculated.

31. All of the following are evidence-based risk factors for periodontal disease EXCEPT one. Which one is the EXCEPTION?
    A. Age
    B. Tobacco use
    C. Retained biofilm
    D. Compromised immune system
    E. Diabetes controlled with insulin

ANS: C

Vasovagal syncope (C), or fainting, is the most common dental emergency situation triggered by anxiety and dental fears. Exercise-induced asthma (A) could also be induced by stress or by allergy to dental office environmental substances, but this reaction is not as common as syncope. Although tonic-clonic seizures (B) may be triggered by stress, failure to take antiseizure medications would be a more common finding.

8. According to the *Fourth Report on the Diagnosis, Evaluation, and Treatment of High Blood Pressure in Children and Adolescents*, at which age should a child's blood pressure be measured at health care appointments?

ANS: A

The most recent guidelines call for the measurement of blood pressure in children older than age 3 years (A) when presenting at any health care facility; an appropriate-sized cuff that accommodates the child's arm size should be used. Children who are >6 years (B), >10 years (C), or >12 years (D), should have blood pressure measurements taken at healthcare appointments.

9. All of the following medical conditions are associated with hypertension EXCEPT one. Which one is the EXCEPTION?

ANS: D

When an individual experiences a type I hypersensitivity reaction (D), blood pressure falls, and this condition is referred to as *anaphylactic shock*. Heart failure (A), hyperthyroidism (B), and diabetes mellitus (C) are all related to complications of hypertension.

10. Under which category does a blood pressure reading of 126/86 mm Hg fall?

ANS: A

Prehypertension (A) occurs with levels from 120/80 mm Hg to less than 139/89 mm Hg. Normal blood pressure is less than 120/80 mm Hg (B). Stage 1 hypertension (C) occurs with levels from 140/90 mm Hg to 159/99 mm Hg. Stage 2 hypertension (D) is 160/100 mm Hg and higher.

11. When evaluating respiration, the clinician should observe all of the following factors EXCEPT one. Which one is the EXCEPTION?

ANS: E

The patient's pulse rate is not evaluated at the same time as respiration (E). Assessment of respiration

includes the rate (A), depth (B), and quality (C). Normal respiration is noiseless, and sounds during respiration indicate a degree of airway obstruction. Patients who have difficulty breathing (orthopnea) in the supine position (D) may have medical conditions such as congestive heart failure that require treatment modification.

12. When nasal congestion is present, which oral procedure would MOST compromise the airway?

ANS: A

Of these procedures, the water lavage produced in ultrasonic scaling (A) will have the most effect on the airway, since breathing through the nose is more difficult. Periodontal probing (B), taking dental images (C), periodontal scaling (D), or intraoral or extraoral examination (E) will affect patient comfort and efficiency of the procedure, and adaptations may need to be made but are less likely to affect the airway compared with ultrasonic scaling.

13. The patient is a 10-year-old who presents with a body temperature of 100.5°F. Treatment considerations for this patient include

ANS: C

The best course of action would involve immediate referral to a physician (C) for further medical evaluation and to minimize further exposure to others. Elevated temperature in children often indicates development of a contagious "childhood illness" (measles, mumps, chickenpox) in which elevation of body temperature is an initial symptom. Although a preprocedural rinse (A) reduces microbial contamination, it would not be sufficient to reduce the risk of infection from someone with an actively infectious disease. Questioning the parent about exposure to others with infectious conditions (B) may not obtain important information if the parent is unaware of exposure.

14. During a medical emergency, the pulse should be taken from which artery?

ANS: B

The cardiopulmonary resuscitation (CPR) guidelines recommend that during a medical emergency, the pulse should be taken from the carotid artery (B). The radial artery (A) is used to take the pulse in normal treatment situations, whereas the brachial artery (C) or the femoral artery (D) would only be used if trauma would not allow access to the carotid artery.

15. All of the following are risk factors in the development of type II diabetes mellitus (T2DM) EXCEPT one. Which one is the EXCEPTION?

ANS: B
Smoking is a risk factor for periodontitis, not T2DM (B). Obesity (A) is strongly correlated to T2DM, or insulin-resistant diabetes. There is a genetic component (C) to T2DM, which places some populations such as African Americans and Latinos and subpopulations such as the Pima Indians at higher risk for developing the disease. T2DM has traditionally been termed "adult-onset diabetes" because the majority of persons developing this disease are middle-aged or older adults (D), although this is changing as the prevalence of obesity increases. A sedentary lifestyle (E) is strongly linked to T2DM.

16. Your client presents with a blood pressure (BP) of 165/102 mm Hg, right arm, sitting. Treatment considerations include all of the following EXCEPT one. Which one is the EXCEPTION?

ANS: B
Treatment does not need to be delayed; delay of treatment is NOT recommended unless BP measurements are 180/110 mm Hg or greater (B). Oral procedures can be provided safely (A) provided the client is not overstressed, generally in a short appointment, and has good pain control (C, E). The client should be advised to see a physician within 1 month for assessment of BP (D).

17. Blood pressure classifications in pediatric individuals are based on all of these factors EXCEPT one. Which one is the EXCEPTION?

ANS: D
Weight (D) is not used in the statistical calculations for categories such as normal, prehypertension, stage 1 hypertension, and stage 2 hypertension. The factors used by the *Fourth Report on the Diagnosis, Evaluation, and Treatment of High Blood Pressure in Children and Adolescents* are age (A), gender (B), and height (C), with seven height levels quantifying various levels according to year of age. Routine BP readings are recommended in children age 3 years and older.

18. Indurated, movable retroauricular lymph nodes suggest examination of which area for etiology?

ANS: A
The scalp behind the ear (A) drains into the retroauricular lymph nodes. The auricular tragus is drained by the anterior auricular glands or preauricular glands (B). The zygomatic region (C) is drained by the buccal, malar, mandibular, and submandibular glands. Maxillary posterior teeth (D) are primarily drained by the submandibular lymph nodes, and maxillary third molars are drained by the superior deep cervical lymph nodes.

19. Submandibular lymph nodes are best examined by

ANS: A
To determine whether abnormal nodes are present, they must be pressed against a hard surface. Of the choices provided, only rolling the node over the inferior border of the mandible (A) allows this technique. Neither pushing the node superiorly to contact the mylohyoid muscle (B) nor asking the patient to swallow while palpating the nodes bilaterally (C) would identify indurated submandibular nodes.

20. All of the following techniques will detect the presence of cysts or lymphadenopathy during the extraoral examination of the neck EXCEPT one. Which one is the EXCEPTION?

ANS: A
The medical history (A) would not reveal the presence of cysts or lymphadenopathy, since patients are usually unaware of having enlarged lymph nodes. Rolling the nodes over a hard surface (B), visual observation as the head is turned to the side (C), and palpation (D) are all methods used to detect indurated structures in the head and neck area.

21. The presence of cystic acne indicates the probable finding of which microorganism?

ANS: A
Cysts and boils are associated with *S. aureus* (A), a common skin microorganism. *N. gonorrhoeae* (B) and *T. pallidum* (C) are associated with infection of mucosal surfaces, not skin. *S. sanguis* (D) is associated with oral ecosystems and is not found on skin.

22. A periodontal infection surrounding tooth #24 would be related to which condition?

ANS: A
Mandibular anterior teeth, including tooth #24, drain into the submental lymph node (A). Submandibular nodes (B) receive drainage from maxillary teeth and posterior mandibular teeth. A mucocele (C) occurs from an injury that traumatizes the salivary gland duct. Sublingual ducts (D) are not affected by tooth-related infections in the local area.

23. An objective abnormal finding during the head and neck examination that can be identified by a health care professional is called a *symptom*. A patient report of pain is a good example of a symptom.

ANS: D
The first statement is false, and the second statement is true (D). The definition of a *sign* is an objective finding identified by the health care professional, whereas the definition of a *symptom* is a subjective finding reported by the patient. A patient report of pain is subjective and is a symptom. Both signs and symptoms are valuable patient assessment tools. Choices A, B, and C do not correctly address the question.

24. During examination of the temporomandibular joint (TMJ), all of the following are issues to be considered EXCEPT one. Which one is the EXCEPTION?

ANS: D
The alignment of incisors (D) is used to determine the possibility of occlusal misalignment and not to examine the TMJ. Malocclusion may be a factor in TMJ assessment if the molar or jaw relationship is abnormal. Noises such as clicking or popping (A), tenderness (B), and movement deviations (C) are all characteristics that should be assessed during TMJ examination.

25. When the oral cavity exhibits a reduction of saliva, all of the following are potential findings EXCEPT one. Which one is the EXCEPTION?

ANS: D
Periodontal disease (D) is a multifactorial disease unrelated to *xerostomia,* which is the clinical term for dry mouth. Caries (A) and a coated tongue (C) may be results of chronic dry mouth. Candidiasis (B) may occur when reduced saliva flow allows opportunistic fungi to flourish.

26. Examination of breath odors is a component of all of the following conditions EXCEPT one. Which one is the EXCEPTION?

ANS: B
Carcinoma (B) presents as a nonhealing ulceration or red-to-white nodule and is not associated with breath odor. Alcoholism (A) may be suspected by the smell of alcohol on the breath. Uncontrolled diabetes (D) may present as a sweet odor of the breath. Tobacco use (C) is often identified by breath odors.

27. Which area of the tongue has the greatest predisposition to development of carcinoma?

ANS: B
The most common location of oral carcinoma on the tongue is the lateral border area (B). The tongue's dorsal (A) and ventral (C) surfaces and the area of foramen cecum (D) are less likely to undergo malignant changes.

28. Palpation of the lymph nodes during the head and neck examination reveals all of the following conditions EXCEPT one. Which one is the EXCEPTION?

ANS: D
Latent TB infection (D) is not detectable from lymphadenopathy. TB bacteria are contained in lung tissue, not in the lymph nodes of the head and neck. Chronically inflamed lymph nodes may form fibrous hyperplasia (B) or fibrous connective scar tissue, and acutely inflamed nodes (C) may fill with fluid, producing edema. Malignant tissue of epithelium metastasizes (A) via the lymphatic system and can be detected by indurated, fixed lymph nodes of the head and neck.

29. During oral examination, the patient is asked to occlude the teeth and swallow. What is the reason for this?

ANS: D
The patient is asked to occlude the teeth and swallow to determine whether tongue thrusting is a habit from reverse swallowing (D). The tongue should go backward during the swallow and should not protrude through the front teeth. Assessment for fremitus (A) requires the tapping of teeth while feeling digitally for tooth movement. Assessment for centric occlusion (B) does not involve swallowing while teeth are in occlusion. Assessment for mouth breathing (C) is done by visually examining the mouth while open.

30. A lesion that is attached by a stemlike or stalklike base is described as

ANS: E
A pedunculated (E) lesion is attached by a stemlike or stalklike base to the tissue surface. Sessile (A) lesions have a broad flat base. Diffuse (B) lesions have borders that are not well defined. Papillary (C) lesions are clusters of small, nipplelike projections or elevations. Corrugated (D) lesions have a wrinkled surface.

31. All of the following are evidence-based risk factors for periodontal disease EXCEPT one. Which one is the EXCEPTION?

ANS: E
Uncontrolled diabetes is associated with increased infection, but individuals with diabetes controlled with medications such as insulin (E) have no greater risk for periodontal disease than do individuals without diabetes. According to surveys of oral health in populations, the risk for periodontal disease increases with age (A). Tobacco use (B) is a documented risk factor associated with periodontal

disease. Retained biofilm (C) becomes more pathogenic the longer it is undisturbed and may cause periodontal inflammation and infection. Any condition that reduces the host response (D) increases the risk of periodontal disease.

32. Periodontal disease is associated with the following obligate, anaerobic, gram-negative bacteria EXCEPT one. Which one is the EXCEPTION?

ANS: A
S. mutans (A) is a gram-positive, not a gram-negative, facultative anaerobic bacterium associated with dental caries. *T. forsythensis* (B), *P. gingivalis* (C), and *A. actinomycetemcomitans* (D) are all gram-negative, obligate, anaerobic bacteria that have strong links to periodontal disease.

33. Which drug has been associated with improved periodontal tissue health?

ANS: D
Doxycycline (Atridox) (D), an antibacterial drug in the tetracycline classification, has been shown to suppress and kill periodontal microorganisms. Nifedipine (Procardia) (A), cyclosporine (Sandimmune) (B), and phenytoin (Dilantin) (C) all are associated with gingival hyperplasia, which makes the periodontal area difficult to clean and predisposes an individual to periodontal inflammation.

34. Which factor is the STRONGEST predictor of future clinical attachment loss?

ANS: B
A history of prior periodontal disease (B) is the strongest predictor of future clinical attachment loss. Individuals are never *cured* of periodontal disease, and frequent maintenance is needed to prevent recurrence. Bleeding on probing (A) is an indicator of active inflammation but does not necessarily predict progression of inflammation into the periodontal ligament. Lack of bleeding on probing (C) is an indicator of low risk of future clinical attachment loss. Bone loss on dental images (D) indicates past disease activity but is not predictive of future clinical attachment loss.

35. Current salivary genetic deoxyribonucleic acid (DNA) tests for periodontal disease (PD) are prognostic tests. These tests can be used to diagnose PD.

ANS: C
The first statement is true, and the second statement is false (C). The DNA test identifies inflammatory markers such as interleukin-1 in saliva and may indicate increased susceptibility to PD. However, the test is used only as a prognostic test and not for diagnosis of PD. Some individuals with a positive test have not developed PD, and others without the DNA indicator have developed PD. Choices A, B, and D do not correctly address the question.

36. Examination of the periodontium reveals localized probe depths between 4 and 5 millimeters (mm), but the tissue do not bleed on probing. All of the following factors should be considered in any determination of this finding EXCEPT one. Which one is the EXCEPTION?

ANS: D
The type of probe used to obtain readings (D) or lack of bleeding on probing should not factor into the readings. Research shows that tobacco use (A) may constrict vasculature of the periodontium, in which case tissues do not bleed easily. When clinicians do not use sufficient pressure in their probing technique (B), it may result in inaccurate readings or failure to reach the base of the ulcerated junctional epithelium where bleeding originates. Periodontal disease is characterized by exacerbation and remission. During remission, the disease is not in an active state (C), so the stable tissue may not bleed although increased probing depths are present due to past disease. Not all microorganisms (E) are capable of causing periodontal infection or inflammation, and anaerobic, gram-negative bacteria are more strongly related to active infection and bleeding.

37. All of the following are components of a periodontal examination EXCEPT one. Which one is the EXCEPTION?

ANS: B
Nutritional evaluation (B) is not part of a thorough periodontal examination, although it may be indicated in some cases. Adequate lighting (A) is important for accurate observation of tissue color and consistency during periodontal examination. A specific probe to measure furcation involvement during periodontal examination is the Nabors probe (C). Compressed air to dry tissues (D) improves observation of tissue. Tooth movement during occlusion, or fremitus (E), is one procedure used to identify mobile teeth.

38. Which of the following instruments is used to assess implants for peri-implantitis?

ANS: A
A plastic probe (A) is used to prevent damage to the titanium implant surface, and it can help assess implants for peri-implantitis. The Williams probe (B), the Florida probe (C), and the Marquis probe

54. Which of the following poses an increased risk for root caries?

ANS: B
Lack of saliva (B) increases the risk for caries of any type. Acidic food consumption (C) is linked to erosion, not caries. Increased salivation (A) assists remineralization and is not a risk factor for caries. Toothbrushing is the primary form of mechanical disruption of biofilm, and the back-and-forth toothbrushing technique (D) has not been linked to caries risk.

55. A patient who displays the typical signs of traumatic occlusion is likely to have radiographic and clinical signs that demonstrate all of the following characteristics EXCEPT one. Which one is the EXCEPTION?

ANS: B
Horizontal bone loss (B) is associated with the slow bone loss seen in chronic periodontal disease. Tooth mobility (A) is often associated with excessive occlusal forces. Widening of the periodontal ligament space (C) is usually the first radiographic sign of occlusal trauma. Angular or vertical bone destruction (D) is found when excessive occlusal forces occur in the presence of inflammation, causing rapid bone loss.

56. All of the following statements about smoking and periodontal disease are true EXCEPT one. Which one is the EXCEPTION?

ANS: C
Smokers may have less bleeding on probing and inflammation compared with nonsmokers (C) because of the vasoconstrictive properties of nicotine and a suppressed immune response to plaque biofilm. Smoking cessation is extremely beneficial to periodontal health (A) because tobacco use puts patients at high risk for development of periodontal disease. Tobacco users have higher levels of pathogenic bacteria compared with nonsmokers (B), even with good oral hygiene. A positive correlation exists between the amount smoked and the severity of periodontal disease (D), with heavy smokers displaying more severe exacerbations of periodontal disease.

57. When a patient is identified as being at high risk for caries during oral examination, which of the following strategies is NOT recommended by the American Dental Association (ADA) for primary prevention of caries?

ANS: D
Although research indicates that xylitol gum chewed after meals (D) reduces caries activity, it has not received a recommendation from the ADA. According to the 2011 ADA clinical practice recommendations, only sealants (A), fluoride (B), and dietary practices (C) are primary caries-preventive strategies.

58. Components of the intraoral examination of the floor of the mouth include assessment of all of the following EXCEPT one. Which one is the EXCEPTION?

ANS: B
The swallowing pattern (B) is examined while teeth are clenched. The flow of saliva (A), the color (C) and surface texture (E) of the mucosa, and the ability to lift the tongue to the palate (D) are all part of the examination of the floor of the mouth.

59. Symptoms of active TB include all of the following EXCEPT one. Which one is the EXCEPTION?

ANS: B
Weight loss, not weight gain (B), is associated with active disease. The Centers for Disease Control and Prevention (CDC) associate flulike symptoms (A), cough that produces blood (C), persistent cough for more than 3 weeks (D) with active TB.

60. Blood in the sputum of an individual infected with TB represents

ANS: B
Violent coughing may cause the blood vessels in the pharyngeal area to rupture (B), mixing blood with sputum. Droplet infection (A) is the method of transmission of TB and is not associated with blood in sputum. Aerosol of the TB organism is the method of transmission (C), which may cause the TB organism to be transmitted in the circulatory system, but does not produce blood in sputum. TB bacteria cannot directly infect or damage blood vessels (D) and do not cause blood in sputum.

61. All of the following are examples of an elevated lesion EXCEPT one. Which one is the EXCEPTION?

ANS: A
A macule (A) is a flat lesion distinguished by a color different from that of surrounding tissues. All of the other lesions are raised lesions. A bulla (B) is a circumscribed elevated lesion more than 5 mm in diameter and is usually filled with serous fluid. Vesicles (C) are small elevated lesions less than 1 cm in diameter and contain serous fluid. Pustules (D) are raised lesions of various sizes that are filled with purulent exudates. A nodule (E) is a solid palpable lesion up to 1 cm in diameter.

62. Which term characterizes an outward growth?

ANS: D

An exophytic (D) lesion is defined as an outgrowing lesion. An ulcer (A) is a break or depression in the surface continuity of the epithelium. A fissure (B) is a cleft or groove in tissue. An induration (C) is an abnormal hardening of tissue, often associated with cancerous growths. Coalescence (E) is the process of joining together, with loss of borders.

63. A radiographically evident lesion or mass that extends beyond the boundaries of one distinct area and has many parts is called

ANS: D

A multilocular (D) lesion is a radiographically evident lesion extending beyond the boundaries of one distinct area and has many parts. The radiographic image of a sclerotic (A) lesion shows a definite radiopaque border because of the highest density, and such a lesion is usually a longstanding one. Radiolucent lesions with scalloped (B) borders extending between the roots of multiple teeth are seen in some types of cysts and neoplasms. Unilocular (C) is a radiographically descriptive term of the appearance of a single, rounded compartment.

64. A cytologic smear of the oral mucosa is a technique used to histologically examine

ANS: A

The cytologic smear examines only surface cells (A) removed for microscopic examination. A biopsy specimen (B) removes all cell layers for microscopic preparation and examination. Keratinized tissue (C) will not always identify a pathologic process, as surface keratin covers potential abnormal tissues underneath. Erythematous nodules (D) are examined when the tissue is removed and glass slides of shaved tissue are made for dye preparation and microscopic examination.

65. Given a history of bruxism and the dental examination revealing flat occlusal surfaces, which muscle would be expected to be prominent when examining the face?

ANS: B

The masseter (B) muscle is overworked and hypertrophies with chronic bruxism. The facial (A), buccinator (C), and pterygomandibular (D) muscles are not activated during occlusion.

66. The presence of extra teeth beyond the normal complement is known as

ANS: C

Hyperdontia (C) refers to the presence of extra teeth beyond the normal complement, or supernumerary teeth. Anodontia (A) refers to the total absence of teeth. Hypodontia (B) refers to the absence of some teeth so that a normal complement is lacking. Macrodontia (D) refers to larger-than-normal teeth.

67. Which of the following is a supernumerary tooth?

ANS: B

The most common supernumerary tooth is the mesiodens (B), found at the midline of the maxillary arch. Dens in dente (A) are an invagination of the pulp canal, literally a "tooth within a tooth." A macrodont (C) is a larger-than-normal tooth. A peg lateral (D) is a smaller-than-normal tooth, or a microdont.

68. A tooth with a normal crown but wide and elongated pulp extending into the root is an example of

ANS: A

A tooth with a normal crown but wide and elongated pulp extending into the root is an example of taurodontism (A). Dentin dysplasia (B) is a developmental disturbance of dentin covered by normal enamel. Dens evaginatus (C) is a cusplike elevation of enamel in the central groove or lingual ridge of the buccal cusp of posterior teeth.

69. A cervical stress-related defect manifesting as a wedge-shaped defect is called an

ANS: D

Occlusal stress forces at the CEJ are speculated to be a cause of abfraction (D), which results in a wedge-shaped defect. Erosion (A) is dissolution of tooth structure caused by chemical contact. Attrition (B) is loss of tooth structure from tooth-to-tooth contact. Abrasion (C) results from abrasive substances.

70. The MOST effective means for detecting occlusal caries is the

ANS: C

Use of visual inspection after drying the enamel surface with air (C) is considered the most effective method for detecting occlusal caries. Use of a thin explorer (A) may damage enamel integrity. Transillumination (B) is used to detect interproximal caries in anterior teeth, not for detection of occlusal caries. Laser detection technology (D), such as Diagnodent, requires calibration, and the efficacy of this technology has not been proven by extensive research.

71. In an assessment of the deciduous dentition, tooth #E is the

ANS: B
Deciduous teeth are designated by the alphabet, beginning at the maxillary right second molar. The maxillary right central incisor (B) is tooth #E. The maxillary right canine (A) is tooth #C, the mandibular right lateral incisor (C) is tooth #Q, and the mandibular right central incisor (D) is tooth #P.

72. The relationship of occlusal surfaces that provide for maximal intercuspation when teeth are occluded is

ANS: A
Centric occlusion (A) refers to the relationship of occlusal surfaces that provide for maximal intercuspation when teeth are occluded. Class I occlusion (B) reflects the location of the maxillary canines and that the first molar relationships are in normal occlusion but there is malpositioning of individual or groups of teeth. Anterior open bite (C) is when the anterior teeth are not in contact but posterior teeth are in normal occlusion. End-to-end occlusion (D) occurs when the molars are in a cusp-to-cusp relationship rather than an intercuspal relationship.

73. According to Black's classification, occlusal caries on cusp tips is an example of what class of caries?

ANS: E
Class VI caries (E) occurs on the incisal edges of anterior teeth or the cusp tips of posterior teeth. Class I caries (A) occurs in pits and fissures. Class II caries (B) occurs on the proximal surfaces of posterior teeth. Class III caries (C) occurs on the proximal surfaces of anterior teeth. Class IV caries (D) occurs on the incisal edge of anterior teeth.

74. Signs of occlusal trauma include all of the following EXCEPT one. Which one is the EXCEPTION?

ANS: D
Widening of periodontal ligament, not narrowing (D), is a sign of occlusal trauma. Fremitus (A), which is the movement of teeth during occlusion, the presence of wear facets (B), pain when teeth are percussed (C), or pain when teeth are in occlusal contact during chewing (E) are additional signs of occlusal trauma.

75. Directing a strong light through tooth surfaces for diagnostic information is an example of

ANS: B
Transillumination (B) involves the direction of light through a tissue to see shadows and is a useful diagnostic tool for detection of proximal caries in anterior teeth. Percussion (A) is a diagnostic procedure in which a tooth is tapped to gauge pain or other response from the patient. The visual examination (C) is used for detection of abnormal findings by direct observation. Auscultation (D) involves the use of sounds to obtain information.

76. An examination of the occlusion reveals a normal canine-to-molar relationship and crowded mandibular anterior teeth. This is described as

ANS: B
Class I, or mesognathic, occlusion (B) involves a normal canine-to-molar relationship, but some other tooth position is incorrect. In a normal occlusion (A), all teeth relationships are correct. In class II, or retrognathic, malocclusion (C), the maxilla is prominent, and the mandible is posterior to its normal relationship. Class III, or prognathic, malocclusion (D) involves a prominent, protruded mandible, and the maxilla is usually in a normal position.

77. Hypoplasia of the enamel is associated with which congenital condition or disease?

ANS: B
Transmission of syphilis (B) from mother to fetus after the 16th week of gestation may alter the development of specific teeth germs, leading to notched incisors and mulberry molars. Aplasia (A) is the lack of development of salivary glands, leading to dry mouth. Cleft palate (C) is a congenital condition involving the development of the palate but does not affect enamel formation. Tetracycline ingestion (D) during tooth formation results in staining of dentin, not enamel.

78. Grooves or pits in enamel corresponding with the stage of tooth development is a condition described as

ANS: B
Hypoplasia (B) is the most common abnormality of tooth development and mineralization. It presents as defective enamel with pits or grooves in enamel, and patterns often are linear, corresponding to the time of tooth development. Attrition (A) is a wearing away of tooth surfaces from tooth-to-tooth contact.

Hyperplasia (C) is the abnormal increase in the number of normal cells, resulting in thickening or enlargement of a tissue or organ but is not a term used to describe teeth. Hypercalcification (D) may occur in areas of enamel and dentin if severe fluorosis occurs, causing changes in tooth color, not in the surface integrity of enamel.

79. In class II, division 1 occlusion, which teeth are protruded?

ANS: C
In class II, division I malocclusion, the mandible is retruded and all maxillary anterior incisors (C) are protruded or flared. In class II malocclusion, all mandibular anterior teeth (A) are retruded. In class II, division II malocclusion, some maxillary anterior teeth (B) are protruded, and some maxillary anterior teeth (D) are retruded, and the entire mandibular arch is retruded.

80. Attrition of tooth surfaces is influenced by which habit?

ANS: A
Bruxism (A) is a parafunctional habit of grinding teeth, which may result in excessive wear on the occlusal and incisal tooth surfaces. Sucking on lemons (B) may result in acidic erosion of enamel but usually occurs on the facial rather than occlusal or incisal surfaces. Reverse swallowing (C) may result in protrusion of anterior teeth. Wearing a bite guard or mouthpiece (D) separates tooth surfaces to prevent excessive wear.

81. White spot lesions are described as

ANS: B
White spot lesions are caused by initial enamel demineralization without breakthrough to enamel surface (B). Hypercalcified areas (A) would not be clinically detectable. In phase II caries, demineralization spreads along the dentinal tubules (C).

82. Factors that increase the risk for development of early childhood caries includes all of the following EXCEPT one. Which one is the EXCEPTION?

ANS: E
Streptococcus mutans is the bacterial species associated with caries, not *S. salivarius* (E). Milk taken at bedtime (A), prolonged breastfeeding (B), high levels of lactobacilli (C), and pacifiers dipped in honey (D) may all be risk factors for early childhood caries.

83. Which teeth are generally affected first in early childhood caries?

ANS: C
Primary mandibular molars along with maxillary anterior teeth (C) are generally affected first in cases of early childhood caries. Maxillary molars (A) are usually not affected in the early disease process, and likewise mandibular anterior teeth are not affected until later in the disease process (B).

84. Parafunctional habits include all of the following EXCEPT one. Which one is the EXCEPTION?

ANS: D
A parafunctional habit is any habit that moves the mandible or rocks teeth beyond normal function. Mouth breathing (D) is not associated with tooth movement. Bruxism (A), clenching (B), and thumbsucking (C) all may affect tooth movement.

85. Blood pressure levels are determined by which mode of examination?

ANS: C
Auscultation (C) is defined as the act of listening to sounds for information, for example, the use of a stethoscope for detection of blood pressure. Olfaction (A) involves using the sense of smell for detection of certain conditions, for example, "juicy fruit" smell being associated with ketoacidosis in severe hyperglycemia. Palpation (B) is the use of the sense of touch for detection of certain conditions, for example, palpating the lymph nodes for pathology. Observation (D) is visual inspection to determine abnormalities.

86. An epithelium-lined sac is referred to as a

ANS: A
A cyst (A) is an epithelium-lined, fluid-filled sac. A bulla (B) is a fluid-filled blister without an epithelial lining. A nodule (C) is a solid elevated lesion. A granuloma (D) is a lesion filled with immature vascular connective tissue.

87. Screening is a type of examination procedure that includes all of the following characteristics EXCEPT one. Which one is the EXCEPTION?

ANS: C
Screening encompasses more than only intraoral and extraoral examinations (C), although they are some of the components of screening. A screening examination includes a brief examination for a specific purpose (A), is used as a component of triage (B), and is used to survey a group for prevalence of a specific condition (D).

88. The pulp testing device is an example of which method of tooth examination?

    ANS: B
    The pulp testing device, or vitalometer, produces an electrical wave (B) that is transmitted through enamel to the pulp, and living pulp tissues may or may not respond with a sensation. Typically, nonvital teeth have no response to the electrical stimuli, whereas vital teeth respond with sensation, although false-positives may occur. Ideally, more than one type of testing should be used to verify pulpal status before performing any nonreversible procedures. Thermal (A) testing involves use of cold and heat for a response to test nerve vitality. Percussion (C) involves tapping on teeth with a metal instrument to test patient response. Auscultation (D) is a listening technique that is not used for pulp testing.

89. Which statement BEST describes a dental office worker who presents with a positive Mantoux skin test and no symptoms of active TB?

    ANS: A
    Because no symptoms are present in this employee, the CDC considers this individual noninfectious, and he or she may continue working in the dental office (A). Some persons exposed to the TB bacteria may develop antibodies that cause a positive Mantoux skin test, although the disease is not active. In the absence of symptoms, the employee is not contagious (C, D), and his or her noninfectious status carries with it no restrictions on work (B).

90. Which of the following terms refers to a lesion limited to a focal area?

    ANS: B
    A localized (B) lesion is limited to one place. A diffuse (A) lesion is spreading from one area to another. Confluent (C) lesions run together or are joined. Generalized (D) lesions are spread over a large area.

91. Signs of a positive Mantoux skin test include all of the following EXCEPT one. Which one is the EXCEPTION?

    ANS: D
    The Mantoux skin test is an example of a type IV hypersensitivity, or delayed hypersensitivity, reaction; that is, a change within 12 to 24 hours (D) is extremely unlikely. Redness (A), induration or hardness (B), the size of the skin reaction (C), and changes to the site within 48 to 72 hours (E) are all included in the CDC guidelines for skin test results indicating exposure to the TB bacillus.

92. If a client has been diagnosed with active TB and reports taking appropriate medication for treating the infection, how long should the clinician wait before providing preventive oral services?

    ANS: C
    The CDC suggests that a client with active TB who has been taking medication is no longer contagious if anti-TB drugs are taken for at least 3 weeks (C). Waiting 1 (A) or 2 (B) weeks would not be sufficient to ensure that the infection would not be spread; waiting 6 months (D) would be erring on the side of caution.

93. Screening questions on the health history concerning active TB are recommended by which health-related agency?

    ANS: C
    The CDC (C) is the governmental agency formulating guidelines for TB prevention and safety practices in health care locations. The NIH (A) is primarily responsible for research and does not develop guidelines to prevent the spread of TB. The FDA (B) regulates safe manufacturing and processing of food, drugs, and medical devices, not TB prevention and safety practices. The NIOSH (D) is the part of the CDC responsible for conducting research and making recommendations on workplace safety.

94. Nonvital teeth may have all of the following characteristics EXCEPT one. Which one is the EXCEPTION?

    ANS: A
    Nonvital teeth have no living nerve, so they are not sensitive (A). Radiolucency at the apex of a tooth (B) indicates inflammation or necrosis of the pulp, so pulp testing should be performed. Intrinsic discoloration (C) is an indication to examine for pulp vitality. Nonvital teeth have no active blood supply and become brittle over time, with increasing susceptibility to fracture (D), which is why endodontically treated teeth are often covered with full crowns.

95. Which of the following terms refers to tissue or mucosa having a blue color?

    ANS: A
    Mucosa or tissue having a bluish color are said to be cyanotic (A). Melanotic (B) tissue has excessive melanin pigmentation and is of a darker hue than expected. Leukoplakia (C) refers to white plaque on skin or the mucosa that cannot be scraped off. Erythroplakia (D) refers to a reddish colored area of tissue or mucosa.

96. Which of the following lymph node findings would have the MOST negative prognosis?

ANS: C
Lymph nodes that are indurated, nonmovable, and nonpainful (C) have the least favorable prognosis because of the high possibility of malignancy. Rapidly dividing cancer cells invading the lymph node form an indurated or hard mass that infiltrates into the underlying connective tissue making the lymph node nonmovable or "fixed." Cancer is often nonpainful until it is widespread. Palpable, tender, movable lymph nodes (A) are indicative of active infection. Palpable, nontender, movable lymph nodes (B) are indicative of past infection and healed scar tissue.

97. Excessive space between two adjacent teeth in the same arch is called

ANS: A
A diastema (A) is defined as excessive space between adjacent teeth in the same arch. An open bite (B) is an open area between opposing arches of teeth. A wear facet (C) involves a wear pattern on the incisal or occlusal surfaces of a tooth. Primate space (D) is the normal space between primary teeth allowing for skeletal growth and the larger size of permanent teeth.

98. Static occlusion can be identified with which tool?

ANS: A
Static occlusion is the relationship between the maxillary and mandibular arches when the jaw is closed and stationary. Study casts (A), placed together, help identify static occlusion. Radiographs (B) will not identify static occlusion due to the positioning of the bite block or sensor. Percussion (C) is a test performed by tapping on teeth with a dental instrument, but it is not a test used to determine occlusion. An examination for fremitus (D) is performed by having the patient tap his or her teeth together and observe movement to determine loss of periodontal support and is unrelated to static occlusion.

99. Malpositioned teeth, overhanging margins of restorations, and abnormal tooth morphology may cause increased accumulation of dental plaque in specific areas. These factors may be the primary etiologic factor in periodontal disease.

ANS: C
The first statement is true, and the second statement is false (C). Malpositioned teeth, overhanging margins of restorations, and abnormal tooth morphology allow increased accumulation of dental plaque in those areas if extraordinary plaque control measures are not taken, but they contribute to, rather than cause,

periodontal disease. The plaque biofilm is the primary etiologic agent in periodontal disease. Choices A, B, and D do not correctly address the question.

100. When the incisal edges of maxillary incisors are within the incisal half of mandibular incisors, the condition is referred to as

ANS: D
Moderate overbite (D) is defined as the incisal edge of maxillary teeth being within the incisal half of mandibular incisors. In open bite (A), the incisal edges of maxillary incisors are not in contact with the incisal edges of mandibular incisors. Deep or severe overbite (B) occurs when maxillary incisors completely cover mandibular incisors and the incisal edges touch the mandibular gingival margin. Normal overbite (C) occurs when maxillary incisors contact the first third of the incisal edges of mandibular teeth.

101. Formation of which connective tissue may cause the pulp chambers and canals to narrow over time?

ANS: D
Secondary dentin (D) forms within the pulp and canals and narrows the inner surfaces of the tooth to protect the pulp in response to the lifelong process of attrition. Mantle dentin (A) is the first product laid of primary dentin produced during odontogenesis. Primary dentin (B) is the first type of dentin formed and makes up the majority of the tooth. Sclerotic dentin (C) is the calcification of open dentinal tubules and does not affect the size of the pulp chamber or canals.

102. Formation of biofilm involves a series of stages. Which of the following is the beginning stage?

ANS: A
The first step in biofilm formation is when a pellicle forms on the tooth surface (A). The initial multiplication of bacterial species (C), the aggregation of bacteria into organized colonies (D), and the differentiation of bacteria into species (B) are the next steps in biofilm formation and maturation.

103. Populations at high risk of contracting TB include all of the following EXCEPT one. Which one is the EXCEPTION?

ANS: A
Dental health care workers (A) are not among the groups listed as being at high risk for TB infection by the CDC. Groups listed as being at high risk for TB infection are individuals with HIV infection (B), immigrants from developing countries (C), and individuals living in environments where active TB exists (D).

## CHAPTER 8

Obtaining and Interpreting Radiographs

Leslie Koberna, Cynthia A. Stegeman, Jean Frahm, Debra K. Arver, Elizabeth Odom Carr

QUESTIONS

1. A periapical (PA) image is needed on the maxillary left premolar area. The patient presents with a large maxillary torus. Using the paralleling, or right-angle, technique, the image receptor film or sensor is to be placed
    A. distal to the maxillary premolar area.
    B. mesial to the maxillary premolar area.
    C. as close to the maxillary left premolar as possible.
    D. on the far side of the torus.

2. A periapical image of the maxillary right molar area is needed, but patient has a shallow palate, and the first image taken misses the apices of the teeth. To correct this error, using the paralleling technique, an acceptable image can be obtained by moving the position indicating device (PID) in a
    A. 20-degree difference in the horizontal angulation toward the mesial surfaces.
    B. 20-degree difference in the horizontal angulation toward the distal surfaces.
    C. positive 20-degree difference in the vertical angulation.
    D. negative 20-degree difference in the vertical angulation.
    E. direction in which the central ray is perpendicular to the image receptor.

3. When taking a premolar bitewing image, which error in the position of the PID is seen in the photograph shown?

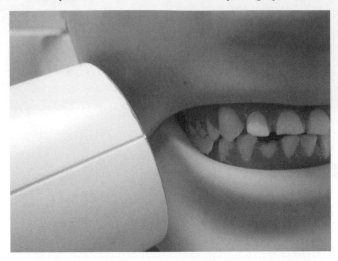

A. Greater horizontal angulation than required
B. Greater positive vertical angulation than required
C. Greater negative vertical angulation than required
D. The PID is correctly positioned for a premolar bitewing

4. The error that will occur to the premolar bitewing image as a result of the PID positioning will be

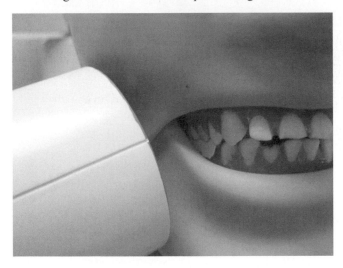

A. unequal distribution of maxillary and mandibular teeth. There will be more coverage of maxillary teeth and fewer mandibular teeth.
B. unequal distribution of maxillary and mandibular teeth. There will be more coverage of mandibular teeth and fewer maxillary teeth.
C. distal overlap.
D. mesial overlap.

5. In the molar bitewing image, the error that will occur as a result of the PID positioning will be distal overlap. Distal overlap is corrected by repositioning the horizontal angulation of the PID more mesiodistally.

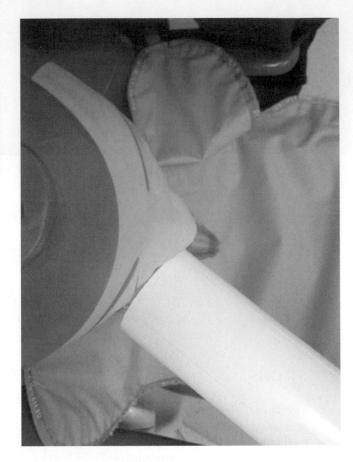

A. Both statements are true.
B. Both statements are false.
C. The first statement is true, and the second statement is false.
D. The first statement is false, and the second statement is true.

6. Considering exposure time during the production of x-rays, how many impulses are equivalent to ¼ second?
A. 1
B. 6
C. 15
D. 30
E. 240

7. Order the steps for the manual processing of x-ray films. Match each letter with its proper sequence number.

Sequence Number	Steps
1. _____	A. Rinsing in water for 30 seconds
2. _____	B. Washing in water for 20 minutes
3. _____	C. Developing
4. _____	D. Fixing
5. _____	E. Drying

8. From the following list, select the three elements used in the x-ray tube.
   A. Bromine
   B. Copper
   C. Iron
   D. Molybdenum
   E. Nickel
   F. Silver
   G. Tungsten

9. Which of the following is the unit used to measure radiation exposure?
   A. Gray (Gy)
   B. Radiation absorbed dose (rad)
   C. Roentgen (R)
   D. Roentgen equivalent in man (rem)
   E. Sievert (Sv)

10. A radiographic image will have increased density if the operator
    A. increases the kVp.
    B. decreases the kVp.
    C. decreases the milliampere (mA).
    D. increases the distance of the x-ray source to the image receptor.

11. The smaller the silver halide crystals in the emulsion of an intraoral film, the faster the film speed. Faster film speed reduces radiation exposure to the patient.
    A. Both statements are true.
    B. Both statements are false.
    C. The first statement is true, and the second statement is false.
    D. The first statement is false, and the second statement is true.

12. Which ingredient of the developing solution in the manual processing of x-ray films is alkaline and aids in the softening of the emulsion?
    A. Potassium bromide
    B. Potassium alum
    C. Sodium carbonate
    D. Sodium sulfite
    E. Sodium thiosulfate

13. In which anomaly is cementum of two adjacent teeth joined together?
    A. Concrescence
    B. Fusion
    C. Gemination
    D. Hypercementosis

14. Which structure or material will appear the MOST radiopaque on a dental image?
    A. Airspace
    B. Amalgam restoration

C. Periodontal ligament space
D. Composite restoration
E. Pulp

15. Which structure appears as a radiopaque line surrounding the root of the tooth?
    A. Trabecular bone
    B. Cancellous bone
    C. Lamina dura
    D. Periodontal ligament space
    E. Pulp

16. Which of the following describes the appearance of a carious lesion on the buccal or lingual surface of a molar on a dental image?
    A. Triangular, radiolucent
    B. Triangular, radiopaque
    C. Circular, radiolucent
    D. Circular, radiopaque

17. Which mandibular anatomic landmark can be seen as a radiolucent area on a mandibular premolar periapical (PA) image?
    A. Genial tubercles
    B. Internal oblique ridge
    C. Mental foramen
    D. Lingual foramen
    E. Mental ridge

18. All of the following are descriptions of a ghost image on a panoramic image EXCEPT one. Which one is the EXCEPTION?
    A. It is a similar sharpness as the original artifact.
    B. It is a similar shape to the original artifact.
    C. It is on the opposite side of the original artifact.
    D. It is located higher than the original artifact.
    E. It is larger than the original artifact.

19. Cone cutting has occurred on the coronal portion of a mandibular anterior PA image. The operator will correct this error by
    A. moving the image receptor more superiorly.
    B. moving the image receptor more inferiorly.
    C. moving the PID to completely cover the image receptor.
    D. adding more solution to the developer.
    E. adding more solution to the fixer.

20. The tubehead of the panoramic unit is angled so that the x-ray beam is directed
    A. in a slightly positive vertical angulation.
    B. in a strong positive vertical angulation.
    C. in a slightly negative vertical angulation.
    D. in a strong negative vertical angulation.
    E. at zero angulation.

21. From the following list, select the three statements associated with digital imaging.
    A. Sensors cannot be sterilized.
    B. A digital image is a two-dimensional representation of a three-dimensional object.
    C. Exposure times are 50% to 90% more than in traditional radiography.
    D. Digital imaging must be wired to function correctly.
    E. Assembled pictorial information with each gray value is assigned a digit in binary code.

22. The tubehead is a component of the x-ray machine that helps limit radiation to the patient in all of the following functions EXCEPT one. Which one is the EXCEPTION?
    A. Inherent filtration within glass tube, insulating oil, and tubehead
    B. Added aluminum disk filtration
    C. Production of both long-wavelength and short-wavelength x-rays
    D. Collimation with lead disk placed in the pathway of the x-ray beam
    E. Rectangular collimated PID

23. Erythema, nausea, diarrhea, hemorrhage, and loss of hair are signs and symptoms seen with
    A. chronic radiation exposure.
    B. acute radiation exposure.
    C. stochastic effects of radiation exposure.
    D. nonstochastic effects of radiation exposure.
    E. A and C
    F. B and D

24. Which statement BEST describes changes to the atom during the ionizing process?
    A. The atom gains an electron and will have a negative charge.
    B. The atom gains an electron and will have a positive charge.
    C. The atom loses an electron and will have a negative charge.
    D. The atom loses an electron and will have a positive charge.

25. For each numbered anatomic landmark, select the BEST associated radiographic description.

Anatomic Landmark	Description of Radiographic Presentation
___1. Median palatine suture	A. Ring-shaped radiopacity noted apical to mandibular incisors
___2. Genial tubercles	B. Dense radiopaque band extending from the molar region downward toward the premolar area of the mandible

___3. Incisive foramen — C. Thin radiolucent line between maxillary central incisors
___4. Mylohyoid ridge — D. Triangular-shaped radiopacity superimposed over or seen inferior to the maxillary tuberosity area
___5. Mental foramen — E. Small oval or round radiolucency seen in the apical region of mandibular premolars
___6. Floor of nasal cavity — F. Dense radiopaque band of bone seen apical to maxillary incisors
___7. Coronoid process — G. Small oval or round radiolucency seen between the roots of maxillary central incisors

26. Order each tissue in order of radiosensitivity, from most sensitive to least sensitive. Match each letter with its proper sequence number.

1. _____   A. Skin
2. _____   B. Oral mucosal epithelium
3. _____   C. Nervous tissue
4. _____   D. Reproductive tissue
5. _____   E. Lymphatic tissue and bone marrow
6. _____   F. Mature bone and cartilage

27. Which factor affects contrast?
    A. Distance
    B. kVp
    C. Exposure time
    D. mA

28. For each numbered x-radiation interaction, select the BEST description.

X-Radiation Interaction	Description
_____ 1. X-ray photon passed through atom unchanged; no interaction	A. Electrons stop suddenly as they hit the anode.
_____ 2. Coherent scatter	B. Ionization takes place when the photon ejects an outer shell electron. This results in the loss of energy for the photon and a negative charged electron. The low energy photon changes direction.
_____ 3. Photoelectric effect	C. An unstable atom releases energy.

X-Radiation Interaction	Description
_____ 4. Compton scatter	D. This is responsible for producing the densities on the receptor or film.
_____ 5. Bremsstrahlung radiation	E. Ionization takes place when photons are absorbed by patient tissues.
_____ 6. Radioactivity	F. No loss of energy and no ionization occur when this low-energy photon interacts with an outer shell electron. The unaffected photon changes direction.

29. Order the steps in the production of x-radiation. Match each letter with its proper sequence number.

1. _____
2. _____
3. _____
4. _____

A. Electrons travel across to the anode when the high voltage circuit is activated.
B. Thermionic emission occurs.
C. 110 or 220 line voltage is reduced to 3 to 5 volts.
D. Kinetic energy is converted to x-ray energy and heat.

30. For each numbered term listed below, select the BEST description from the list provided.

Term	Description
_____ 1. Anode	A. Produces electrons
_____ 2. Cathode	B. Controls the number of electrons
_____ 3. Kilovoltage	C. Decreases voltage
_____ 4. Milliamperage	D. Narrows the beam and controls the direction of the beam
_____ 5. Molybdenum cup	E. Release of electrons from the tungsten filament when the electrical current passes through it and heats the filament
_____ 6. Tungsten filament	F. Spot where the electrons are converted into x-ray photons
_____ 7. Tungsten target	G. Positive electrode
_____ 8. Thermionic emission	H. Restricts the size and shape of the x-ray beam to reduce patient exposure
_____ 9. Step-down transformer	I. Controls the force of the electrons
_____ 10. Collimator	J. Negative electrode

31. In the formation of x-radiation, electrons that strike the nucleus of a tungsten atom produce which type of x-ray?
    A. Low-energy
    B. High-energy
    C. Both high-energy and low-energy

32. You wish to compare your patient's current images with images that were taken 2 years ago. The images from 2 years ago have a yellowish-brown color. Which of the following is the cause of the yellow-brown stains?
    A. Temperature of the water bath is colder than the developer temperature
    B. Insufficient fixing
    C. High developer temperature
    D. Prolonged rinsing

33. Which of the following is the receptor that captures computerized images as discrete units of information?
    A. Sensor
    B. Film
    C. Pixel
    D. Bit-depth image

34. It is acknowledged that the routine performance of radiography is not recommended. Using sound professional judgment, for each numbered type of patient listed, select the recommended prescription of radiography based on the Guidelines for Prescribing Radiographs established by the U.S. Food and Drug Administration (FDA) from the list provided. Not all guidelines will be used.

Type of Patient	Guideline for Prescribing Radiography
_____ 1. Recall patient: adult patient with no sign of clinical caries; presents with no caries risk	A. Posterior bitewings; every 6 to 18 months
_____ 2. Recall patient: child with no significant clinical caries; presents with no caries risk	B. Clinical judgment based on patient needs
_____ 3. New patient: 14-year-old with clinical caries in select areas	C. Every 3 to 6 months
_____ 4. Recall patient: adult with clinical caries or caries risk	D. Every 12 to 24 months if proximal contacts are not visible and cannot be checked with probe

56. Which of the following statements BEST describes the anomaly in the image shown below?

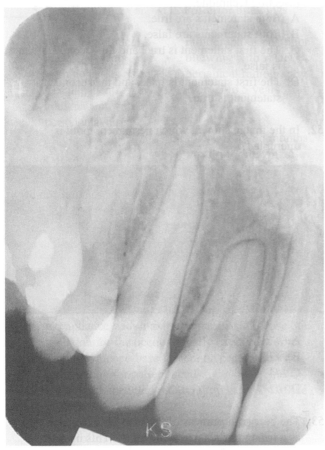

From Haring JI, Lind LJ: Radiographic interpretation for the dental hygienist, *Philadelphia, PA, 1993, Saunders.*

   A. Foreshortening of the root, vertical angle too great
   B. Foreshortening of the root, vertical angle not enough
   C. Incomplete apical development of the root
   D. Internal resorption of the root
   E. External resorption of the root

57. The device that restricts the size of the x-ray beam is called a/an
   A. dosimeter.
   B. aluminum filter.
   C. collimator.
   D. focusing cup.
   E. inherent filtration.

58. All of the following structures could be seen on a maxillary molar periapical image EXCEPT one. Which one is the EXCEPTION?
   A. Coronoid process of the mandible
   B. Mandibular condyle
   C. Maxillary tuberosity
   D. Hamulus
   E. Floor of the maxillary sinus

59. Radiography provides the most accurate measurements for assessment of periodontal disease and its progression. This is because radiographs record both historical and current disease activity.
   A. Both statements are true.
   B. Both statements are false.
   C. The first statement is true, and the second statement is false.
   D. The first statement is false, and the second statement is true.

60. Which statement BEST describes a principle of radiographic image magnification?
   A. Greater target–receptor distance increases greater image magnification.
   B. Less target–receptor distance reduces image magnification.
   C. Greater target–receptor distance reduces image magnification.
   D. Target–receptor distance does not affect magnification.

61. In a darkroom, the correct lighting and distance from the working surface should be
   A. a 60-watt bulb placed 6 feet away.
   B. a 75-watt bulb placed 6 feet away.
   C. a 7.5-watt bulb place 6 feet away.
   D. a 30-watt bulb placed 8 feet away.

62. An impulse is equal to
   A. 1 second.
   B. $\frac{1}{6}$ of a second.
   C. $\frac{1}{60}$ of a second.
   D. $\frac{1}{600}$ of a second.

63. Which statement BEST describes the kVp rule?
   A. When the kVp is decreased by half, the exposure time is increased by 15.
   B. When the kVp is decreased by 15, the exposure time is decreased by half.
   C. When the kVp is doubled, the exposure time is decreased by half.
   D. When the kVp is increased by 15, the exposure time is decreased by half.

64. To maintain the same image density when increasing the mA, which of the following actions should be taken?
    A. Increase kVp
    B. Decrease exposure time
    C. Increase film speed
    D. Decrease distance from source to object

65. An x-ray beam has a half-value layer (HVL) of 6 mm. How many millimeters of aluminum are required to reduce the x-ray beam intensity by half?
    A. 2 mm
    B. 3 mm
    C. 6 mm
    D. 12 mm

66. The indirect theory of radiation injury suggests that cell damage occurs when ionizing radiation hits critical areas within the cell. The direct theory of radiation injury suggests that x-ray photons are absorbed within the cell and cause the formation of toxins that in turn damage the cell.
    A. Both statements are true.
    B. Both statements are false.
    C. The first statement is true, and the second statement is false.
    D. The first statement is false, and the second statement is true.

67. The kVp setting is the only exposure factor that has direct influence on the contrast of a dental radiograph. High kVp settings result in high contrast images.
    A. Both statements are true.
    B. Both statements are false.
    C. The first statement is true, and the second statement is false.
    D. The first statement is false, and the second statement is true.

68. Which of the following terms refers to the majority of scatter radiation produced in dental imaging?
    A. Coherent scatter
    B. Compton scatter
    C. Primary scatter
    D. Secondary scatter

69. The penetrating quality of the x-ray beam is controlled by the
    A. film speed.
    B. exposure time.
    C. source-to-film distance.
    D. wavelength.

70. All of the following factors increase image sharpness EXCEPT one. Which one is the EXCEPTION?
    A. Slower film speed
    B. Small focal spot
    C. Decreased penumbra
    D. Movement

71. Which of the following BEST describes the purpose of the lead foil contained within a radiograph film packet?
    A. Shield the film from backscattered radiation
    B. Protect the film from light
    C. Protect the oral tissues and teeth from excess radiation
    D. Reduce the amount of radiation received by the patient

72. Which statement BEST describes the relationship of the image receptor and the tooth in the paralleling technique?
    A. The image receptor is parallel to the long axis of the tooth.
    B. The image receptor is slightly angled toward the long axis of the tooth.
    C. The central ray of the x-ray beam is directed perpendicular to the receptor and the long axis of the tooth.
    D. Both A and C
    E. Both B and C

73. According to the SLOB rule, the position of objects can be determined if the tubehead is shifted in a mesial direction. The lingual object moves distally, and the buccal object moves mesially.
    A. Both statements are true.
    B. Both statements are false.
    C. The first statement is true, and the second statement is false.
    D. The first statement is false, and the second statement is true.

74. For each description of a radiograph's appearance listed, select the most closely linked error. Each answer will only be used once.

Appearance	Error
____ 1. Clear	A. Film was developed in weak developer
____ 2. Light	B. Film was exposed to white light
____ 3. Light film with "tire tracks"	C. Film was placed backward
____ 4. Fogged	D. Film was developed in a dark room with a crack in the safelight cover
____ 5. Black	E. Film was not exposed to x-rays

for 30 seconds (A); the third step is fixing (D); the fourth step is washing in water for 20 minutes (B); and the fifth step is drying (E).

8. From the following list, select the three elements used in the x-ray tube.

   ANS: B, D, G
   The copper (B) stem, the molybdenum (D) cup, and the tungsten (G) filament and target are parts of the x-ray tube. Bromine (A), iron (C), nickel (E), and silver (F) are not present in the x-ray tube.

9. Which of the following is the unit used to measure radiation exposure?

   ANS: C
   In the traditional unit of radiation measurement, the roentgen (R) is the unit used to measure radiation exposure (C). Within this same system, the rad (B), and the rem (D) are other units of measurement. In the newer SI system (International System of Units), there is no unit for exposure that is equivalent to the roentgen. Instead, gray (A) is the unit equivalent to the rad, and Sievert (E) is the unit equivalent to the rem.

10. A radiographic image will have increased density if the operator

    ANS: A
    Increasing the kVp (A) will increase the density (darkness) of the image. Decreasing either the kVp (B) or mA (C) decreases the density of the image. The distance of the x-ray source to the image affects the intensity of the beam, and increasing this distance (D) lowers beam intensity, resulting in an image with decreased density.

11. The smaller the silver halide crystals in the emulsion of an intraoral film, the faster the film speed. Faster film speed reduces radiation exposure to the patient.

    ANS: D
    The first statement is false, and the second statement is true (D). The smaller the silver halide crystals, the longer the exposure time required to create an image. Larger silver halide crystals require a shorter exposure time, reducing radiation exposure to the patient. Choices A, B, and C do not accurately reflect the statements.

12. Which ingredient of the developing solution in the manual processing of x-ray films is alkaline and aids in the softening of the emulsion?

    ANS: C
    Sodium carbonate (C) provides the necessary alkaline environment in the developing solution to aid in the

developing solution and aids in the softening of the emulsion. Potassium bromide (A) is a restrainer in the developing solution. Potassium alum (B) is a hardening agent in the fixing solution. Sodium sulfite (D) is a preservative in both the fixing and developing solutions. Sodium thiosulfate (E) is a fixing agent in the fixing solution.

13. In which anomaly is cementum of two adjacent teeth joined together?

    ANS: A
    Concrescence (A) is the condition in which cementum of two adjacent teeth is joined together. Fusion (B) can be complete, involving dentin, or incomplete, involving only the crown or the root of two adjacent teeth, depending on the stage of tooth development at the time of contact. Gemination (C), or twinning, is an anomaly in which one tooth bud divides into two incomplete teeth with one pulp with a shared root and root canal. Hypercementosis (D) is excessive cementum on the root of a tooth.

14. Which structure or material will appear the MOST radiopaque on a dental image?

    ANS: B
    An amalgam restoration (B) will appear the most radiopaque of the given structures or materials. It is the densest structure and will absorb or block the most radiation, and the area of the amalgam on the image receptor will not be exposed, resulting in an image that appears white or radiopaque. Airspace (A) appears mostly radiolucent. The periodontal ligament space (C) appears as a thin radiolucent line around the root of the tooth. Composite restorations (D) may appear radiolucent to slightly radiopaque, depending on the composition of the material. Pulp (E) appears relatively radiolucent.

15. Which structure appears as a radiopaque line surrounding the root of the tooth?

    ANS: C
    The lamina dura (C) is cortical bone surrounding the root of the tooth and appears radiopaque. Cancellous bone (B) is composed of numerous trabecular spaces (A) and appears predominantly radiolucent. The periodontal ligament space (D) appears as a thin radiolucent line around the root of the tooth. The entire pulp cavity (E) appears relatively radiolucent.

16. Which of the following describes the appearance of a carious lesion on the buccal or lingual surface of a molar on a dental image?

ANS: C
A carious lesion on the buccal or lingual surface of a molar will appear as a radiolucent circle (C) on a dental image. Depending on the depth, an interproximal carious lesion appears as a radiolucent triangle (A). Carious lesions appear radiolucent, not radiopaque (B, D).

17. Which mandibular anatomic landmark can be seen as a radiolucent area on a mandibular premolar periapical (PA) image?

ANS: C
The mental foramen (C) is a radiolucent, circular structure that appears on the mandibular premolar PA image. The genial tubercles (A) are the mandibular anatomic landmarks that appear as a radiopaque area on a mandibular central incisor PA image. The internal oblique ridge (B) is a mandibular anatomic landmark that cannot be seen on a maxillary premolar PA image. The lingual foramen (D) is a small, ring-shaped radiopacity inferior to the mandibular central incisors and does not appear on the premolar view. The mental ridge (E) appears as a radiopaque band in the premolar and incisor region.

18. All of the following are descriptions of a ghost image on a panoramic image EXCEPT one. Which one is the EXCEPTION?

ANS: A
The ghost image does not have similar sharpness but is more blurred compared with the original artifact (A). When comparing the original artifact with the ghost image, the ghost image appears to have a similar shape (B), is located on the opposite side (C), is higher (D), and is larger (E) than the original artifact.

19. Cone cutting has occurred on the coronal portion of a mandibular anterior PA image. The operator will correct this error by

ANS: C
Moving the PID to completely cover the image receptor will allow the x-ray beam to reach each part of the image receptor. Adjusting the PID to cover the entire image receptor (C) corrects the error of cone cutting. Proper placement of the image receptor more superiorly or inferiorly (A, B) to cover the area intended to be radiographed is imperative and should not be overlooked. Adding solution to the developer (D) or fixer (E) has no impact on cone cutting.

20. The tubehead of the panoramic unit is angled so that the x-ray beam is directed

ANS: C
The tubehead of a panoramic unit is stationary so that the x-ray beam is directed in an upward or

slightly negative vertical angulation (C), −4 to −7 degrees. This allows the x-ray beam to emerge from the panoramic tubehead through the collimator as a narrow band that passes through the patient and exposes the receptor through another vertical slit in the cassette. This narrow collimated beam greatly reduces the amount of patient radiation exposure. The panoramic unit also has a head position that aligns the patient's teeth in the focal trough as accurately as possible. If the x-ray beam is directed in a slightly positive vertical (A), strong positive vertical (B), strong negative vertical (D), or zero (E) angulation, the x-ray beam will not be in the proper position to expose the receptor.

21. From the following list, select the three statements associated with digital imaging.

ANS: A, B, E
Digital sensors cannot be sterilized (A) by traditional methods of sterilization used in dental offices and must be covered with a disposable barrier or sleeve. The image produced in digital radiography is a two-dimensional representation of a three-dimensional object (B). To form the image, each pixel in the image is assigned a binary code to represent a shade of gray (E). Digital imaging uses 50% to 90% *less* radiation than traditional imaging (C). Digital imaging may be either wired or wireless (D).

22. The tubehead is a component of the x-ray machine that helps limit radiation to the patient in all of the following functions EXCEPT one. Which one is the EXCEPTION?

ANS: C
Production of both long-wavelength and short-wavelength x-rays (C) occurs during patient exposure, and is NOT a component of tubehead radiation safety. Long-wavelength x-rays cannot penetrate tissue and are stopped by the patient's skin, increasing unnecessary radiation exposure. Radiation safety is increased by the addition of inherent filtration (A) and aluminum disks (B) within the tubehead to filter out some of the long, nonpenetrating wavelength x-rays, increasing radiation safety. Collimation with a lead disk (D) restricts the size of the x-ray beam, reducing the amount of tissue exposed to radiation. Use of a rectangular collimated PID (E) reduces the size of the primary beam, reducing patient radiation.

23. Erythema, nausea, diarrhea, hemorrhage, and loss of hair are signs and symptoms seen with

ANS: F
Erythema, nausea, diarrhea, hemorrhage, and loss of hair are all symptoms of acute radiation syndrome

not recommended radiographic prescriptions for any of the types of patients described above.

35. Which of the following concepts are examples of the ALARA concept? (Select all that apply.)

ANS: A, B, E, F
The ALARA concept is the concept that individuals working with radiation should attempt to keep all radiation *as low as reasonably achievable*. Compliance with the maximum permissible dose (MPD) for occupational exposure received by the dental personnel working with radiation (A) means that no more than 50 millisievert (mSv) or 5000 millirem (mrem) is permitted. The use of evidence-based criteria for patient radiographic needs reduces unnecessary exposure (B). Use of a film holder (E) increases the diagnostic quality of images and reduces additional exposure required by retakes. Shielding reproductive system tissues and the thyroid gland with lead collars and aprons (F) protects sensitive areas from secondary radiation. Routinely, scheduled images based on office protocol (C) do not take the individual needs of the patient into account and could result in unnecessary exposure. Use of the fastest image receptor would indicate use of "F" speed film or digital sensors; these options would result in less radiation exposure than slower "D" speed film (D).

36. From the following list, select the four characteristics that describe properties of dental x-radiation.

ANS: A, B, E, F
X-radiation is absorbed by matter (A); may cause certain substances to fluoresce (B); is capable of penetrating matter (E); and travels in a straight line (F). X-radiation *does not* travel at the speed of sound (C) but instead at the speed of light. It has no charge or weight (D), and it cannot be focused to a point (G).

37. Radiation may damage cells indirectly by damaging the cell nucleus. Direct cellular damage occurs when ionization causes radiolysis of water producing hydrogen peroxide.

ANS: B
Both statements are false (B). The nucleus of the cell is most sensitive to ionizing effects and damage to the nucleus is termed *direct*, not *indirect*. It is indirect cellular damage that occurs when x-ray photons are absorbed with the cell, causing the formation of toxins (e.g., hydrogen peroxide [H_2O_2]), which, in turn, damages the cell. Choices A, C, and D do not accurately reflect the statements.

38. When an x-ray photon passes through matter, which of the following situations is MOST likely to occur?

ANS: B
Although all of the situations shown may occur when an x-ray photon passes through matter, the most common scenario is the creation of Compton scatter (B), which occurs about 62% of the time. In Compton scatter, the x-ray photon collides with the loosely bound, outer shell electron and gives up part of its energy to dislodge the electron from the shell. The lower-energy photon loses energy and continues in another direction or scatters until its energy is depleted. The ejected electron is termed a *Compton (or recoil)* electron and has a negative charge, whereas the atom remains positively charged. An x-ray photon collides with a tightly bound, inner-shell electron and gives up all of its energy to eject the electron from its orbit. All of the photon's energy is absorbed into the orbital electron, which is called a *photoelectron*, and has a negative charge (A). This occurs about in about 30% of the interactions of matter with the dental x-ray beam. The photoelectric effect occurs when absorption occurs at the atomic level. *Coherent (or unmodified)* scatter (C) occurs when the path of the low-energy x-ray photon interacts with an outer shell electron. The atom does not change, and an x-ray photon of scattered radiation is produced, which moves in a different direction from that of the original photon. No energy loss or ionization occurs, so the x-ray photon is unmodified. This happens to about 8% of the interactions of matter with the x-ray beam. Characteristic radiation (D) is created when the high-speed electrons dislodge electrons from the K-shell of the atoms at the anode. This occurs in the x-ray tube. General/Bremsstrahlung radiation (E) is responsible for the formation of x-ray photons. They are produced when the high-speed electrons strike the nucleus of the atoms at the anode. This occurs in the x-ray tube. In some cases, the x-ray photon has no interaction (F) with matter, but this is not the most common scenario.

39. From the following list, select examples of stochastic effects of radiation exposure. (Select all that apply.)

ANS: B, D
Stochastic effects have no dose threshold, do not follow the dose–response curve, and often the effects of exposure are delayed. Examples include cancer (B) and genetic mutations (D). Nonstochastic effects have a dose threshold, a clear relationship between exposure and dose, and generally occur from an acute radiation exposure. Examples include erythema (A), hair loss (C), and decreased fertility (E).

40. Radiation exposure is not of concern when it occurs in small doses. The cumulative effect of radiation exposure may lead to health problems such as cancer.

ANS: D
The first statement is false, and the second statement is true (D). All radiation exposure causes damage, even in small doses. Repeated doses of radiation are cumulative; health problems such as cancer may occur. Choices A, B, and C do not accurately reflect the statements.

41. All of the following are examples of radiosensitive cells EXCEPT one. Which one is the EXCEPTION?

ANS: C
A cell that is resistant to changes induced by radiation is termed *radioresistant*. Older, mature cells divide infrequently, have a lower metabolism, and are considered radioresistant (C). Examples of radioresistant cells include cells of bones, muscles, and nerves. *Radiosensitive* cells, or cells that are sensitive to radiation, include cells with a higher metabolism (A), cells that frequently undergo mitotic activity or division (B), and cells that are primitive or nonspecialized (D). Examples include blood cells, immature reproductive cells, and young bone cells. The small lymphocyte is the cell that is most sensitive to radiation.

42. Failing to follow radiation exposure patient guidelines would put a fetus at greatest risk in which trimester?

ANS: A
Although failure to use appropriate patient safeguards such as a lead apron could potentially risk the unborn child during any trimester, the greatest risk for embryologic damage is during the first trimester (A) because of the increased mitotic activity, immature cells, and increased cell metabolism. There is less risk during the second (B) and third (C) trimesters, but it prudent to refrain from taking x-rays until after delivery, if possible. The American Dental Association (ADA) and FDA *Guidelines for Prescribing Dental Radiographs* state that the recommended guidelines do not need to be altered because of pregnancy because no detectable exposure to the embryo or fetus occurs with the use of the lead apron (E).

43. Which of the following BEST describes the process of heating the cathode wire until it is red hot and "boiling off" of electrons?

ANS: C
As the tungsten filament of the cathode portion of the x-ray tube heats up after activation of the filament circuit, the release or "boiling off" of electrons is defined as *thermionic emission* (C). The cathode ray

(A) is a stream of high-speed electrons that originates from the cathode in an x-ray tube. Beta-particles (B) are fast-moving electrons emitted from the nucleus of radioactive atoms. A recoil electron (or Compton electron; D) is a negative outer-shell electron that is ejected from its orbit during Compton scatter. Rectification (E) is the conversion of alternating current to direct current.

44. All of the following decrease radiation exposure to the patient EXCEPT one. Which one is the EXCEPTION?

ANS: C
The 8-inch PID creates more divergence of the x-ray beam compared with the 16-inch PID, creating more radiation exposure (C). The thyroid collar (A) is a flexible lead shield that protects the thyroid from scatter radiation. F-speed film (B), the fastest intraoral film available, reduces the patient's exposure to x-radiation. A rectangular PID (D) is the most effective PID in reducing patient exposure as it restricts the size of the x-ray beam to an area slightly larger than a size 2 intraoral film. A collimator (E) is a diaphragm (commonly made of lead) used to restrict the size and shape of the x-ray beam to reduce patient exposure.

45. Which of the following is (are) the maximum permissible dose (MPD) for a dental hygienist? (Select all that apply)

ANS: B, D
The maximum permissible dose for occupationally exposed persons such as dental hygienists is 5 rems per year (B), according to the traditional radiation measurement system, or 50 mSv (D), according to the International System of Units (SI); 0.5 rems a year (A) is significantly *lower* than 5 rems per year, the maximum permissible dose for occupationally exposed persons according to the traditional radiation measurement system; 50 rems a year (C) is significantly *higher* than 5 rems per year, the maximum permissible dose for occupationally exposed persons according to the traditional radiation measurement system; and 5 mSv (E) is significantly *lower* than 50 mSv, the maximum permissible dose for occupationally exposed persons according to the International System of Units (SI).

46. A radiograph that has many shades of grade is considered to have

ANS: D
Contrast is the difference among the shades of gray in the radiograph. A low-contrast (D) image has *long-scale contrast* or many shades of gray. Density is the amount of darkness or black in the radiograph.

reduces image magnification) are incorrect. Further, less target–receptor distance does NOT reduce image magnification (B).

61. In a darkroom, the correct lighting and distance from the working surface should be

ANS: C
A safelight consists of a lamp of 7.5 to 15 watts (C) and a safelight filter, which permits the passage of light in the red-orange wavelength range and removes those in the blue-green portion responsible for exposing and damaging x-ray film. A minimum distance of 4 feet must exist between the safelight and the film and work area. The bulb choices of 60 watt (A); 75-watt (B); and 30-watt (D) are too high a wattage and could cause film fog.

62. An impulse is equal to

ANS: C
Because x-rays are created in a series of bursts, exposure time is measured in impulses. One impulse occurs every $\frac{1}{60}$ of a second; therefore, 60 impulses occur in 1 second (C). Choices A (1 second), B ($\frac{1}{6}$ of a second), and D ($\frac{1}{600}$ of a second) do not correctly represent an impulse.

63. Which statement BEST describes the kVp rule?

ANS: D
The kVp rule states that when the kVp is increased by 15, the exposure time should be decreased by half (D); conversely, when the kVp is decreased by 15, the exposure time should be doubled. Choices A, B, and C do not accurately define the kVp rule.

64. To maintain the same image density when increasing the mA, which of the following actions should be taken?

ANS: B
mA and exposure time directly influence the number of electrons produced by the cathode filament, affecting film density. The product of mA and exposure times is termed *milliampere-second* (mAs) and is calculated by multiplying the two variables. When mA is increased, the exposure time must be decreased (B) and vice versa if the density of the exposed radiograph is to remain the same. Increasing kVp (A) would increase film density. Film speed (C) has no effect on image density. Decreasing the distance from source to object (D) would decrease film density.

65. An x-ray beam has a half-value layer (HVL) of 6 mm. How many millimeters of aluminum are required to reduce the x-ray beam intensity by half?

ANS: C
When placed in the path of the x-ray beam, the thickness of a specified material that reduces the x-ray beam intensity by half is termed the *half-value layer* (HVL). An HVL of 6 mm would require a 6 mm (C) thickness of aluminum to decrease the x-ray beam intensity by half. Measuring the HVL determines the penetrating quality of the beam. Aluminum that is 2 mm thick (A) and 3 mm thick (B) would be too thin to reduce the x-ray beam intensity by half. Aluminum that is 12 mm thick (D) is too thick and would reduce the x-ray beam intensity by more than half.

66. The indirect theory of radiation injury suggests that cell damage occurs when ionizing radiation hits critical areas within the cell. The direct theory of radiation injury suggests that x-ray photons are absorbed within the cell and cause the formation of toxins that in turn damage the cell.

ANS: B
Both statements are false (B). The *indirect theory* suggests that x-ray photons are absorbed within the cell and cause the formation of free radicals, which damages the cell. The *direct theory* of radiation injury suggests that cell damage results when ionizing radiation directly hits critical areas, such as the cell nucleus, within the cell. Choices A, C, and D do not accurately reflect the statements.

67. The kVp setting is the only exposure factor that has direct influence on the contrast of a dental radiograph. High kVp settings result in high contrast images.

ANS: C
The first statement is true, and the second statement is false (C). The only factor that influences film contrast is the kVp. Increasing the kVp increases the average energy of the x-rays, producing x-rays better able to penetrate the tissue and resulting in low-contrast films. Lowering the kVp produces images with increased or high contrast. Choices A, B, and D do not accurately reflect the statements.

68. Which of the following terms refers to the majority of scatter radiation produced in dental imaging?

ANS: B
Compton scatter (B) accounts for the majority of the scatter that occurs in dental radiography. Ionization in Compton scatter takes place when an x-ray photon collides with a loosely bound, outer-shell electron, which gives up part of its energy. The x-ray photon continues, or "scatters," in a different direction at lower energy. Coherent scatter (A) occurs when x-rays interact with an outer shell electron. No atomic change

occurs and an x-ray photon of scattered radiation is produced, going in a different direction. Coherent scatter occurs about 8% of the time when matter interacts with dental x-rays. Primary scatter (C) and secondary scatter (D) are not terms used in association with scatter radiation.

69. The penetrating quality of the x-ray beam is controlled by the

ANS: D
Wavelength (D) determines the energy and penetrating power of the radiation, making it the main factor in x-ray penetration. Although film speed (A), exposure time (B), and source-to-film distance (C) all are contributing factors to consider in the exposure of dental radiographs, they are not the main factor in x-ray penetration. Film speed (A) is the amount of radiation required to produce a standard density radiograph. Exposure time (B) is the interval during which x-rays are produced. Source-to-film distance (C) is the distance from the focal spot of the radiograph tube to the radiographic image.

70. All of the following factors increase image sharpness EXCEPT one. Which one is the EXCEPTION?

ANS: D
Even slight movement (D) of the tubehead, the image receptor, or the patient will result in an unclear image. The size of the crystals in the film emulsion influences image sharpness. Fast-speed film (A) contains larger crystals that produce less image sharpness because the large crystals do not show the outlines of the object as clearly as smaller crystals do. Limiting the size of the focal spot (B) concentrates the bombarding electrons into an x-ray photon, and the smaller the focal spot, the sharper is the image. The fuzzy, unclear area surrounding the radiographic image is defined as *penumbra,* so decreasing the penumbra (C) would increase film sharpness.

71. Which of the following BEST describes the purpose of the lead foil contained within a radiograph film packet?

ANS: A
The thin lead foil sheet is positioned behind the film to shield the film from backscattered (secondary) radiation (A) that results in fogging of the film. The paper film wrapper and outer package wrapping serve to protect the film from light (B). Film speed and other protective measures outside the physical film packet determine how much radiation the patient receives (C, D).

72. Which statement BEST describes the relationship of the image receptor and the tooth in the paralleling technique?

ANS: D
Both Choices A and C are correct (D). In the paralleling technique, the central x-ray beam is directed perpendicular (at a right angle) to the receptor and long access of the tooth (C) and the receptor is placed in the mouth parallel to the long axis of the tooth (A). In bisecting angle technique, the clinician must bisect the angle formed by the image receptor and the long axis of the tooth (B).

73. According to the SLOB rule, the position of objects can be determined if the tubehead is shifted in a mesial direction. The lingual object moves distally, and the buccal object moves mesially.

ANS: B
Both statements are false (B). SLOB (Same=Lingual; Opposite=Buccal) is a mnemonic used to help remember the buccal object rule to determine the position of an object portrayed in two radiographs exposed at different angulations. When the two objects are compared, the object that lies to the *lingual* appears to have moved in the *same* direction as the PID, and the object that lies to the *buccal* appears to have moved in the opposite direction as the PID. Choices A, C, and D do not accurately reflect the statements.

74. For each description of a radiograph's appearance listed, select the most closely linked error. Each answer will only be used once.

ANS: 1E; 2A; 3C; 4D; 5B
A clear radiograph (1) occurs when the film was not exposed to x-rays (E). A light radiograph (2) occurs if the film was developed in weak developer or given inadequate developer time (A). If the radiograph is light and has a herringbone or "tire track" pattern (3), the film was placed in the mouth backward and then exposed (C). A fogged radiograph (4) occurs with improper safe lighting (D). A black radiograph (5) will result if the film was exposed to white light (B).

75. Identify the structure to which the arrows are pointing in the image shown.

ANS: D
The zygoma (D) appears as a radiopaque band that extends distally from the zygomatic process of the maxilla. The maxillary sinus (A) is in the radiograph but is the radiolucent image above the teeth. The maxillary tuberosity (B) is posterior to the maxillary molars and is not seen in this radiograph. The genial tubercles (C) are found on a mandibular central incisor periapical radiograph, not on a maxillary molar periapical radiograph.

76. Identify the almond-shaped radiolucent area in the image shown.

   ANS: E
   The incisive foramen (E) is an almond-shaped radiolucency located between maxillary central incisors. The infraorbital foramen (A) is seen as as a small, oval radiolucency representing an opening in the maxillary bone located below the infraorbital margin of the orbit that allows the passage of the infraorbital artery, vein, and nerve. The nasal cavity (B) appears as a large radiolucent area above the maxilla. The median palatal suture (C) is a radiolucency marking the union of the horizontal plates of the palatine bones. The maxillary sinus (D) appears as radiolucent paired cavities of bone located within the maxilla and located superior to maxillary posterior teeth.

77. Identify the radiolucent area indicated in the radiograph shown.

   ANS: B
   The arrows point to the anterior portion of the maxillary sinus (B). The maxillary sinus is located in the premolar and molar region. An abscess (A) appears as a circular radiolucency, not as the radiopaque border shown in the radiograph. The nasal fossa (C) is the nasal cavity and is found on radiographs containing the maxillary central incisors. The nasal septum (D) separates the nasal fossa and is found on radiographs containing the maxillary central incisors.

## CHAPTER 9

Planning and Managing Dental Hygiene Care

Joanna Campbell, Jamie Collins,
Demetra Daskalos Logothetis, Laura J. Webb

QUESTIONS

1. A program for tobacco use cessation is an essential component of the dental hygiene care plan for appropriate patients. The first step for tobacco dependence intervention is to:
   A. advise users about using tobacco products.
   B. ask patients about their current tobacco use habits.
   C. suggest the use of a nicotine replacement gum or lozenges.
   D. educate patients about the risks of tobacco use to themselves and others.

2. The normal respiration rate range, in breaths per minute, for an adult is
   A. 8–10.
   B. 12–20.
   C. 22–27.
   D. 28–32.

3. A blood pressure reading of 146/90 mm Hg would be classified as
   A. normal.
   B. prehypertension.
   C. hypertension, stage 1.
   D. hypertension, stage 2.

4. The first course of action in the dental hygiene process of care is to
   A. recognize any deviations or abnormalities.
   B. identify the presence of plaque deposits.
   C. obtain medical and dental histories.
   D. classify the extent of periodontal disease.

5. Which of the following is another name for hypoglycemia?
   A. Low blood sugar
   B. High blood sugar
   C. High cholesterol
   D. Low blood pressure
   E. Underactive thyroid

6. During an epileptic seizure, the patient should be placed in which position in the dental chair?
   A. Upright
   B. Supine
   C. Trendelenburg
   D. Semi-upright

7. Body core temperature exceeding 37.5 °C (99.1 °F) but less than 41.0 °C (105.8 °F) is termed
   A. pyrexia.
   B. anorexia.
   C. hypothermia.
   D. hyperthermia.

8. All of these factors are associated with increased respiration, pulse, and blood pressure EXCEPT one. Which one is the EXCEPTION?
   A. Strong emotions
   B. Physical exertion
   C. Nitrous oxide inhalation
   D. Consumption of caffeine
   E. Decongestant medications

9. Caries management by risk assessment (CAMBRA) is an evidence-based approach to the prevention and management of caries, which assesses levels of risk and serves as a guideline for interventions. Current research indicates that the most important factor in dental caries prevention and treatment is to modify and correct the dental biofilm and transform oral factors to favor dental health.
   A. Both statements are true.
   B. Both statements are false.
   C. The first statement is true, and the second statement is false.
   D. The first statement is false, and the second statement is true.

10. The highest pH level at which demineralization occurs in enamel is between
    A. 2.5 and 3.5.
    B. 3.5 and 4.5.
    C. 4.5 and 5.5.
    D. 6.0 and 6.7.
    E. 7.0 and 7.2.

11. A caries management by risk assessment (CAMBRA) protocol for enamel remineralization involves chewing of xylitol gum or mints because xylitol reduces the levels of *Streptococcus mutans* and promotes remineralization.
    A. Both the statement and reason are correct and related.
    B. Both the statement and reason are correct and NOT related.
    C. The statement is correct, but the reason is NOT.
    D. The statement is NOT correct, but the reason is correct.
    E. NEITHER the statement NOR the reason is correct.

12. Dental caries is a(n)
    A. hereditary disease.
    B. autoimmune disease.
    C. communicable disease.
    D. nontransmissible disease.

13. If a patient is taking phenytoin (Dilantin), it is usually an indication that he or she is being treated for
    A. diabetes.
    B. epilepsy.
    C. tuberculosis.
    D. hypertension.

14. For a patient who is classified as being at moderate to extreme risk for caries, all of the following are recommended risk-reduction and treatment strategies EXCEPT one. Which one is the EXCEPTION?
    A. Topical and systemic fluoride use
    B. Chewing an antacid before bedtime
    C. Using a 0.12% chlorhexidine gluconate rinse
    D. Substituting xylitol mints for sugared mints
    E. Brushing with a calcium phosphate paste daily

15. Hyposalivation may develop into all of these oral conditions EXCEPT one. Which one is the EXCEPTION?
    A. Dysgeusia
    B. Dysphagia
    C. Xerostomia
    D. Rampant caries
    E. Periodontal disease

16. Hand washing is recommended after removal of gloves because
    A. regloving is easier with damp hands.
    B. hand washing prevents allergic reactions with gloves.
    C. microorganisms can penetrate the glove after a certain amount of time.
    D. organisms on the hand multiply rapidly inside the warm, moist environment of the glove.

17. Which percentage of ethanol or isopropanol should an alcohol-based hand rub contain to be effective in removing transient microorganisms and reducing resident flora?
    A. 10%–20%
    B. 20%–30%
    C. 40%–50%
    D. 50%–60%
    E. 60%–70%

18. Which type of modifications should be made when scheduling dental appointments for a patient with significant manifestation of autism spectrum disorder?
    A. Longer appointments in the morning
    B. Every 2 weeks until the patient is familiar with the staff
    C. Several short, frequent appointments with the same staff members
    D. Frequent appointments with different members of the dental team

19. Biologic monitoring tests evaluate the effectiveness of the sterilization cycle. These monitoring tests should be performed monthly to verify effective functioning of the sterilization equipment.
    A. Both statements are true.
    B. Both statements are false.
    C. The first statement is true, and the second statement is false.
    D. The first statement is false, and the second statement is true.

20. Which is the MOST effective test for a steam under pressure sterilization unit?
    A. Biologic monitor
    B. External heat indicator
    C. External chemical indicator
    D. Internal chemical indicator

21. A patient who indicates a food allergy to avocados, chestnuts, and papayas may be at risk for which type of sensitivity?
    A. Latex
    B. Aspirin
    C. Penicillin
    D. Epinephrine

22. Which is the MOST commonly administered agent for a patient in a hypoglycemia emergency?
    A. Sugar
    B. Aspirin
    C. Oxygen
    D. Epinephrine

23. Which pulse is palpated to check for circulation during administration of adult cardiopulmonary resuscitation (CPR)?
    A. Radial
    B. Carotid
    C. Brachial
    D. Temporal

24. The vestibular mucosa exhibits superficial anesthesia from a topical anesthetic agent more rapidly than the hard palate because nonkeratinized tissues absorb the drug more rapidly.
    A. Both the statement and reason are correct and related.
    B. Both the statement and reason are correct and NOT related.
    C. The statement is correct, but the reason is NOT.
    D. The statement is NOT correct, but the reason is correct.
    E. NEITHER the statement NOR the reason is correct.

25. Which topical anesthetic would be MOST effective and offer the longest duration during scaling and root planing procedures?
    A. 20% benzocaine gel
    B. 2.5% lidocaine spray
    C. 2.5% lidocaine ointment
    D. 2.5% lidocaine and prilocaine gel

26. An apparently healthy 35-year-old female presents for her first restorative appointment in 7 years. After placing topical anesthetic, prior to the injection, the patient complains of a racing heart rate and is breathing rapidly and perspiring. Which is the likely cause?
    A. Nausea
    B. Anxiety
    C. Allergic reaction
    D. Myocardial infarction (MI)

27. A patient does not want to undergo dental radiography because of a hypersensitive gag reflex and expresses anxiety related to dental procedures. Which of the following is the optimal way to suppress the gag reflex to obtain a periapical dental image?
    A. Local anesthetic
    B. Enteral conscious sedation
    C. Parenteral conscious sedation
    D. Nitrous oxide or oxygen sedation

28. The most comprehensive infection control procedures used to ensure the safe delivery of oral care are commonly referred to as
    A. standard precautions.
    B. universal precautions.
    C. hazardous materials standard.
    D. bloodborne pathogens standard.

51. Which of the following is the primary concern when a patient experiencing blurred vision, light headedness, slurred speech, anxiety, bradycardia, tachypnea, and tinnitus after administration of four carpules of local anesthesia?
    A. Shock
    B. Hemorrhage
    C. Adrenal crisis
    D. Local anesthesia toxicity
    E. Anaphylaxis

52. Which of the following options is MOST appropriate for a patient experiencing severe dentinal hypersensitivity during instrumentation at the prophylaxis appointment?
    A. Fluoride varnish
    B. Local anesthesia
    C. Home fluoride trays
    D. Desensitizing toothpaste

53. Each of the following agents may be effective in relieving dentinal hypersensitivity EXCEPT one. Which one is the EXCEPTION?
    A. Stannous fluoride
    B. Potassium oxalate
    C. Potassium nitrate
    D. Sodium bicarbonate
    E. Amorphous calcium phosphate (ACP)

54. In individuals with Down syndrome, conditions that may require special care include all of the following oral manifestations EXCEPT one. Which one is the EXCEPTION?
    A. Dens in dente
    B. Malocclusion
    C. Fissured tongue
    D. Periodontal disease
    E. Congenitally missing teeth

55. The need for antibiotic premedication should be considered for an individual with a history of intravenous (IV) drug use. Damage to the tricuspid valve of the heart between the right atrium and ventricle may be associated with substance abuse.
    A. Both statements are true.
    B. Both statements are false.
    C. The first statement is true, and the second statement is false.
    D. The first statement is false, and the second statement is true.

56. Which of the following is the BEST choice for a prescribed postoperative pain medication for a recovering chemically dependent patient who is experiencing moderate pain?
    A. Ibuprofen (Motrin)
    B. Meperidine (Demerol)
    C. Hydrocodone (Vicodin)
    D. Oxycodone combined with aspirin (Percodan)
    E. Oxycodone combined with acetaminophen (Percocet)

57. Candidiasis is the most common oral characteristic of
    A. bulimia nervosa.
    B. anorexia nervosa.
    C. Human immunodeficiency virus (HIV) infection.

58. Parotid enlargement, xerostomia, commissure lesions, and perimolysis are common oral characteristics of which condition?
    A. Epilepsy
    B. Cleft palate
    C. Eating disorders
    D. Intravenous (IV) drug abuse
    E. Acquired immunodeficiency syndrome (AIDS)

59. Planning a home care routine for a patient with an eating disorder may include all of the following suggestions EXCEPT one. Which one is the EXCEPTION?
    A. Chlorhexidine rinse
    B. Home fluoride therapy
    C. Rehydrating the mouth with saliva substitute
    D. Rinsing with water before toothbrushing after purging

60. Pregnant women with poor oral health are at increased risk of
    A. caries.
    B. pyogenic granuloma.
    C. low-birthweight babies.
    D. B and C only.
    E. A, B and C.

61. Recommendations for a patient with burning mouth syndrome include all of the following suggestions EXCEPT one. Which one is the EXCEPTION?
    A. Acetaminophen daily
    B. Dietary modifications
    C. Xylitol-containing gum and mints
    D. Avoid toothpaste containing sodium lauryl sulfate

62. Individuals who have undergone radiation to the head and neck are at increased risk for all of the following conditions EXCEPT one. Which one is the EXCEPTION?
    A. Candidiasis
    B. Muscle fibrosis
    C. Kaposi sarcoma
    D. Osteoradionecrosis
    E. Salivary gland dysfunction

63. Health care workers diagnosed with any of the following conditions, EXCEPT one, should refrain from direct patient contact. Which one is the EXCEPTION?
    A. Mumps
    B. Diphtheria
    C. Hepatitis A
    D. Oral candidiasis
    E. Upper respiratory illness

64. During disinfection of the treatment room the light handles should be disinfected. Semicritical items penetrate tissue and should be autoclavable.
    A. Both statements are true.
    B. Both statements are false.
    C. The first statement is true, and the second statement is false.
    D. The first statement is false, and the second statement is true.

65. The most common method of sterilization in a dental office is the autoclave. An autoclave uses steam sterilization under pressure to destroy all potentially infectious disease and spores.
    A. Both statements are true.
    B. Both statements are false.
    C. The first statement is true, and the second statement is false.
    D. The first statement is false, and the second statement is true.

66. Limiting the risk of bloodborne pathogen exposure includes all of the following actions EXCEPT one. Which one is the EXCEPTION?
    A. Recapping needles by hand
    B. Using a disposable needle system
    C. Creating a neutral zone for sharps
    D. Avoid wiping instrument with gauze in hand
    E. Disposing of sharps in appropriate container

67. A severely anxious patient may show all of the following signs and symptoms EXCEPT one. Which one is the EXCEPTION?
    A. Trembling
    B. Dilated pupils
    C. Excessive sweating
    D. Decreased heart rate
    E. Increased blood pressure

68. All of the following actions may be demonstrated by a moderately anxious patient EXCEPT one. Which one is the EXCEPTION?
    A. Unnatural stiff posture
    B. Nervously plays with object in hand
    C. History of emergency dental care only
    D. Unnatural long pause before answering questions

69. Early defibrillation is important to restore a normal heart rhythm in an individual experiencing cardiac arrest. Each minute that it is delayed, the patient's chance of survival diminishes by 10%.
    A. Both statements are true.
    B. Both statements are false.
    C. The first statement is true, and the second statement is false.
    D. The first statement is false, and the second statement is true.

70. During a medical emergency, the individual may need 100% positive-pressure oxygen at a high flow rate. One condition requiring this level of oxygen administration is chronic obstructive pulmonary disease (COPD).
    A. Both statements are true.
    B. Both statements are false.
    C. The first statement is true, and the second statement is false.
    D. The first statement is false, and the second statement is true.

71. A patient suddenly sits upright and then stands and is perspiring, wheezing, and coughing. The respiratory rate is greater than 30 respirations per minute. The patient complains of inability to breathe and exhibits nasal flaring. The likely cause of these signs and symptoms is
    A. an acute asthma attack.
    B. tuberculosis.
    C. cardiac arrest.
    D. emphysema.
    E. angina pectoris.

72. Use of a rubber dam is contraindicated in an individual with COPD because the rubber dam may transmit pathogens to the lungs.
    A. Both the statement and reason are correct and related.
    B. Both the statement and reason are correct but NOT related.
    C. The statement is correct but the reason is NOT.
    D. The statement is NOT correct, but the reason is correct.
    E. NEITHER the statement NOR the reason is correct.

73. Use of the ultrasonic scaler in an individual with asthma is controversial because the pathogens found in bacterial plaque and periodontal pockets may be aspirated into the lungs.
    A. Both the statement and reason are correct and related.
    B. Both the statement and reason are correct but NOT related.
    C. The statement is correct, but the reason is NOT.
    D. The statement is NOT correct, but the reason is correct.
    E. NEITHER the statement NOR the reason is correct.

101. The Environmental Protection Agency (EPA) states that the maximum number of colony-forming units per milliliter (CFU/mL) of microbes in a dental water line used during patient treatment should be less than
    A. 500.
    B. 1000.
    C. 5000.
    D. 7000.

102. Which time frame BEST describes the frequency of how often dental water and air lines with high-speed handpiece attachments is flushed to meet the CDC recommendation?
    A. Once a month
    B. After every patient
    C. At the end of the day
    D. At the end of the week

103. When an impression is sensitive to immersion into a disinfectant, which is the proper disinfection procedure for that impression after rinsing and shaking off the excess water?
    A. Sterilizing in dry heat
    B. Sterilizing in a steam sterilizer
    C. Air drying and wrapping in a paper towel
    D. Spraying with a disinfectant and wrapping in a paper towel

104. Which of the following statements regarding the handling of sharps is correct?
    A. The clinician should recap a needle using the scoop method.
    B. The clinician may throw an unused needle into the regular trash.
    C. The clinician's assistant may hold the needle cap after an injection for ease of capping the needle.
    D. The clinician may recap the needle using both hands if the needle has not been contaminated.

105. All of the following are modes of transmission of HIV EXCEPT one. Which one is the EXECPTION?
    A. Inhalation
    B. Percutaneous contact
    C. Sexual contact
    D. Blood transfusion
    E. Mother-to-fetus transmission

106. Which of the following concentrations of anesthetic drug in milligrams per cartridge (mg/mL) is contained in 0.5% bupivacaine (Marcaine) 1:200,000 epinephrine?
    A. 9
    B. 36
    C. 54
    D. 72

107. A dental hygienist administered additional anesthesia for a procedure that lasted longer than expected, and the patient is beginning to experience discomfort in the area of treatment. The dental hygienist administers additional anesthesia, but the patient is still experiencing pain. Which of the following is the MOST likely explanation for the anesthesia failure?
    A. Polarization
    B. Drug toxicity
    C. Depolarization
    D. Tachyphylaxis
    E. Absolute refractory period

108. During the posterosuperior alveolar (PSA) anesthesia block, incorrect penetration of the needle into which location could result in a hematoma?
    A. Mandibular artery
    B. Infraorbital artery
    C. Parotid salivary gland
    D. Pterygoid plexus of veins

109. Which of the following local anesthetics would provide the MOST effective hemostasis?
    A. Lidocaine 2%, 1:50,000 epinephrine
    B. Lidocaine 2%, 1:100,000 epinephrine
    C. Articaine 4%, 1:200,000 epinephrine
    D. Mepivacaine 2%, 1:20,000 levonordefrin

110. Methemoglobinemia is caused by which topical anesthetic?
    A. Procaine
    B. Prilocaine
    C. Articaine
    D. Mepivacaine

111. Which of the following is an initial symptom of a toxic overdose from a vasoconstrictor drug in local anesthetic preparation?
    A. Euphoria
    B. Hypotension
    C. Hypertension
    D. Swelling of hands and feet

112. The dental hygienist injects one full 1.8 mL cartridge of articaine 4%. Which is the accurate amount in milligrams per milliliter (mg/mL) of local anesthetic administered?
    A. 9
    B. 36
    C. 54
    D. 72

113. Epinephrine is added to local anesthetic cartridges to produce all of the following effects EXCEPT one. Which one is the EXCEPTION?
    A. Decrease the risk of toxicity
    B. Provide hemostasis on the area of treatment

C. Prolong the duration of action of the local anesthetic

D. Increase the vasodilatory effects of the local anesthetic

114. Paraesthesia may be caused during an anesthetic injection if the clinician
A. injects into a muscle.
B. injects the anesthetic without aspirating.
C. injects several cartridges in the same location.
D. injects a cartridge contaminated by alcohol or other disinfectant.

115. Which of the following topical anesthetics is considered an eutectic mixture?
A. Oraqix
B. Benzocaine
C. Dyclonine hydrochloride
D. Transdermal lidocaine patches

116. The concentration of topical anesthetics is greater than those of their injectable counterparts. Topical anesthetics do not contain vasoconstrictors.
A. Both statements are true.
B. Both statements are false.
C. The first statement is true, and the second statement is false.
D. The first statement is false, and the second statement is true.

117. Before administration of nitrous oxide sedation, it is important for the clinician to consider the
A. patient's weight.
B. patient's liver function.
C. patient's pregnancy status.
D. patient's stomach contents.

118. Which of the following topical anesthetics is classified as an amide?
A. Lidocaine
B. Benzocaine
C. Tetracaine
D. Dyclonine

119. At the termination of administration of nitrous oxide–oxygen (N_2O/O_2) sedation, the clinician should terminate the N_2O–O_2 flow; and administer what percentage of oxygen for 5 minutes postoperatively?
A. 70%
B. 80%
C. 90%
D. 100%

120. Spasms of the muscles, soreness, and difficulty opening the mouth after a local anesthetic injection is referred to as
A. trismus.
B. hematoma.

C. paraesthesia.
D. nerve paralysis.

121. In which of the following toothbrushing methods are the bristles directed away from the gingiva toward the occlusal or incisal edge?
A. Bass
B. Charters
C. Stillman
D. Roll stroke

122. A score on a plaque index (PI) of a 1.0 to 1.9 means that the patient has which type of oral hygiene?
A. Poor
B. Fair
C. Good
D. Excellent

123. What is the patient's score on the O'Leary's Plaque Control Record if he or she has plaque at the gingival margin of 40 surfaces and a total of 28 teeth?
A. 28%
B. 40%
C. 60%
D. 100%

124. Which ingredient prevents drying and separation of a dentifrice?
A. Fluorides
B. Detergents
C. Humectants
D. Preservatives
E. Sweetening agents

125. Which of the following is the MOST effective tool for cleaning the embrasure space in a patient with missing interdental papillae?
A. Floss
B. Toothpicks
C. Proxy brush
D. Oral irrigator
E. Rubber tip stimulator

126. Which type of toothbrush should the dental hygienist recommend to a patient with generalized toothbrush abrasion caused by aggressive brushing technique with a hard toothbrush?
A. Power toothbrush
B. Extra-soft toothbrush
C. Medium-bristle toothbrush
D. A only
E. A or B

154. A 63-year-old male patient presents with cirrhosis of the liver. Which of the following should be a consideration before periodontal surgical treatment begins?
    A. Need for premedication
    B. Use of benzocaine topical
    C. Administration of an amide local anesthetic
    D. Administration of alcohol-free chlorhexidine gluconate (CHG)

155. A patient indicates a history of myocardial infarction (MI) 2 years ago. What is the implication of this with regard to periodontal therapy?
    A. Antibiotic premedication is required.
    B. The patient may not be placed in the supine position.
    C. Excessive bleeding can be expected during periodontal therapy.
    D. Cognitive function is impaired from oxygen deprivation to the brain.

156. The MOST dangerous side effect of opioid drug use is
    A. seizures.
    B. tinnitus.
    C. stomach ulcers.
    D. respiratory depression.

157. When treating a patient with hemophilia, the clinician should
    A. determine the clotting status of the patient.
    B. prescribe prophylactic antibiotic premedication.
    C. watch for pallor of the mucosa and provide a referral when seen.
    D. discontinue all medications 2 days before treatment.

158. All of the following are important considerations directly related to a dental hygiene treatment for the patient with asthma EXCEPT one. Which one is the EXCEPTION?
    A. Triggers for asthma attacks
    B. Use of antidepressant medication
    C. Use of aerosol-producing instrument
    D. Use of a local anesthetic with a vasoconstrictor

159. A 10-year-old patient with seizure disorder may present with which of the following oral health issues?
    A. Rampant caries
    B. Anterior open bite
    C. Periodontal disease
    D. Delayed tooth eruption

160. A patient undergoing a solid organ transplantation may have oral and facial complications associated with immunosuppressive drugs. A medical consultation is the best way to ensure appropriate modifications are taken.
    A. Both statements are true.
    B. Both statements are false.
    C. The first statement is true, and the second statement is false.
    D. The first statement is false, and the second statement is true.

161. Untreated inflammation around an implant could cause the following conditions to progress EXCEPT one. Which one is the EXCEPTION?
    A. Implant failure
    B. Peri-implantitis
    C. Implant mucositis
    D. Implant osseointegration

162. Which of the following microorganisms is the primary colonizer in generalized aggressive periodontitis?
    A. *Treponema denticola*
    B. *Prevotella intermedia*
    C. *Porphyromonas gingivalis*
    D. *Aggregatibacter actinomycetemcomitans*

163. Which of the following is the major role of prostaglandins in the inflammatory process?
    A. Bacterial lysis
    B. Cessation of the inflammation
    C. Initiation of alveolar bone destruction
    D. Degradation of epithelial cells and the periodontal ligament

164. The extension of the periodontal lesion from the gingiva into the supporting alveolar bone is characteristic of which lesion?
    A. Initial lesion
    B. Early lesion
    C. Established lesion
    D. Advanced lesion

165. What is the role of subgingival calculus in the development of periodontal disease?
    A. Prime etiologic factor
    B. Environmental factor
    C. Local contributing factor
    D. Systemic contributing factor

166. All of the following adjunctive antimicrobials contain an antibiotic EXCEPT one. Which one is the EXCEPTION?
    A. Arrestin
    B. Periostat
    C. PerioChip
    D. Atridox gel

167. The antimicrobial agents commonly utilized in controlled release local site application are
A. amoxicillin, erythromycin, and ampicillin.
B. ampicillin, cephalosporin, and tetracycline.
C. penicillin, metronidazole, and chlorhexidine.
D. minocycline, doxycycline, and chlorhexidine.

168. A major advantage of locally delivered antimicrobial agents over systemically delivered agents is the lowered dose of drug in blood plasma. This means that the active agent is also present in a much lower dose at the site of infection.
A. Both statements are true.
B. Both statements are false.
C. The first statement is true, and the second statement is false.
D. The first statement is false, and the second statement is true.

169. All of the following conditions have oral manifestations EXCEPT one. Which one is the EXCEPTION?
A. Cherubism
B. Laband syndrome
C. Cyclic neutropenia
D. Congestive heart failure
E. Papillon-Lefèvre syndrome

170. A patient is experiencing an acute periodontal abscess. In this instance, the patient would be expected to present with all of the following signs and symptoms EXCEPT one. Which one is the EXCEPTION?
A. Severe pain
B. Tooth mobility
C. Absence of pain
D. Tooth discoloration
E. Swelling of the gingiva

171. Immunofluorescence technique could be used to assist in the diagnosis of all of the following EXCEPT one. Which one is the EXCEPTION?
A. Pemphigoid
B. Lichen planus
C. Squamous cell carcinoma
D. Systemic lupus erythematosus (SLE)

172. All of the following are indications of an endodontic abscess EXCEPT one. Which one is the EXCEPTION?
A. Positive vitality test
B. Swelling and suppuration.
C. Tooth sensitivity to pressure
D. Asymptomatic to slight report of pain

173. Malpositioned teeth, overhanging margins of restorations, and abnormal tooth morphology may cause increased accumulation of oral biofilm in those areas. This may contribute to the development of gingivitis.
A. Both statements are true.
B. Both statements are false.
C. The first statement is true, and the second statement is false.
D. The first statement is false, and the second statement is true.

174. Bleeding on probing is an indication of active inflammation. It can be used to develop a periodontal diagnosis
A. Both statements are true.
B. Both statements are false.
C. The first statement is true, and the second statement is false.
D. The first statement is false, and the second statement is true.

175. Following reevaluation of periodontal therapy, which of the following would be the MOST appropriate time frame for the periodontal maintenance appointment?
A. 2 weeks
B. 4 weeks
C. 3 months
D. 6 months

176. A dental hygiene treatment plan indicates two quadrants of nonsurgical periodontal therapy (NSPT) with the use of local anesthesia. Which of the following is the MOST appropriate plan of treatment for the first appointment?
A. Maxillary right and left quadrants
B. Mandibular right and left quadrants
C. Maxillary and mandibular right quadrants
D. Maxillary right and mandibular left quadrants

177. Which of the following should be avoided when the dental hygienist is preparing a dental hygiene diagnosis statement?
A. Unmet need
B. Etiology of disease
C. Signs and symptoms
D. Attitudes or judgments

178. The dental hygiene care plan is a blueprint that should be developed between which individuals?
A. Dentist and patient
B. Dental hygienist and patient
C. Dental hygienist and dentist
D. Dental hygienist independently

179. The dental hygiene patient is informed that nonsurgical periodontal therapy (NSPT) is required. The patient is knowledgeable regarding the need for treatment but declines the care. Which legal term describes the patient's decision?
    A. Implied refusal
    B. Informed refusal
    C. Implied consent
    D. Informed consent

180. All of the following management strategies will benefit the anxious patient EXCEPT one. Which one is the EXCEPTION?
    A. Utilizing the tell-show-do method
    B. Scheduling the appointment at the end of the day
    C. Communicating with the patient throughout the appointment
    D. Considering premedication with diazepam (Valium) before the appointment

181. The presence of visible exudate around the gingival margins is an indication of
    A. active disease.
    B. periodontal disease.
    C. low patient motivation.
    D. completion of the disease cycle.

182. An isotonic sodium chloride solution is an aqueous mixture that has the same salinity as natural human cellular fluids. An isotonic solution is made of one half teaspoon of salt (sodium chloride) to one half cup of water.
    A. Both statements are true.
    B. Both statements are false.
    C. The first statement is true, and the second statement is false.
    D. The first statement is false, and the second statement is true.

183. Oral irrigation is an adjunctive method to periodontal therapy for the removal of oral biofilm. Oral irrigation effectively targets attached oral biofilm, unattached oral biofilm, and loosely adherent oral biofilm.
    A. Both statements are true.
    B. Both statements are false.
    C. The first statement is true, and the second statement is false.
    D. The first statement is false, and the second statement is true.

184. Which is the FIRST clinical feature of plaque-induced gingivitis?
    A. Edema
    B. Redness
    C. Exudate
    D. Loss of function
    E. Bleeding on probing

185. The "nonspecific plaque hypothesis" theory is valid for both gingivitis and periodontitis. This is because everyone who develops gingivitis will develop periodontitis.
    A. Both statements are true.
    B. Both statements are false.
    C. The first statement is true, and the second statement is false.
    D. The first statement is false, and the second statement is true.

186. Lipopolysaccharide is
    A. a component of normal saliva.
    B. the causative agent of root caries.
    C. easily degraded by salivary enzymes.
    D. a component of the cell wall of gram-negative rods.
    E. a component of the cell wall of gram-positive cocci.

187. A-delta sensory nerve fibers are myelinated and responsible for well-localized, short-duration sensations. C-fibers are unmyelinated fibers characterized by poorly localized, aching pain.
    A. Both statements are true.
    B. Both statements are false.
    C. The first statement is true, and the second statement is false.
    D. The first statement is false, and the second statement is true.

188. Which of the following dosages of epinephrine is preloaded in an adult EpiPen?
    A. 30 mg
    B. 0.3 mg
    C. 0.15 mg
    D. 15 mg

189. "Dental fear" is an unpleasant mental, emotional, or physiologic sensation caused by a specific tooth-related stimulus. "Dental fear" is a strong motivator for utilization of oral health care.
    A. Both statements are true.
    B. Both statements are false.
    C. The first statement is true, and the second statement is false.
    D. The first statement is false, and the second statement is true.

190. Instruments that are classified as critical must be sterilized between each use. Instruments that are classified as semicritical may be disinfected with an EPA-registered low-level to intermediate-level disinfectant.
    A. Both statements are true.
    B. Both statements are false.

C. The first statement is true, and the second statement is false.

D. The first statement is false, and the second statement is true.

191. Nitrous oxide–oxygen (N_2O/O_2) sedation is not recommended for a patient who has
A. asthma.
B. hypertension.
C. dental fear.
D. a seizure disorder.
E. a history of substance abuse.

192. Pregnant women and women taking oral contraceptives are at risk for increased gingival inflammation. The etiologic factor in the gingival inflammation is the elevated hormonal levels.
A. Both statements are true.
B. Both statements are false.
C. The first statement is true, and the second statement is false.
D. The first statement is false, and the second statement is true.

193. Which of the following is the primary bacterium implicated in pregnancy gingivitis and other hormonal periodontal diseases?
A. *Treponema denticola*
B. *Porphyromonas gingivalis*
C. *Tannerella forsythia*
D. *Prevotella intermedia*
E. *Aggregatibacter actinomycetemcomitans*

194. Rampant caries and advanced periodontal disease are common intraoral findings in patients who abuse
A. Lysergic acid diethylamide (LSD).
B. cocaine.
C. cannabis.
D. methamphetamine.

195. Type 1 diabetes mellitus (DM) is the most common form of DM. The primary risk factor for type I diabetes mellitus is obesity.
A. Both statements are true.
B. Both statements are false.
C. The first statement is true, and the second statement is false.
D. The first statement is false, and the second statement is true.

196. Transosteal implants are the most frequently used implants. They are used most often in patients who have a narrow mandible.
A. Both statements are true.
B. Both statements are false.
C. The first statement is true, and the second statement is false.
D. The first statement is false, and the second statement is true.

197. All of the following are current over-the-counter nicotine replacement products EXCEPT one. Which one is the EXCEPTION?
A. Gum
B. Spray
C. Lozenge
D. Transdermal patch

198. Bisphosphonates are a class of drugs used to reduce the risk of fracture in patients with osteoporosis. Oral bisphosphonates are most strongly linked with the development of bisphosphonate osteonecrosis of the jaw.
A. Both statements are true.
B. Both statements are false.
C. The first statement is true, and the second statement is false.
D. The first statement is false, and the second statement is true.

199. Most denture-related infections are caused by
A. ill-fitting dentures.
B. riboflavin deficiency.
C. chemical agent irritation.
D. chronic candidiasis infection.

200. "A desired end result, in terms of knowledge that the client is to achieve through specific dental hygiene actions" describes what type of patient-centered goal?
A. Affective
B. Cognitive
C. Psychomotor
D. Oral health status

201. All of the following may be included as part of the dental hygiene care plan EXCEPT one. Which one is the EXCEPTION?
A. Removal of caries
B. Administration of fluoride
C. Placement of pit and fissure sealants
D. Therapeutic periodontal debridement

15. Hyposalivation may develop into all of these oral conditions EXCEPT one. Which one is the EXCEPTION?

    ANS: E
    Periodontal disease (E) is a multifactorial disease that has its primary etiology in oral biofilm, not hyposalivation. Hyposalivation is a salivary gland dysfunction in which salivary flow is reduced, which puts the patient at risk for the development of dysgeusia (A), or taste impairment, and dysphagia (B), or difficulty swallowing. Xerostomia (C), or dryness of the mouth, and rampant caries (D) are also linked to hyposalivation.

16. Hand washing is recommended after removal of gloves because

    ANS: D
    Hand washing is recommended promptly after removal of gloves because organisms on the hand multiply rapidly inside the warm, moist environment of the glove (D), even when no external contamination has occurred. Hands should always be thoroughly dried before regloving (A), since moisture inside the gloves can promote the regrowth of bacteria on the skin and cause skin irritation. Allergic reaction to gloves may develop in spite of washing the hands after removal (B). Time is not a factor in loss of glove integrity (C).

17. Which percentage of ethanol or isopropanol should an alcohol-based hand rub contain to be effective in removing transient microorganisms and reducing resident flora?

    ANS: E
    Alcohol-based hand rubs should contain concentrations of between 60% and 95% (E) ethanol or isopropanol to be effective in removing transient microorganisms and reducing resident flora concentrations to below 60% (A, B, C, and D) are not considered adequately effective for clinical use.

18. Which type of modifications should be made when scheduling dental appointments for a patient with significant manifestation of autism spectrum disorder?

    ANS: C
    When scheduling an appointment for a patient with autism, plan several short orientation and familiarization appointments with no more than 1 week between visits with the same staff members (C). Appointments should be kept short and be scheduled at the time of day when the child is at his or her best (A). There should be no more than 1 week between visits (B). The same members of the dental staff should be involved at each appointment to prevent distressing the patient and losing time for reorientation (D).

19. Biologic monitoring tests evaluate the effectiveness of the sterilization cycle. These monitoring tests should be performed monthly to verify effective functioning of the sterilization equipment.

    ANS: C
    The first statement is true, and the second statement is false (C). A biologic monitoring test does evaluate the effective functioning of the sterilizing equipment. The second statement is false. The monitoring tests should be performed weekly, not monthly, to verify effective functioning of the sterilization equipment. Choices A, B, and D do not accurately reflect the statements.

20. Which is the MOST effective test for a steam under pressure sterilization unit?

    ANS: A
    Sterilization is the process by which all forms of life are destroyed. Only biologic monitors (A) such as the live spore test provides reliable proof of sterilization and are used to evaluate steam under pressure, dry heat, and chemical vapor sterilization equipment. External heat indicators (B), external chemical indicators (C), and internal chemical indicators (D) only provide indicators that the parameters of sterilization such as temperature and pressure have or have not been met.

21. A patient who indicates a food allergy to avocados, chestnuts, and papayas may be at risk for which type of sensitivity?

    ANS: A
    Patients who indicate a food allergy to avocados, bananas, kiwi fruits, chestnuts, papayas, or peanuts may be at risk for a latex sensitivity (A) because the proteins found in latex that cause latex sensitivity are also present in these foods. Sensitivity to penicillin (C), epinephrine (D), and aspirin (B) are not indicated by any specific food allergy.

22. Which is the MOST commonly administered agent for a patient in a hypoglycemia emergency?

    ANS: A
    Hypoglycemia (low blood sugar) is found predominately in patients with diabetes. Sugar (A) or sugared drinks such as orange juice or nondiet soft drinks are commonly administered to the conscious patient in an emergency situation. Aspirin (B) is used

for mild-to-moderate pain control, fever control, treatment of inflammatory conditions, and unwanted clotting and may be chewed and swallowed if a myocardial infarction (MI) is suspected. Oxygen (C) is administered to patients who are experiencing syncope, cardiac problems, and cardiac difficulties. Epinephrine (D), administered in emergency situations, is used to treat cardiac arrest, anaphylaxis, or acute asthmatic attack.

23. Which pulse is palpated to check for circulation during administration of adult cardiopulmonary resuscitation (CPR)?

ANS: B
The carotid pulse (B) in the neck is used for the pulse check in both the adult and child patients because the body delivers blood to the brain for as long as possible. The radial pulse (A) should not be checked, as peripheral blood supply may decline in emergency situations. The brachial pulse (C) of the upper arm is used for the pulse check in an infant, as it is easier to find. The temporal pulse (D) may be checked it trauma prevents checking of the carotid pulse.

24. The vestibular mucosa exhibits superficial anesthesia from a topical anesthetic agent more rapidly than the hard palate because nonkeratinized tissues absorb the drug more rapidly.

ANS: A
Both the statement and reason are correct and related (A). The anesthesia produced by a topical anesthetic is related to the amount of absorption of the drug by the tissue and varies with the thickness of squamous epithelia covering and the degree of keratinization. Tissues without keratinization absorb the anesthetic more rapidly. Choices B, C, D, and E do not accurately reflect the statement.

25. Which topical anesthetic would be MOST effective and offer the longest duration during scaling and root planing procedures?

ANS: D
2.5% lidocaine and prilocaine gel (D) provide anesthesia to soft tissue and sometimes a slight loss of sensation to teeth. The duration of the anesthesia is usually 20 minutes after a 2-minute onset period and provides effective anesthesia for scaling procedures because of the subgingival delivery system. Benzocaine gel (A) anesthetizes soft tissue for only 5 to 15 minutes. Lidocaine sprays (B) typically last for 20 minutes. Lidocaine ointment (C) may be effective for 15 minutes.

26. An apparently healthy 35-year-old female presents for her first restorative appointment in 7 years. After placing topical anesthetic, prior to the injection, the patient complains of a racing heart rate and is breathing rapidly and perspiring. Which is the likely cause?

ANS: B
Rapid breathing, perspiration, and increased heart rate are signs commonly associated with fear or anxiety (B), and the length of time since last dental treatment suggests "dental fear." Symptoms are not congruent with nausea (A) or an allergic reaction (C). Myocardial infarction (D) would be an unlikely reaction in an apparently healthy 35-year-old female.

27. A patient does not want to undergo dental radiography because of a hypersensitive gag reflex and expresses anxiety related to dental procedures. Which of the following is the optimal way to suppress the gag reflex to obtain a periapical dental image?

ANS: D
Nitrous oxide or oxygen sedation (D) will suppress the gag reflex and reduce anxiety and has very few drug interactions. Nitrous oxide or oxygen sedation will also be expelled from the body after 3 to 5 minutes of oxygenation, with no long-term effect, making it the best choice. Local anesthesia (A), enteral conscious sedation (B) with an agent such as diazepam (Valium), and parenteral conscious sedation (C) with an agent such as midazolam (Versed) are not indicated for suppression of the gag reflex.

28. The most comprehensive infection control procedures used to ensure the safe delivery of oral care are commonly referred to as

ANS: A
Standard precautions (A) are designed to protect health care providers from pathogens that can be spread via blood or any body fluid, excretion, or secretion except sweat; they integrate and expand on the concept of universal precautions. Universal precautions (B) were the original concept based on the theory that all human blood and blood contaminated body fluids are to be treated as if they are infected with a bloodborne disease. They were incorporated into Standard Precautions by the Centers for Disease Control and Prevention (CDC). The Hazardous Materials Standards (C) are the CDC guidelines for handling of potentially hazardous materials in the workplace. The Occupational Safety and Health Association (OSHA) Blood-Borne Pathogens Standard (D) is the infection control policy created by the CDC and provides guidelines for health care and is designed to protect employees from occupational exposure to bloodborne, disease-causing organisms.

29. The CDC has identified four principles of infection control to protect all individuals. Which of the following principles is the EXCEPTION?

    ANS: B
    Instruments that have been autoclaved do not need to be thrown away (B) since sterilization kills all living organisms. Only instruments that are disposable after single use or are autoclavable should be used with any patient, especially after they come in contact with an infectious patient. The CDC has identified the following principles of infection control: taking action to stay healthy (A), limiting the spread of blood and other body substances that can transmit infection (C), avoiding contact with blood and other body substances that can transmit infection (D), and making client care items safe for use (E).

30. As identified by the CDC, which category falls under transmission-based precautions?

    ANS: E
    Droplet precautions (A), airborne precautions (B), and contact precautions (C) are all of the choices listed that are part of transmission-based precautions. Transmission-based precautions are used when the route of transmission is not completely interrupted using only standard precautions.

31. Parents of infants with high caries risk should use a xylitol-containing gum four to five times daily. Use of xylitol gum by the parent will reduce the transfer of caries-causing bacteria to the infant.

    ANS: A
    Both statements are true (A). Xylitol, a sweetener found in certain brands of gum, inhibits attachment and transmission of bacteria and is an effective anticaries therapeutic measure. In addition, it inhibits the transfer of bacteria from person to person by altering the way it sticks to surfaces. Choices B, C, and D do not accurately reflect the statements.

32. All of the following are symptoms of myocardial infarction EXCEPT one. Which one is the EXCEPTION?

    ANS: B
    Headache (B) is not a symptom of MI. Nausea (A), clammy skin (C), pain in the left arm or jaw (D), and burning feelings of indigestion (E) are all symptoms of myocardial infarction. A patient may also experience a cold feeling, anxiety, and shortness of breath, weakness, or perspiration.

33. If a patient is hyperventilating at the dental appointment, the provider should reassure the patient and encourage him or her to take slow, deep breaths. Hundred-percent oxygen should be quickly administered to a patient who is hyperventilating.

    ANS: C
    The first statement is true, and the second statement is false (C). The provider should have the patient breathe slowly into a paper bag or cupped hands. The second statement is false because oxygen is not necessary since a patient who is hyperventilating has an excess of oxygen in his or her system already and needs carbon dioxide. Choices A, B, D, and E do not accurately reflect the statements.

34. All of the following are symptoms of hypoglycemia EXCEPT one. Which one is the EXCEPTION?

    ANS: E
    Acetone breath (E) is a symptom associated with hyperglycemia, not hypoglycemia. Hunger (A), nausea (B), confusion (C), and perspiration (D), are all symptoms of hypoglycemia (low blood sugar). Other symptoms of hypoglycemia include headache, irritation, mood changes, dizziness or weakness, increased anxiety, and possible unconsciousness.

35. After the active phase of periodontal treatment is completed, the patient's needs are assessed and timed intervals for which procedure are planned?

    ANS: E
    Periodontal maintenance (E), also known as *recall*, *recare*, or *continuing care*, is planned after the active phase of periodontal treatment is completed. Maintenance is performed at timed intervals for the life of the dentition or implant replacements to assist the patient in maintaining oral health. Intervals of periodontal maintenance include treatment multiple times in a 12-month period. A periodic examination is usually indicated once to twice a year (A), with a medical update (B) performed at each appointment. Restorative treatment (C) and radiographic images (D) should be provided when they are needed to maintain oral health.

36. Chronic periodontitis typically responds predictably to periodontal treatment. Treatment response is unpredictable in the case of aggressive periodontitis.

    ANS: A
    Both statements are true (A). Treatment of a chronic disease will often respond predictably as the disease-causing bacteria are reduced. An aggressive disease response is unpredictable because the amount of disease-causing bacteria is less important than the host response to inflammation and the immune

response to the pathogen. Choices B, C, and D do not accurately reflect the statements.

37. A patient presents with necrotizing ulcerative periodontitis (NUP) and complains of pain. Each of the following procedures should take place on the first appointment EXCEPT one. Which one is the EXCEPTION?

ANS: A
Restorative treatment (A) should be postponed until the pain and NUP are controlled or resolved. Home plaque control instruction (B), scaling and debridement of the mouth (C), a review of the health history (D), and having the patient rinse with a 3% mixture of hydrogen peroxide and water until the infection is resolved (E) are all indicated for oral therapy at the initial appointment. In addition, the use of an antibiotic may be indicated if the patient presents with a fever or cervical lymphadenopathy.

38. To control high levels of *Streptococcus mutans* in an individual with existing decay and high caries activity, which of the following protocols is recommended to control the microorganisms?

ANS: B
Use of 0.12% chlorhexidine rinse for 1 minute per day for a 2-week period every 2 to 3 months will eliminate the microorganisms that initiate the caries process (B). A lidocaine oral rinse (A) is used to control oral pain and will not eliminate bacteria. Amoxicillin (C) is not widely used over the long term to eliminate *S. mutans* for caries management. A weekly debridement appointment (D) is not an optimal option.

39. Chlorhexidine gluconate rinse is effective in the reduction of caries-causing bacteria along with the pathogens associated with periodontal disease. Chlorhexidine gluconate is a broad-spectrum antibacterial agent.

ANS: A
Both statements are true (A). Chlorhexidine gluconate may be used to prevent caries in high-risk populations by reducing oral biofilm. It is a chemical antiseptic effective against both gram-positive and gram-negative bacteria, as well as fungi and enveloped viruses. Its primary disadvantage is staining with prolonged use. Choices B, C, and D do not accurately define the statements.

40. Recaldent is a complex of casein phosphopeptide (CPP) and amorphous calcium phosphate (ACP) that precipitates the calcium and phosphate ions needed to remineralize teeth. CPP and ACP are used in place of fluoride products.

ANS: C
The first statement is true, and the second statement is false (C). In an amorphous state, calcium and phosphate ions may enter tooth enamel. The high concentration of calcium and phosphate ions in dental plaque after exposure to CPP and ACP has been shown to reduce the risk of enamel demineralization and promote enamel remineralization. The second statement, however, is false because CPP and ACP should be used in conjunction with fluoride treatment, as CCP and ACP enhance fluoride's ability to provide an increased effect for remineralization. Choices A, B, and D do not accurately define the statements.

41. Which of the following conditions presents as a contraindication for the use of nitrous oxide/oxygen conscious sedation?

ANS: D
Nitrous oxide sedation is NOT indicated for patients with a history of substance abuse (D). Nitrous oxide may be abused and should be avoided in patients with susceptibility to substance abuse. Nitrous oxide analgesia is beneficial for patients with asthma (B) because during sedation the patient receives more oxygen than is normally available. Nitrous oxide analgesia is indicated for patients with apprehension (A) because it relaxes them and lessens their apprehension. Nitrous oxide analgesia is beneficial for patients with cardiac conditions (C) because it decreases stress and exposes the patient to more oxygen than is normally available.

42. Which of the following items can be adapted to aid in oral care for a patient who has difficulty holding objects because of severe arthritis? (Choose all that apply.)

ANS: A, D, E
Bicycle grips (A), soft rubber balls (D), and quick-cure acrylic molds (E) may be used to build up the handle of a device, making it easier for the patient to grip. The universal cuff (C) may be used when a patient cannot hold devices on his or her own. The cuff straps to the patient's hand or wrist, and the device is attached. A mouth stick (B) is most commonly used by tetraplegic patients, who cannot move their hands at all.

43. A patient with an unshielded cardiac pacemaker requires antibiotic premedication before treatment. Ultrasonic scaling systems are safe in patients with an unshielded cardiac pacemaker.

ANS: B
Both statements are false (B). Antibiotic premedication prior to dental treatment is NOT

indicated for patients with a cardiac pacemaker. The use of an ultrasonic scaling system with an individual with an unprotected cardiac pacemaker could cause interference and is therefore contraindicated. Choices A, C, and D do not accurately reflect the statements.

44. Patients with uncontrolled diabetes mellitus are at increased risk for all of the following oral conditions EXCEPT one. Which one is the EXCEPTION?

ANS: B
Uncontrolled diabetes is not a risk factor for oral cancer. Caries (A), glossodynia (C), or pain in the tongue, fungal infections (D), and periodontal disease (E) are all oral conditions related to uncontrolled diabetes mellitus.

45. Which of the following emergency situations is the primary concern when a patient with diabetes presents with confusion, pallor, hunger, fatigue, blurred vision, headache, and irritability?

ANS: B
Confusion, pallor, hunger, fatigue, blurred vision, headache, and irritability are all symptoms of hypoglycemia (B) associated with diabetes mellitus. Other symptoms such as paraesthesias, stupor, convulsions, unconsciousness, impaired concentration, somnolence, transient memory, or motor defects may be present. Symptoms of angina (A) include crushing, burning, or squeezing chest pain radiating to left shoulder, arms, neck, or mandible and lasting 2 to 15 minutes; shortness of breath; and sweating. Symptoms of hyperglycemia (C) include excessive thirst, urination, or hunger; labored respirations; nausea; dry, flushed skin; low blood pressure; weak, rapid pulse; acetone breath; blurred vision; headache; and unconsciousness. Symptoms of MI (D) include mild to severe chest pain; pain in the left arm or jaw (not relieved by rest and nitroglycerin); cold, clammy skin; nausea; anxiety; shortness of breath; weakness; perspiration; and a burning feeling of indigestion. Symptoms of a cerebrovascular accident (E) include sudden weakness on one side, difficulty speaking, temporary loss of vision, dizziness, change in mental status, nausea, severe headache, and convulsions.

46. Chemotherapeutic drugs used in the treatment of cancer may cause mucositis in the oral cavity. Mucositis can be prevented or lessened by the use of sodium bicarbonate and saline water rinses to hydrate and soothe the tissue.

ANS: A
Both statements are true (A). Mucositis, characterized by edema, inflammation, and ulcerations of the oral cavity, is related to the toxicity of the chemotherapeutic drugs. Bicarbonate and saline water rinses or alcohol-free rinse will soothe and hydrate the oral cavity as well as neutralize pH and aid in biofilm removal. Choices B, C, and D do not accurately reflect the statements.

47. For a patient undergoing cancer treatment and has demineralization and xerostomia, which strategy would be MOST effective for caries management?

ANS: C
Patients undergoing cancer treatment often experience chronic dry mouth (xerostomia), which increases the risk of demineralization and subsequent caries. Use of home fluoride trays for daily application of fluoride gel (C) is the most effective measure for caries management because frequent fluoride uptake is the best way to enhance remineralization. Xylitol-containing chewing gum (A) would be helpful to reduce cariogenic bacteria but does not address demineralization. Oral fluoride supplements (B) provide systemic fluoride delivery, which is not helpful in remineralization. Professional fluoride varnish (D) would certainly be helpful, but a single delivery is not as effective as frequent delivery in reducing caries. Prophylaxis with fluoride prophylaxis paste (E) has no significant effect on remineralization or caries reduction.

48. Oral candidiasis is the most common oral lesion associated with human immunodeficiency virus (HIV). An individual with HIV should be instructed to rinse with hydrogen peroxide daily to lessen the chance that he or she will develop candidiasis.

ANS: C
The first statement is true, and the second statement is false (C). The common strains of candidiasis in individuals with HIV include pseudomembranous, atrophic or erythematous, hyperplastic, and angular cheilitis. The second statement is false. Hydrogen peroxide rinses may actually increase the risk of oral candidiasis in an immunocompromised individual. Choices A, B, and D do not accurately reflect the statements.

49. Which of the following emergency situations is the primary concern when an individual reports a feeling of warmth, flushing of skin, and nausea and starts to perspire?

ANS: B
Skin flushing, warm feeling, nausea, rapid heart rate, perspiration, and pallor are all symptoms of syncope (B). Symptoms of shock (A) include pale and clammy skin, a change in mental status and

eventual unconsciousness if untreated, drop in blood pressure, and increases in pulse and respiratory rate. Symptoms of cardiac arrest (C) include ashen, cold clammy skin; no pulse, heart sounds, or respirations; and unconsciousness. Symptoms of angina pectoris (D) include crushing, burning, or squeezing chest pain radiating to the left shoulder, arms, neck, or mandible and lasting 2 to 15 minutes; shortness of breath; and sweating. Symptoms of hyperglycemia (E) include excessive thirst, urination, and hunger; labored respirations; nausea; dry, flushed skin; low blood pressure; weak, rapid pulse; acetone breath; blurred vision; headache; and unconsciousness.

50. Which of the following actions would be MOST appropriate for the patient with a history of seizures who is experiencing an aura?

ANS: D
The clinician's correct course of action is to terminate the procedure and clear the area of objects that may injure the patient during an epileptic seizure. The patient should not be restrained (D), although it is important that the clinician be prepared to prevent injury, maintain adequate ventilation, and reassure the patient. It may be necessary to activate the emergency medical services (EMS). Doing nothing (A) could place the patient in danger. The clinician should always remain with the patient (B) to make sure that he or she does not injure himself or herself, to maintain adequate ventilation, and to reassure the patient. The clinician should NOT attempt to restrain the patient (C) or place anything in the mouth (E), as it may cause injury to the patient or the clinician.

51. Which of the following is the primary concern when a patient experiencing blurred vision, light headedness, slurred speech, anxiety, bradycardia, tachypnea, and tinnitus after administration of four carpules of local anesthesia?

ANS: D
Blurred vision, lightheadedness, slurred speech, anxiety, bradycardia, tachypnea, and tinnitus are all symptoms of toxicity from local anesthesia (D). In this type of emergency, the dental team members should assess airway, breathing, and circulation; administer oxygen; and activate the EMS. Symptoms of shock (A) include pale and clammy skin; change in mental status and eventual unconsciousness, if untreated; drop in blood pressure; and increase in pulse and respiratory rate. Symptoms of hemorrhage (B) include spurting or oozing blood. Symptoms of an adrenal crisis (C) include confusion, weakness, lethargy, respiratory depression, hypercalcemia,

shocklike symptoms, abdominal pain, and loss of consciousness. Symptoms of anaphylaxis (E) include hives; swelling of lips, tongue, larynx, and pharynx; respiratory distress; wheezing; laryngeal edema; weak pulse; and low blood pressure; these may progress to unconsciousness and cardiovascular collapse.

52. Which of the following options is MOST appropriate for a patient experiencing severe dentinal hypersensitivity during instrumentation at the prophylaxis appointment?

ANS: A
Fluoride varnish (A) has the U.S. Food and Drug Administration (FDA) approval for treatment of severe dentinal hypersensitivity. Local anesthesia (B), although effective, would be impractical, since the entire mouth would need to be anesthetized. The individual may be instructed to use home fluoride gel trays (C) or desensitizing toothpastes (D) to decrease hypersensitivity for future appointments but this would not provide immediate relief.

53. Each of the following agents may be effective in relieving dentinal hypersensitivity EXCEPT one. Which one is the EXCEPTION?

ANS: D
Sodium bicarbonate (D) has antibacterial properties and is used with individuals who are at high risk for caries and dry mouth. It does not relieve hypersensitivity. Stannous fluoride (A), potassium oxalate (B), potassium nitrate (C), and ACP (E) all reduce dentin tubule hypersensitivity.

54. In individuals with Down syndrome, conditions that may require special care include all of the following oral manifestations EXCEPT one. Which one is the EXCEPTION?

ANS: A
Dens in dente (A) is not an increased risk for individuals with Down syndrome. Manifestations present in individuals with Down syndrome often include malocclusion (B) and fissured tongue (C). Periodontal disease (D) is prevalent among individuals with Down syndrome because of neutrophil dysfunction. Individuals with Down syndrome often present with congenitally missing teeth (E).

55. The need for antibiotic premedication should be considered for an individual with a history of intravenous (IV) drug use. Damage to the tricuspid valve of the heart between the right atrium and ventricle may be associated with substance abuse.

ANS: A

Both statements are true (A). A physician should evaluate the individual before any treatment to determine whether premedication is needed for the risk of venous thrombosis, organic valvular disease, and endocarditis (caused by *Staphylococcus aureus* on nonsterile needles). Damage to the tricuspid valve of the heart is a possible result of drug abuse. Choices B, C, and D do not accurately reflect the statements.

56. Which of the following is the BEST choice for a prescribed postoperative pain medication for a recovering chemically dependent patient who is experiencing moderate pain?

ANS: A

Ibuprofen (Motrin) (A) is in the class of nonsteroidal antiinflammatory drugs (NSAIDs). These drugs reduce inflammation and do not have addictive properties, so prescribing these drugs will not trigger a relapse into addiction. Meperidine (Demerol) (B), hydrocodone (Vicodin) (C), oxycodone combined with aspirin (Percodan) (D), and oxycodone combined with acetaminophen (Percocet) (E) are all drugs with potential for addiction and abuse.

57. Candidiasis is the most common oral characteristic of

ANS: C

Candidiasis is the most common oral lesion associated with HIV infection (C). Common oral characteristics of bulimia nervosa (A) include enamel erosion (the most common dental finding), xerostomia, dentinal hypersensitivity, caries, periodontal disease, and intraoral trauma. The most common oral characteristic of anorexia nervosa (B) is xerostomia caused by lack of nutrients. Over 50% of patients with anorexia nervosa also have bulimia nervosa, with the additional oral symptoms described above.

58. Parotid enlargement, xerostomia, commissure lesions, and perimolysis are common oral characteristics of which condition?

ANS: C

Parotid enlargement, xerostomia, commissure lesions, and perimolysis (enamel erosion) all are clinical findings associated with the eating disorders (C) anorexia and bulimia nervosa. The individual may also experience dehydration, dentinal hypersensitivity, and diminished taste acuity. Seizures (A) are the most common sign of epilepsy. A cleft palate (B) occurs when the palatal shelves fail to fuse with the primary palate. Common signs of IV drug abuse (D) include unreliability, carelessness in appearance and personal

hygiene, memory lapses, needle marks, mood swings, constricted pupils, and nonreactivity to light. Common signs and symptoms of AIDS (E) include fever, lymph node enlargement, headache, rash, sore throat, aching muscles and joints, erythematous patches on the hard and soft palates, angular cheilitis, hairy leukoplakia, and oral ulcers.

59. Planning a home care routine for a patient with an eating disorder may include all of the following suggestions EXCEPT one. Which one is the EXCEPTION?

ANS: A

Chlorhexidine rinses (A) are NOT recommended for individuals with eating disorders because their alcohol content may cause irritation and may also alter taste perception. Home fluoride therapy (B), in addition to professional fluoride applications, is recommended for individuals with eating disorders to help remineralize fragile dentition. Rehydrating the mouth (C) is recommended as decreased salivary flow may predispose the patient to increased dental caries. It is important that the individual who purges rinse with water before brushing (D) to avoid increasing acid erosion by brushing the acid into teeth.

60. Pregnant women with poor oral health are at increased risk of

ANS: D

Pyogenic granulomas (B) are tumorlike soft tissue growths that appear on the interdental papillae. They are related to poor oral care and increased levels of estrogen and progesterone, which accompany pregnancy, although they may also occur in men and nonpregnant women. They are pedunculated, painless, deep-red to purple in color, and resolve after pregnancy. Women with periodontal disease are more likely to have preterm, low-birthweight babies (C). Pregnancy has not been correlated to an increase in caries (A, E).

61. Recommendations for a patient with burning mouth syndrome include all of the following suggestions EXCEPT one. Which one is the EXCEPTION?

ANS: A

Acetaminophen (A) is not a recommended treatment for burning mouth syndrome, which is believed to be neuropathic in origin, and acetaminophen is not effective with this type of pain. Dietary modifications (B) such as avoiding spicy and acidic foods may help to alleviate symptoms of burning mouth syndrome. Changes in diet may also address any nutritional deficiencies that may be causing the symptoms. Xylitol-containing gum and mints (C) stimulate salivary secretion and may help individuals with burning mouth syndrome. It is possible the patient's symptoms may be caused by sensitivity to sodium lauryl sulfate (D), which has been linked to oral mucosal inflammation.

62. Individuals who have undergone radiation to the head and neck are at increased risk for all of the following conditions EXCEPT one. Which one is the EXCEPTION?

ANS: C
Kaposi sarcoma (C) is related to HIV infection and AIDS. All of the other choices are possible effects of radiation therapy to the head and neck. Radiation may cause an increase in opportunistic infections such as candidiasis (A) from salivary gland dysfunction (E). Radiation damage to the small capillaries of the radiated area increases the risk of muscle fibrosis (B) and osteoradionecrosis (D).

63. Health care workers diagnosed with any of the following conditions, EXCEPT one, should refrain from direct patient contact. Which one is the EXCEPTION?

ANS: D
There are no specific precautions for health care workers with oral candidiasis (D) to abstain from patient contact, as oral candidiasis is normally not contagious. The U.S. Public Health Service recommends that health care workers with mumps (A) refrain from working during the acute illness phase, those with diphtheria (B) refrain from working until the illness resolves, and those with hepatitis A (D) refrain from direct patient contact. Individuals and health care workers with upper respiratory illnesses (E) should avoid contact with medically compromised persons. Choices A, B, C, and E are all contagious diseases.

64. During disinfection of the treatment room the light handles should be disinfected. Semicritical items penetrate tissue and should be autoclavable.

ANS: C
The first statement is true, and the second statement is false (C). Light handles are noncritical items and cannot be sterilized; they are disinfected using a registered low-level to intermediate-level disinfectant. Semicritical items do not penetrate tissue; however, they should be autoclaved. Choices A, B, and D do not accurately reflect the statements.

65. The most common method of sterilization in a dental office is the autoclave. An autoclave uses steam sterilization under pressure to destroy all potentially infectious disease and spores.

ANS: A
Both statements are true (A). The autoclave, the most common method of heat sterilization in the dental office, sterilizes by the use of steam under pressure. Distilled water is heated to generate steam to produce moist heat, which rapidly kills microorganisms. Choices B, C, and D do not accurately reflect the statements.

66. Limiting the risk of bloodborne pathogen exposure includes all of the following actions EXCEPT one. Which one is the EXCEPTION?

ANS: A
The CDC's guidelines for handling needles recommend that needles never be recapped using hands (A) or any other technique that involves directing the point of a needle toward any part of the body to prevent percutaneous injuries. The clinician should use the scoop method or a mechanical device (such as a needle sheath prop or a shield) to diminish the risk of exposure. A disposable needle system (B) is engineered with safety features designed to prevent percutaneous injuries. A neutral zone (C) limits exposure potential by allowing health care workers to avoid passing directly between other health care workers who may be using sharps. Instruments should never be wiped on gauze in the hand (D) or wrapped around the finger. Sharps should be disposed of in an appropriate puncture-resistant, reclosable, leakproof, and color-coded container (E), which should be labeled with the biohazard symbol.

67. A severely anxious patient may show all of the following signs and symptoms EXCEPT one. Which one is the EXCEPTION?

ANS: D
The heart rate is usually increased, not decreased (D), in an anxious individual. Trembling (A), dilated pupils (B), excessive sweating (C), and increased blood pressure (E) are all symptoms and signs that may be exhibited by the severely anxious patient.

68. All of the following actions may be demonstrated by a moderately anxious patient EXCEPT one. Which one is the EXCEPTION?

ANS: D
An anxious patient typically provides very quick answers to a question (D). An unnaturally stiff posture (A), nervously playing with objects (B), and a history of only emergency dental care (C) are all signs that may be demonstrated by a moderately anxious patient.

toothpaste (C) are all important factors in caries prevention, but they all require patient compliance to be effective in caries prevention.

141. Which of the following statements about leukocytosis is true?

    ANS: D
    Leukocytosis is an increase in WBC count and is the body's attempt to provide more neutrophils in response to an infection (D). Leukocytosis is a systemic, not local (A), sign of inflammation. Leukocytosis is an increase, not decrease, in circulating neutrophils (B). A normal WBC count is 4000 to 10,000, and a count of 1000 (C) is too low.

142. Acute inflammation is characterized by a large number of macrophages and plasma cells. Chronic inflammation is characterized by an increased amount of polymorphonuclear leukocytes (PMNs).

    ANS: B
    Both statements are false (B). The two types of white blood cells involved initially in the inflammatory response are neutrophils and monocytes. The neutrophil or PMN is the most prevalent WBC in acute inflammation. The second statement is false. The most prevalent cell in chronic inflammation is the macrophage, characterized by granulomas, or microscopic groupings of macrophages. Choices A, C, and D do not accurately reflect the statements.

143. Which of the following terms describes the bluish-purple coloration of the mucous membrane that results from a deficient supply of oxygenation?

    ANS: B
    Cyanosis (B) is blue or purple discoloration of skin or mucosal tissues. Pallor (A) describes a paleness of skin or mucosal tissues. Hyperemia (C) is the component of the inflammatory response that sends an excess of blood to the injured area. Hyperkeratosis (D) is a thickening of the stratum corneum, with a qualitative abnormality of keratin, or a response to trauma.

144. Which of the following dental conditions could be mistaken for amelogenesis imperfecta?

    ANS: A
    Fluorosis (A) appears as change in the enamel that range from barely noticeable white spots to staining to dark brown staining and pitting. Amelogenesis imperfecta is a group of genetic autosomal defects in enamel formation, resulting in a variety of clinical manifestations. The white mottled appearance of the "snow-capped" variety of amelogenesis imperfecta resembles the white spots often seen in fluorosis. Tetracycline stain (B) in teeth is brown or grayish in color, usually being darker on the center of the tooth. Osteogenesis imperfecta (C) is an autosomal genetic disease that results in defective collage and abnormal bones that fracture easily. Dentition in this condition may have a dentinogenesis imperfecta–like condition, with small crowns, roots, and pulp chambers. At eruption, teeth appear translucent or opalescent, but darken with time. The abnormal dentin does not adequately support enamel, which is often lost. Dentinogenesis imperfecta (D) is an autosomal genetic disease that results in defective dentin formation, with small or absent pulp chambers and dentin that appears translucent or opalescent. The soft underlying dentin leads to chipping and loss of enamel.

145. Which of the following recommendations should the dental hygienist make to the patient with black hairy tongue?

    ANS: A
    The dental hygienist should recommend improved oral hygiene and the use of a tongue scraper to treat black hairy tongue (A). Black hairy tongue is caused by the buildup of oral bacteria or oral fungi on the filiform papilla. Instead of normal exfoliation, the papilla lengthens and becomes stained with pigments from food, drink, and even chromogenic bacteria. There is no evidence to support the use of an antifungal medication (B) to treat this condition. Oxygenating mouth rinses (C) such as peroxide also have been identified as an etiologic agent in hairy tongue. The use of antibacterial medications (D), especially broad-spectrum antibiotics such as penicillin, is often associated with black hairy tongue. Other factors associated with the development of black hairy tongue are smoking, medications containing bismuth such as Pepto-Bismol, heavy intake of coffee or tea, and severe xerostomia.

146. Which of the following terms describes the histopathologic change demonstrated within tissues affected by morsicatio buccarum?

    ANS: C
    Morsicatio buccarum, or chronic cheek biting, is a thickening of the stratum corneum within the buccal mucosa precipitated by chronic irritation or injury from repetitive chewing, biting, or nibbling. Hyperkeratosis (C) is a response to chronic physical trauma to tissues, as with check biting. *Dysplasia* (A) is a term used in pathology to refer to an

abnormality of development. Carcinoma (B) is a malignant epithelial tumor, and the common type of cancer occurring in humans. Carcinoma in situ (D) is defined as the absence of invasion of tumor cells into surrounding tissue, usually before penetration through the basement membrane.

147. What is the MOST desired outcome in wound healing?

ANS: B
Regeneration (B) is the most desired outcome of inflammation, returning the damaged tissue to its identical preinflammatory structure and function. Repair (A) of damaged tissue occurs when the damage has been so great that functioning cells and tissues are replaced with nonfunctioning scar tissue. Granulation tissue (C) is immature connective tissue with numerous capillaries and fibroblasts. Granulation tissue may interfere with healing and may require surgical removal. Healing by secondary intention (D) involves injury in which a large amount of tissue is lost, preventing the edges of the injury from becoming joined. Healing starts with the formation of a large clot, increased formation of granulation tissue, and scar tissue.

148. The patient presents with a 2 × 2 mm, white-yellowish, flat lesion that has a slight erythematous halo on the buccal mucosa adjacent to tooth #28. Which of the following lesions is described here?

ANS: B
Aphthous ulcers (B) are often triggered from some form of trauma such as cheek biting. Mucositis (A) is generalized mucosal inflammation. Irritation fibroma (C) is scarlike connective tissue that is a result of chronic trauma and contains few blood vessels. Lichenoid reaction (D) resembles lichen planus, presenting as white, plaquelike, lacy lesions on skin and the oral mucosa. This reaction is often linked to drugs, stress, or dental materials.

149. Contact dermatitis is exemplified by which type of hypersensitivity?

ANS: D
Contact dermatitis is a delayed hypersensitivity, which is type IV (D). Type I (A) hypersensitivity occurs immediately and includes anaphylaxis, hay fever, and asthma. Type II (B) hypersensitivity includes autoimmune hemophilic anemia. In type III (C) hypersensitivity, immune complexes are formed, and they occur in autoimmune diseases.

150. The severe form of erythema multiforme, which involves widespread lesions that may appear in the oral cavity and on the eyes, genitalia, and the thoracic and abdominal regions, is known as

ANS: D
The most severe form of erythema multiforme is called Stevens-Johnson syndrome (D), and it causes extensive and painful lesions. *Sutton disease* (A) is a term used for aphthous ulcerations that are numerous and extensive. Behçet syndrome (B) is an autoimmune disease consisting primarily of oral ulcers, genital ulcers, and ocular inflammation. Marfan syndrome (C) is a genetic disorder of connective tissue.

151. Which of the following levels is a desirable glucose level for an individual with diabetes?

ANS: C
A desirable glucose level for an individual with diabetes should be between 70 and 130 (C). A glucose level of 65 (A) may indicate possible hypoglycemia; a level of 150 may indicate possible hyperglycemia (B). A glucose level of 220 (D) is considered uncontrolled and may indicate problems with management of diabetes.

152. Which of the following factors could be responsible for the high prevalence of periodontal disease in patients with diabetes mellitus (DM)?

ANS: A
The elevated glucose levels in poorly controlled DM reduce the body's resistance to infection, and patients with poorly controlled DM are at increased risk for developing periodontal disease (A). DM, by itself, does not affect the virulence or oral microflora (B), or its levels (C), although once periodontal disease develops, both the levels and virulence of oral microbes increase. There are no intrinsic defects of the periodontal ligament linked to DM (D).

153. A 30-year-old patient has come for a dental hygiene appointment. The patient marks *yes* on the medical history for HIV infection. What should the dental hygienist do next?

ANS: D
Major considerations in safe dental treatment of the patient with HIV are the current CD4+ lymphocyte count and viral load (D). These laboratory values are related to the patient's susceptibility to opportunistic infections. Use of standard precaution is indicated with all patients, so double-gloving and wearing a face shield (A) is not warranted unless this personal

as it does not have to be diffused throughout the bloodstream. Choices A, B, and D do not correctly address the question.

169. All of the following conditions have oral manifestations EXCEPT one. Which one is the EXCEPTION?

    ANS: D
    Congestive heart failure (D) has no oral manifestations, although it may require modifications to dental treatment such as positioning the patient in the upright position. Cherubism (A) involves bilateral facial swelling in either the mandible or the maxilla, and dental images show multilocular radiolucent lesions. Oral characteristics common to patient with Laband syndrome include gingival fibromatosis (B). Cyclic neutropenia's oral characteristics include severe ulcerative gingivitis, and aggressive periodontitis if not carefully managed (C). Papillon-Lefèvre syndrome's oral characteristics include destruction of the periodontal tissues of both dentitions with premature loss of teeth (E).

170. A patient is experiencing an acute periodontal abscess. In this instance, the patient would be expected to present with all of the following signs and symptoms EXCEPT one. Which one is the EXCEPTION?

    ANS: C
    Chronic periodontal abscesses present with varying degrees of pain, and a chronic draining abscess is rarely painful (C). Acute periodontal abscesses present with throbbing and radiating pain (A). Tooth mobility (B), tooth discoloration (D), and localized swelling of the gingiva (E) are all symptoms of an acute periodontal abscess.

171. Immunofluorescence technique could be used to assist in the diagnosis of all of the following EXCEPT one. Which one is the EXCEPTION?

    ANS: C
    Squamous cell carcinoma is diagnosed by biopsy (C). Immunofluorescence is a technique typically used to diagnose the presence of antibodies and, in the case of autoimmune diseases, autoantibodies. Pemphigoid (A), lichen planus (B), and SLE (D) are considered autoimmune in origin, and immunofluorescence may be used to assist in their detection.

172. All of the following are indications of an endodontic abscess EXCEPT one. Which one is the EXCEPTION?

    ANS: A
    Endodontic abscesses respond with a negative response to vitality testing (A), a distinguishing factor

between periodontal and endodontic abscesses. A tooth associated with an endodontic abscess typically presents with swelling and suppuration (B), is sensitive to pressure (C), and as long as the abscess drains into the oral cavity, it is unlikely to be painful (D).

173. Malpositioned teeth, overhanging margins of restorations, and abnormal tooth morphology may cause increased accumulation of oral biofilm in those areas. This may contribute to the development of gingivitis.

    ANS: A
    Both statements are true (A). Malpositioned teeth, overhanging margins of restorations, and abnormal tooth morphology all contribute to the accumulation of oral biofilm and make effective home care more difficult. Accumulation of oral biofilm contributes to the development of gingivitis. Choices B, C, and D do not correctly reflect the statements.

174. Bleeding on probing is an indication of active inflammation. It can be used to develop a periodontal diagnosis

    ANS: C
    The first statement is true, and the second statement is false (C). Bleeding on probing is an indication of inflammation and an important assessment tool, but it cannot be used to develop a periodontal diagnosis. Diagnosis of disease is not based on bleeding on probing because it does not indicate whether the inflammatory state is confined to the gingiva or extends into the deeper periodontium. Other parameters such as attachment loss, radiographic images, and number of sites involved must be assessed before a diagnosis can be made. Choices A, B, and D do not correctly reflect the statements.

175. Following reevaluation of periodontal therapy, which of the following would be the MOST appropriate time frame for the periodontal maintenance appointment?

    ANS: C
    The goal of periodontal maintenance therapy is to preserve clinical attachment levels, control inflammation, and maintain optimal oral health. Maintenance should begin soon after periodontal therapy and occur at 3-month intervals (C) to prevent recolonization by destructive periodontal pathogens and destruction from the host response. Two weeks (A) or 4 weeks (B) after periodontal therapy is too soon for the patient to undergo additional therapy. Six months (D) is too long to wait for periodontal maintenance and may result in further disease progression.

176. A dental hygiene treatment plan indicates two quadrants of nonsurgical periodontal therapy (NSPT) with the use of local anesthesia. Which of the following is the MOST appropriate plan of treatment for the first appointment?

ANS: C
For NSPT using local anesthesia for two quadrants, it is recommended and safest to treat upper and lower quadrants on either the right or the left side (C). This allows the patient to have one side of the mouth free of anesthesia. The dental hygienist should avoid administering local anesthesia to both quadrants in the maxillary (A) or mandibular (B) arches in a single appointment to prevent self-mutilation. The dental hygienist should avoid administering local anesthesia to the maxillary right and mandibular left quadrants (D) in a single treatment because the patient does not have one side of the mouth free of anesthesia.

177. Which of the following should be avoided when the dental hygienist is preparing a dental hygiene diagnosis statement?

ANS: D
The dental hygiene diagnostic statement should not include words that express attitudes or judgments (D). The diagnostic statement should address the unmet needs of the patient (A), the etiology of the disease (B), and signs and symptoms (C).

178. The dental hygiene care plan is a blueprint that should be developed between which individuals?

ANS: B
The dental hygienist should work in collaboration with the patient (B) to encourage participation of the patient in identifying goals, priorities, and unmet needs for the care plan. Collaboration between the dentist and the patient (A) without the input of the dental hygienist is not likely to be as effective as involving the person responsible for creating the dental hygiene care plan. Collaboration between just the dental hygienist and the dentist (C) does not include the patient, and it is important that the patient be involved with the treatment plan. Patient goals established solely by the dental hygienist (D) will fail to establish a collaborative, co-therapeutic relationship with the patient.

179. The dental hygiene patient is informed that NSPT is required. The patient is knowledgeable regarding the need for treatment but declines the care. Which legal term describes the patient's decision?

ANS: B
Informed refusal (B) indicates that the patient is knowledgeable and has been presented with the care plan that describes the services to be rendered and the consequences of no treatment but declines the care. Implied refusal (A) or implied consent (D) is not expressly denied or granted by the patient, but rather inferred from a patient's actions and should be avoided. Informed consent (C) is given when the patient agrees, in writing, to the services to be rendered after proper presentation of and education about the treatment.

180. All of the following management strategies will benefit the anxious patient EXCEPT one. Which one is the EXCEPTION?

ANS: B
It is best to schedule a highly anxious patient in the morning when he or she is rested and less stressed, rather than at the end of the day (B). The tell-show-do method (A), a technique that works with both children and adults, familiarizes the patient with the dental environment and procedure in a nonthreatening way and helps alleviate patient anxiety. Positive and frequent communication during dental hygiene care (C) is important in reassuring the patient and fosters trust and openness between the hygienist and patient. Diazepam (Valium) (D) is an anxiolytic, or antianxiety medication, that is frequently given before dental appointments to fearful patients.

181. The presence of visible exudate around the gingival margins is an indication of

ANS: A
The presence of visible exudate around the gingival margins is an indication of active disease (A). Exudate around the gingival margin is not always indicative of periodontal involvement (B), as the disease may be contained to the gingiva. Exudate around the gingival margin does not necessarily mean low patient motivation (C), as the dental hygienist must assess the patient's oral hygiene techniques, compliance, frequency, and overall health. With completion of the disease cycle (D), visible exudate will not be present, as the area would have already healed.

182. An isotonic sodium chloride solution is an aqueous mixture that has the same salinity as natural human cellular fluids. An isotonic solution is made of one half teaspoon of salt (sodium chloride) to one half cup of water.

ANS: C
The first statement is true, and the second statement is false (C). An isotonic solution has the same salinity as natural human cellular fluids. An example of an isotonic solution could be made with one half teaspoon of salt (sodium chloride) in one cup of water. A hypertonic solution is more salty than natural human cellular fluids and its use is often recommended to reduce swelling. A hypotonic solution is less salty than natural human cellular fluids. Choices A, B, and D do not accurately reflect the statements.

183. Oral irrigation is an adjunctive method to periodontal therapy for the removal of oral biofilm. Oral irrigation effectively targets attached oral biofilm, unattached oral biofilm, and loosely adherent oral biofilm.

ANS: C
The first statement is true, and the second statement is false (C). It is true that oral irrigation is an adjunctive method to periodontal therapy for the removal of oral biofilm. The second statement is false because oral irrigation is most effective in removal of unattached and loosely adherent oral biofilm but does not effectively remove attached oral biofilm, which requires mechanical removal. Choices A, B, and D do not accurately reflect the statements.

184. Which is the FIRST clinical feature of plaque-induced gingivitis?

ANS: E
Bleeding on probing (E) is the first clinical feature of plaque induced gingivitis. Edema (A) and redness (B) are markers of inflammation that occur slightly later than bleeding on probing. Exudate (C) and loss of function (D) are late findings on plaque-induced gingivitis.

185. The "nonspecific plaque hypothesis" theory is valid for both gingivitis and periodontitis. This is because everyone who develops gingivitis will develop periodontitis.

ANS: B
Both statements are false (B). The "nonspecific plaque hypothesis" theory states that all bacteria in oral plaque are harmful and that the amount of plaque is the primary factor in the progression of oral inflammatory conditions. However, research has indicated that specific periodontal pathogens are associated with the development of periodontal diseases. In addition, many patients never progress from gingivitis to periodontitis. Choices A, C, and D do not accurately reflect the statements.

186. Lipopolysaccharide is

ANS: D
Lipopolysaccharide or endotoxin is a component of the cell wall of gram-negative rods (D), and is released on cell lysis by WBCs. Lipopolysaccharide is a primary mediator in the inflammatory process and is responsible for much of the host damage sustained in periodontal disease. Immunoglobulin A, lysozyme, lactoferrin, salivary amylase, lactoperoxidase, and other proteins are normal components of saliva (A), lipopolysaccharide is not. *Streptococcus mutans* and *Actinomyces viscosus* are the microorganisms primarily responsible for root caries (B). Lipopolysaccharide is not easily degraded by salivary enzymes (C). Teichoic acid, not lipopolysaccharide, is a component of the cell wall of gram-positive cocci (E).

187. A-delta sensory nerve fibers are myelinated and responsible for well-localized, short-duration sensations. C-fibers are unmyelinated fibers characterized by poorly localized, aching pain.

ANS: A
Both statements are true (A). Different types of sensory nerve fibers are found to extend from the pulpal side of the dentinal tubule to the dentinoenamel junction (DEJ), resulting in different types of tooth pain when stimulated. A-delta fibers are myelinated fibers that evoke a sensation of well-localized, sharp pain. A-beta fibers respond more sensitively to electrical stimulation, and C-fibers are unmyelinated and stimulation results in a dull, poorly localized, aching type of pain. Choices B, C, and D do not accurately reflect the statements.

188. Which of the following dosages of epinephrine is preloaded in an adult EpiPen?

ANS: B
The usual adult dosage of epinephrine is 0.3 mg (B). An adult EpiPen is available for patients who weigh 60 pounds or more. The usual dosage for children is 0.15 mg (C). The EpiPen Junior is available for patients weighing 40 pounds or less. 30 mg (A) or 15 mg (D) is too high a dosage.

189. "Dental fear" is an unpleasant mental, emotional, or physiologic sensation caused by a specific tooth-related stimulus. "Dental fear" is a strong motivator for utilization of oral health care.

ANS: C
The first statement is true, and the second statement is false (C). It is true that "dental fear" is an unpleasant mental, emotional, or physiologic

sensation caused by a specific tooth-related stimulus. The second statement is false because "dental fear" often prevents patients from seeking much-needed oral health care. Choices A, B, and D do not correctly reflect the statements.

190. Instruments that are classified as critical must be sterilized between each use. Instruments that are classified as semicritical may be disinfected with an EPA-registered low-level to intermediate-level disinfectant.

ANS: C
The first statement is true, and the second statement is false (C). Instruments that are classified as critical are those that penetrate soft tissue or bone and must be sterilized between each use. Semicritical instruments are not intended to penetrate soft tissue or bone but do contact oral fluids. These instruments should also be sterilized between each use. Choices A, B, and D do not correctly reflect the statements.

191. Nitrous oxide-oxygen (N_2O/O_2) sedation is not recommended for a patient who has

ANS: E
N_2O/O_2 sedation is not recommended for patients with a history of substance abuse (E) to avoid triggering addictive behaviors. A patient with asthma is a good candidate for N_2O/O_2 because of the increased O_2 received during sedation (A). A patient with hypertension (B) is a good candidate for N_2O/O_2 sedation because it decreases stress and provides more O_2 during sedation than is normally available. N_2O/O_2 sedation is indicated for patients with dental fear (C) because of its sedative effect. A patient with a seizure disorder (D) is a good candidate for N_2O/O_2 sedation because of the higher levels of oxygen, which reduces the seizure threshold.

192. Pregnant women and women taking oral contraceptives are at risk for increased gingival inflammation. The etiologic factor in the gingival inflammation is the elevated hormonal levels.

ANS: C
The first statement is true, and the second statement is false (C). Pregnant women, women taking oral contraceptives, females at puberty, and women at certain stages of their menstrual cycle are at risk for increased gingival inflammation. The primary etiologic factor in the gingival inflammation is oral biofilm. Elevated hormonal factors increase the risk of inflammation but are not the primary factor. Choices A, B, and D do not correctly reflect the statements.

193. Which of the following is the primary bacterium implicated in pregnancy gingivitis and other hormonal periodontal diseases?

ANS: D
P. intermedia (D) is a primary bacterium implicated in pregnancy gingivitis and other hormonal periodontal diseases. *T. denticola* (A), *P. gingivalis* (B), and *T. forsythia* (C) are periodontal pathogens that make up the "red complex." The red complex is a group of bacteria implicated in chronic periodontitis. *A. actinomycetemcomitans* (E) is the primary periodontal pathogen implicated in aggressive periodontitis.

194. Rampant caries and advanced periodontal disease are common intraoral findings in patients who abuse

ANS: D
The acid content of methamphetamine (D), decreased salivary flow, the craving for high-sugar-containing beverages or food, and lack of oral hygiene care result in "meth mouth," in the form of rampant caries and periodontal disease. Oral findings in patients who abuse LSD (A) include orofacial injuries experienced when under the drug's influence and bruxism. Oral findings in patients who abuse cocaine (B) include perforation of the nasal septum and palate, gingival lesions, and erosion of tooth services. Oral findings in patients who abuse cannabis (C) include leukoplakia, increased incidence of lingual carcinoma, and gingival enlargement.

195. Type 1 diabetes mellitus (DM) is the most common form of DM. The primary risk factor for type I diabetes mellitus is obesity.

ANS: B
Both statements are false (B). Type 1 diabetes mellitus occurs in 5% to 10% of the population with diabetes and is believed to be an autoimmune disease that causes destruction of the insulin-producing cells of the pancreas. Obesity is not a risk factor for type I diabetes mellitus; however, it is strongly associated with type II diabetes mellitus. Choices A, C, and D do not correctly reflect the statements.

196. Transosteal implants are the most frequently used implants. They are used most often in patients who have a narrow mandible.

ANS: D
The first statement is false, and the second statement is true (D). Transosteal or transosseous implants are designed for a patient with a narrow mandible who needs strength and support for chewing, biting,

and grinding. However, transosteal implants are rarely used, as their placement involves an invasive surgical procedure, which increases the probability of infection and implant failure. The most frequently placed implant for oral rehabilitation is the endosteal implant. Choices A, B, and C do not accurately reflect the statements.

197. All of the following are current over-the-counter nicotine replacement products EXCEPT one. Which one is the EXCEPTION?

   ANS: B
   Nicotine spray (B) is available by prescription only because of the rapid absorption of nicotine through nasal membranes and the potential for abuse. Nicotine gum (A), nicotine lozenge (C), and the transdermal patch (D) are all available over the counter for support and assistance with smoking cessation.

198. Bisphosphonates are a class of drugs used to reduce the risk of fracture in patients with osteoporosis. Oral bisphosphonates are most strongly linked with the development of bisphosphonate osteonecrosis of the jaw.

   ANS: C
   The first statement is true, and the second statement is false (C). Bisphosphonates are a class of drugs that alter or inhibit the ability of osteoclasts to resorb bone, thus suppressing bone turnover. They increase bone mass and reduce the risk for fracture in persons with osteoporosis. Intravenous use of bisphosphonates has the strongest risk factor for development of bisphosphonate osteonecrosis of the jaw. Oral bisphosphonates carry a much lower risk of developing this condition. Choices A, B, and D do not correctly reflect the statements.

199. Most denture-related infections are caused by

   ANS: D
   Chronic candidiasis infection (D) is the cause of most denture-related infections, including denture stomatitis, which is the most common. Ill-fitting dentures (A) and chemical agent irritation (C) are more likely to result in traumatic lesions such as ulcers. Riboflavin deficiency (B) may result in angular cheilitis, which often becomes infected with *Candida*.

200. "A desired end result, in terms of knowledge that the client is to achieve through specific dental hygiene actions" describes what type of patient-centered goal?

   ANS: B
   Cognitive (B) goals aim to increase in the client's knowledge to achieve a desired end result through specific dental hygiene actions. Affective (A) goals are desired changes in client values, beliefs, and attitudes as a result of dental hygiene care. Psychomotor (C) goals are those that reflect a client's skill development and skill mastery. Oral health status (D) goals are tangible desired outcomes in the client's oral health status.

201. All of the following may be included as part of the dental hygiene care plan EXCEPT one. Which one is the EXCEPTION?

   ANS: A
   Removal of caries (A) is part of the overall dental care plan but is not included as part of the dental hygiene care plan, as it is not within the scope of dental hygiene practice. Administration of fluoride (B), placement of pit and fissure sealants (C), and therapeutic periodontal debridement (D) may all be included as part of the dental hygiene care plan. They support the overall dental plan and are within the scope of dental hygiene practice.

## CHAPTER 10

Performing Periodontal Procedures

Phyllis L. Beemsterboer, Gwen Essex, Jean Frahm,
Leslie Koberna, Dorothy A. Perry, Laura J. Webb

QUESTIONS

1. The therapeutic end point of periodontal debridement is
   A. restoration of gingival health.
   B. creation of nonretentive root surfaces.
   C. removal of detectable biofilm and calculus.
   D. use of a chemotherapeutic agent.

2. When performing periodontal debridement procedures on multirooted tooth surfaces, it is recommended that each root be instrumented as a separate tooth. The use of longer-shanked, miniature-bladed, area-specific curettes is helpful in accessing these surfaces.
   A. Both statements are true.
   B. Both statements are false.
   C. The first statement is true, and the second statement is false.
   D. The second statement is true, and the first statement is false.

3. Frequent periodontal debridement of subgingival root surfaces for the purpose of removing biofilm is important for the treatment of periodontal disease because most subgingival biofilm is not easily reached during patient self-care.
   A. Both the statement and the reason are correct and related.
   B. Both the statement and reason are correct but NOT related.
   C. The statement is correct, but the reason is NOT.
   D. NEITHER the statement NOR the reason is correct.

4. Each of the following is a common response to successful periodontal debridement EXCEPT one. Which one is the EXCEPTION?
   A. Reduced probing depth
   B. Reduction of tissue swelling
   C. Formation of new alveolar bone
   D. Formation of a long junctional epithelium

5. The "gross scale" technique of removing only the large deposits of supragingival calculus at the first appointment is no longer recommended because of the potential problems from incomplete calculus removal.
   A. Both the statement and the reason are correct and related.
   B. Both the statement and reason are correct but NOT related.
   C. The statement is correct, but the reason is NOT.
   D. NEITHER the statement NOR the reason is correct.

6. Which of the following instruments is designed for removal of fine deposit in a deep, narrow pocket on the distal root surface of tooth #27?
   A. 15/16 Gracey curette
   B. 6/7 anterior sickle scaler
   C. 3/7 Hirschfeld periodontal file
   D. 13/14 micro-miniature Gracey curette

7. Chronic periodontitis may be either localized or generalized. The disease progresses continuously over time.
   A. Both statements are true.
   B. Both statements are false.
   C. The first statement is true, and the second statement is false.
   D. The first statement is false, and the second statement is true.

8. Phase I of periodontal therapy, or the etiologic phase, includes each of the following procedures EXCEPT one. Which one is the EXCEPTION?
   A. Biofilm control
   B. Occlusal therapy
   C. Patient education
   D. Endodontic therapy
   E. Periodontal debridement

9. The severity of periodontal disease is most accurately measured over time by
   A. caries rate.
   B. probing depths.
   C. gingival bleeding.
   D. clinical attachment loss.

10. Which of the following is NOT an underlying objective of periodontal maintenance?
    A. Control of inflammation
    B. Maintenance of alveolar bone height
    C. Preservation of clinical attachment levels
    D. Reduction of periodontal maintenance intervals
    E. Evaluation and reinforcement of patient oral hygiene

11. Probing depth is usually equal to clinical attachment loss. Periodontal surgery is most successful when treating periodontal pockets with probing depths of 5 to 9 mm.
    A. Both statements are true.
    B. Both statements are false.
    C. The first statement is true, and the second statement is false.
    D. The first statement is false, and the second statement is true.

12. Periodontal surgery is not indicated for patients under 30 years old who present with pocket depths exceeding 5 mm and loss of half of their supporting bone because they likely have a slowly progressing form of periodontal disease.
    A. Both the statement and the reason are correct and related.
    B. Both the statement and reason are correct but NOT related.
    C. The statement is correct, but the reason is NOT.
    D. NEITHER the statement NOR the reason is correct.

13. Which of the following is the preferred form of excisional surgery for the treatment of drug-induced gingival enlargement?
    A. Ostectomy
    B. Gingivectomy
    C. Periodontal flap
    D. Guided tissue regeneration

14. The goal of periodontal flap procedures is
    A. access to root surface.
    B. guided tissue regeneration.
    C. improvement of osseous defects.
    D. pocket reduction by apical repositioning.

15. Which of the following is a contraindication to osseous recontouring?
    A. Reverse alveolar bone architecture
    B. Bone defect too deep to allow removal of osseous walls
    C. Thick bony ledges interfering with gingival flap procedures
    D. Periodontal pockets that extend below the level of the osseous crest

16. The surgical procedure which only involves removal of bony ledges or nonsupporting bone is called
    A. ostectomy.
    B. osteoplasty.
    C. apicoectomy.
    D. gingivectomy.

17. The type of periodontal bone grafting created from synthetic bone minerals is a/an
    A. allograft.
    B. alloplast.
    C. autograft.
    D. xenograft.

18. Lasers are considered an adjunct therapy for removal of soft tissue within the periodontal pocket. The Er:YAG laser has been shown to be safe for use around implants.
    A. Both statements are true.
    B. Both statements are false.
    C. The first statement is true, and the second statement is false.
    D. The first statement is false, and the second statement is true.

19. Evaluating mobility is a critical tool in assessment of implant success. Probing is a less useful assessment tool in evaluating implant success.
    A. Both statements are true.
    B. Both statements are false.
    C. The first statement is true, and the second statement is false.
    D. The first statement is false, and the second statement is true.

20. Professionally placed controlled-release local drug delivery is indicated for deep pockets and nonresponsive sites because it routinely provides superior results in reducing pocket depths and attachment levels compared with periodontal debridement.
    A. Both the statement and the reason are correct and related.
    B. Both the statement and reason are correct but NOT related.
    C. The statement is correct, but the reason is NOT.
    D. NEITHER the statement NOR the reason is correct.

21. Which of the following regions of the dentition has the narrowest width of attached gingiva?
    A. Maxillary molars
    B. Maxillary incisors
    C. Mandibular molars
    D. Maxillary premolars
    E. Mandibular premolars

22. Which of the following types of tissue makes up the outer layer of gingival tissue?
    A. Cuboidal cell epithelial
    B. Dense regular connective
    C. Dense irregular connective
    D. Simple squamous epithelial
    E. Stratified squamous epithelial

23. For each numbered term listed, select the most closely associated description.

Term	Definition
____ 1. Interdental gingiva	A. Coronal border of gingiva
____ 2. Mucogingival junction	B. Separates the free and attached gingiva
____ 3. Gingival margin	C. Below mucogingival junction
____ 4. Sulcus	D. Contains two papillae
____ 5. Alveolar mucosa	E. Suspends the tooth
____ 6. Free gingival groove	F. Point where attached gingiva meets alveolar mucosa
____ 7. Col	G. Marks the border of the free gingiva and the attached gingiva
____ 8. Periodontal ligament	H. Gingival depression between two teeth

24. Crevicular fluid increases its flows in the gingival sulcus during gingival health. It decreases in flow in the presence of plaque biofilm and inflammation.
    A. Both statements are true.
    B. Both statements are false.
    C. The first statement is true, and the second statement is false.
    D. The first statement is false, and the second statement is true.

25. Each of the following is a function of the periodontal ligament EXCEPT one. Which one is the EXCEPTION?
    A. Supports the tooth in alveolar bone
    B. Stimulates formation of secondary dentin
    C. Transmits sensations of touch and pressure
    D. Provides nutrition to bone and cementum
    E. Provides regeneration for cementum and bone

26. Order the steps (from first to last) in the spread of inflammation seen with vertical bone loss. Match each letter with its appropriate number.
    1. ____ A. Alveolar bone
    2. ____ B. Gingival connective tissue
    3. ____ C. Periodontal ligament (PDL) space

27. There is a greater prevalence and severity of periodontal disease among the female population in the United States than among the male population. A person in his or her 60s is at greater risk for periodontal disease than an individual in his or her 40s.
   A. Both statements are true.
   B. Both statements are false.
   C. The first statement is true, and the second statement is false.
   D. The first statement is false, and the second statement is true.

28. Which of the following are local contributing factors for periodontal disease? (Select all that apply.)
   A. Smoking
   B. Medications
   C. Biofilm growth
   D. Faulty restorations
   E. Tooth concavities

29. For each numbered component of the immune system listed, select the function that most closely matches it from the list provided. Not all functions will be used.

Immune System Component

_____ 1. B-lymphocyte

_____ 2. Polymorphonuclear neutrophils (PMNs)

_____ 3. T-lymphocytes

_____ 4. Immunoglobulins

_____ 5. Macrophage

_____ 6. Complement system

Function

A. First white blood cell at site of injury; begins phagocytosis; releases cytokines and lysosomes

B. Neutralizes bacterial toxins; activates complement system; coats bacteria for phagocytosis

C. Generates chemotaxis; activates lysis of cell membrane and phagocytosis; recruits phagocytic cells

D. Produces plasma cells, which produce immunoglobulins; make antibodies; destroy antigens

E. Stimulates production of prostaglandins

F. Second inflammatory cell to arrive; ingests and digests microorganisms; releases cytokines, prostaglandins, and lysosomes

G. Further stimulates immune response; secretes cytokines and kills infected cells

H. Proteins that regulate cell activity

30. All the following describe the plaque biofilm overgrowth phase of early gingivitis EXCEPT one. Which one is the EXCEPTION?
   A. Cytokines are released.
   B. Osteoclasts are activated.
   C. Polymorphonuclear neutrophils (PMNs) are recruited by cytokines.
   D. Macrophages are recruited to connective tissue.
   E. PMNs (neutrophils) destroy healthy gingival connective tissue.

31. Which systemic risk factor for periodontitis is characterized by a gradual onset, an inadequate supply of insulin, or the inability to use produced insulin effectively?
   A. Leukemia
   B. Osteoporosis
   C. Type 1 diabetes mellitus (DM)
   D. Type 2 diabetes mellitus
   E. Gestational diabetes mellitus

32. A person with uncontrolled type 2 diabetes mellitus is at greater risk for periodontal disease compared with a person with controlled type 1 diabetes mellitus because the uncontrolled diabetic has an impaired host response, disruption in collagen formation, and higher glucose levels in the gingival crevicular fluid.
   A. Both the statement and reason are correct and related.
   B. Both the statement and reason are correct but NOT related.
   C. The statement is correct, but the reason is NOT.
   D. The statement is NOT correct, but the reason is correct.
   E. NEITHER the statement NOR the reason is correct.

33. Smoking affects the periodontium in all the following ways EXCEPT one. Which one is the EXCEPTION?
   A. Increased bone loss
   B. Increased tissue fibrosis
   C. Decreased bleeding response
   D. Decreased plaque accumulation
   E. Decreased inflammatory response

34. Your patient presents with gingival redness, inflammation, bleeding, sensitivity, and tenderness. There is visible plaque biofilm at the gingival margin. There is no bone loss indicated on dental images. This individual most likely has
   A. chronic periodontitis.
   B. healthy gingival tissue.
   C. aggressive periodontitis.
   D. gingivitis associated with an allergic reaction.
   E. gingivitis associated with dental plaque biofilm.

35. Rapid periodontal destruction, including bone loss, tissue necrosis, severe pain, tissue sloughing, spontaneous bleeding, and fiery red erythematous tissue, all describe which of the following conditions?
    A. Primary herpetic gingivostomatitis
    B. Gingivitis induced by malnutrition
    C. Necrotizing ulcerative gingivitis
    D. Necrotizing ulcerative periodontitis (NUP)

36. For each numbered inherited disease with risk of periodontal disease listed below, select the most closely linked description from the list provided.

Disorder	Characteristics
_____ 1. Leukocyte adhesion deficiency	A. Developmental delay; small head; hyperelasticity of skin; weak muscle tone; short philtrum; vaulted palate; prominent maxillary central incisors
_____ 2. Papillon-Lefévre syndrome	B. Pale-colored hair, eyes, and skin; neutrophil chemotactic defect; early tooth loss in both dentitions; high risk for fatal bacterial infection; extractions recommended to decrease dental infections
_____ 3. Cohen syndrome	C. Disorders that affect the bone marrow and neutrophil levels; possible severe bone and tooth loss; possible early exfoliation of deciduous teeth; permanent teeth exfoliation as soon as they erupt
_____ 4. Chediak-Higashi syndrome	D. Inherited disorder of severe chronic neutropenia; severe bone and tooth loss resulting in exfoliation on deciduous and permanent teeth
_____ 5. Down syndrome	E. Hyperkeratosis of palms of hands and soles of feet (palmoplantar keratoderma); severe periodontal defects; bone and tooth loss; all primary teeth by age 5 years; all permanent teeth by age 15 years
_____ 6. Cyclic neutropenia	F. Additional chromosome 21; mild to moderate retardation; severe early-onset aggressive periodontitis; generalized heavy plaque; deep pocketing; gingival inflammation
_____ 7. Glycogen storage disorder	G. Problem with storage of carbohydrates as glycogen; neutropenia; bone and tooth loss; exfoliation of deciduous and permanent teeth

37. Periodontal disease is associated with coronary heart disease, diabetes mellitus, preeclampsia, hospital-acquired pneumonia, and some types of cancer. Association indicates causation.
    A. Both statements are true.
    B. Both statements are false.
    C. The first statement is true, and the second statement is false.
    D. The first statement is false, and the second statement is true.

38. Which of the following nutrients is MOST critical for wound healing and collagen formation in the periodontium?
    A. Calcium
    B. Protein
    C. Vitamin D
    D. Vitamin C
    E. Antioxidant

39. Order the five phases of therapy in the periodontal treatment plan. Match each letter with its proper sequence number.
    1. _____   A. Surgical
    2. _____   B. Restorative
    3. _____   C. Nonsurgical periodontal
    4. _____   D. Periodontal maintenance
    5. _____   E. Assessment and preliminary

40. Periodontal debridement is beneficial for each of the following conditions EXCEPT one. Which one is the EXCEPTION?
    A. Allergic gingivitis
    B. Chronic periodontitis
    C. Aggressive periodontitis
    D. Dental plaque–induced gingivitis
    E. Necrotizing ulcerative periodontitis (NUP)

41. Most cases of halitosis originate in the oral cavity. Pyridine has been identified as the leading cause of halitosis.
    A. Both statements are true.
    B. Both statements are false.
    C. The first statement is true, and the second statement is false.
    D. The first statement is false, and the second statement is true.

42. Tetracyclines are bacteriocidal. They are broad-spectrum antibiotics that affect gram-positive and gram-negative bacteria.
    A. Both statements are true.
    B. Both statements are false.
    C. The first statement is true, and the second statement is false.
    D. The first statement is false, and the second statement is true.

43. The reestablishment of junctional epithelium after periodontal debridement occurs within
    A. 1–2 weeks.
    B. 4–6 weeks.
    C. 6–8 weeks.
    D. 24–48 hours.
    E. 48–64 hours.

44. All the following are characteristics of chronic periodontitis EXCEPT one. Which one is the EXCEPTION?
    A. Periodontal disease is communicable.
    B. Prevalence and severity increases with age.
    C. Chronic periodontitis is the most common form of periodontitis.
    D. The amount of dental biofilm is disproportionate to the amount of tissue destruction.

45. A patient who has previously had nonsurgical periodontal surgery returns for the 4-month periodontal maintenance appointment. The patient presents with visible plaque, increased pocket depth and clinical attachment loss, inflammation with exudate, and bleeding on probing in the maxillary right molar region. There is also some evidence of increased bone loss on dental images. All other areas have remained stable. Which of the following is the BEST course of action?
    A. Localized periodontal surgery
    B. Evaluation of the patient's systemic condition
    C. Increasing the number of periodontal maintenance appointments
    D. Decreasing the number of periodontal maintenance appointments
    E. Localized nonsurgical periodontal therapy

46. The maintenance interval schedule for the first year after the placement of an implant is
    A. 1 month.
    B. 3 months.
    C. 4 months.
    D. 6 months.

47. Which gram-negative, nonmotile pathogen is found in small numbers in the healthy periodontium and in large numbers in recurrent disease sites with deep periodontal pockets?
    A. *Tannerella forsythia*
    B. *Treponema denticola*
    C. *Porphyromonas gingivalis*
    D. *Aggregatibacter actinomycetemcomitans*

48. Dentinal sensitivity can only be managed with the use of fluoride toothpaste because the sensitivity is more often related to root caries than exposure of root surfaces.
    A. Both the statement and reason are correct and related.
    B. Both the statement and reason are correct but NOT related.
    C. The statement is correct, but the reason is NOT.
    D. The statement is NOT correct, but the reason is correct.
    E. NEITHER the statement NOR the reason is correct.

49. Periodontal disease is almost always preceded by gingivitis. Gingivitis almost always leads to periodontal disease.
    A. Both statements are true.
    B. Both statements are false.
    C. The first statement is true, and the second statement is false.
    D. The first statement is false, and the second statement is true.

50. To determine immediate success of scaling and root planning, the clinician must rely on
    A. tactile evaluation.
    B. visual examination.
    C. microscopic evaluation.
    D. radiographic evaluation.

51. Order the healing events after treatment for gingivitis. Match each letter with its proper sequence number.
    1. _____ A. Stippling reappears.
    2. _____ B. Collagen is deposited.
    3. _____ C. Clinical probing depth is reduced.
    4. _____ D. Tissues return to normal coloration.
    5. _____ E. Inflammatory cells are replaced by fibroblasts.
    6. _____ F. Collagen fibers become functionally oriented.

52. The most common form of gingivitis is plaque-induced gingivitis. The most common symptoms of the disease are pain and bleeding.
    A. Both statements are true.
    B. Both statements are false.
    C. The first statement is true, and the second statement is false.
    D. The first statement is false, and the second statement is true.

53. From the following list, select the three items that characterize gingivitis.
    A. Bone loss
    B. Degree of inflammation
    C. Clinical attachment loss
    D. Localized or generalized involvement
    E. Location in marginal or papillary tissues

54. Systemic factors may modify the patient's reaction to plaque biofilm. The patient's reaction to plaque biofilm may be caused by alterations in the immune system caused by stress, endocrine-related changes, and drug-induced changes.
    A. Both statements are true.
    B. Both statements are false.
    C. The first statement is true, and the second statement is false.
    D. The first statement is false, and the second statement is true.

55. Pregnancy gingivitis is a condition that occurs because the elevation of female hormones cause exaggerated cellular and vascular proliferation, and microvessel leakage in response to oral biofilm. Pregnancy gingivitis is an unavoidable outcome of pregnancy.
    A. Both statements are true.
    B. Both statements are false.
    C. The first statement is true, and the second statement is false.
    D. The first statement is false, and the second statement is true.

56. From the following list, select the three items that are characteristic of the contents of the inflamed periodontal pocket.
    A. Osteoclastic cells
    B. Increased collagen fibers
    C. Increased gingival crevicular fluid
    D. Bacteria, both in biofilm and planktonic motile forms
    E. Purulent exudate made up of dead cells and serum products

57. Periodontal disease activity is
    A. episodic.
    B. continuous.

C. site specific.
D. episodic *and* site specific.
E. continuous *and* site specific.

58. Bleeding on probing is a sign of active periodontal disease. Bleeding sites are indicative of increasing bone loss and soft tissue destruction.
    A. Both statements are true.
    B. Both statements are false.
    C. The first statement is true, and the second statement is false.
    D. The first statement is false, and the second statement is true.

59. Chronic periodontal disease is consistent with the amount of oral biofilm found in the mouth, including the presence of subgingival calculus. Chronic periodontitis progresses at a slow rate, with short bursts of disease progression.
    A. Both statements are true.
    B. Both statements are false.
    C. The first statement is true, and the second statement is false.
    D. The first statement is false, and the second statement is true.

60. Clinical characteristics such as the rate of bone loss and age of onset are the most reliable distinguishing features between aggressive periodontal disease and chronic periodontal disease because both conditions present with a similar bacterial microflora.
    A. Both the statement and the reason are correct and related.
    B. Both the statement and the reason are correct but NOT related.
    C. The statement is correct, but the reason is NOT.
    D. The statement is NOT correct, but the reason is correct.
    E. NEITHER the statement NOR the reason is correct.

61. After periodontal surgery, all of the following postoperative instructions should be given EXCEPT one. Which one is the EXCEPTION?
    A. Eat a soft diet.
    B. Smoking is permitted.
    C. Limit physical activity.
    D. Use light pressure to control any seepage of blood.

62. Which of the following BEST describes the progress of surgical wound healing at the 1-week postoperative visit?
    A. The wound is completely healed.
    B. The wound is completely reepithelialized.
    C. The wound has complete bone regeneration.
    D. The wound has complete connective tissue regeneration.

63. Which of the following is the earliest period after surgery when it is safe to probe the surgical site?
    A. 1 week
    B. 2 weeks
    C. 3 weeks
    D. 4 weeks
    E. 6 weeks

64. In the first few days after periodontal surgery, the dental hygienist is likely to see all of the following clinical signs or symptoms in the periodontal patient EXCEPT one. Which one is the EXCEPTION?
    A. Mobility
    B. New caries
    C. Root sensitivity
    D. Larger spaces between teeth

65. The MOST common type of implant used in clinical dentistry is the
    A. blade implant.
    B. transosteal implant.
    C. endosseous implant.
    D. subperiosteal implant.

66. The formation of an intimate lattice between the implant surface and bone is referred to as
    A. ankylosis.
    B. ossification.
    C. mineralization.
    D. osseointegration.

67. Plaque biofilm and calculus removal for dental implants should be performed with
    A. plastic instruments.
    B. ultrasonic instruments.
    C. stainless steel hand instruments.
    D. polishing cup and regular prophy paste.

68. Home care for patients with implants is very important because they require the same cleaning aids as do patients with natural teeth.
    A. Both the statement and the reason are correct and related.
    B. Both the statement and the reason are correct but NOT related.
    C. The statement is correct, but the reason is NOT.
    D. The statement is NOT correct, but the reason is correct.
    E. NEITHER the statement NOR the reason is correct.

69. Maintenance visits for implant patients should occur every 3 months during the first year. After the first year, recall intervals may be extended to 4 to 6 months if the gingival health is good and home care is excellent.
    A. Both statements are true.
    B. Both statements are false.

C. The first statement is true, and the second is false.
D. The first statement is false, and the second is true.

70. Implant-supported removable prostheses should be removed at home daily by patients because the supporting abutments need to be cleaned thoroughly with soft toothbrushes, single-tufted toothbrushes, and other devices, as needed.
    A. Both the statement and the reason are correct and related.
    B. Both the statement and the reason are correct but NOT related.
    C. The statement is correct, but the reason is NOT.
    D. The statement is NOT correct, but the reason is correct.
    E. NEITHER the statement NOR the reason is correct.

71. The expected outcome after treatment is termed the *overall* or *global prognosis* for the periodontal patient. Risk factors such as diabetes or tobacco use may alter the prognosis for the individual.
    A. Both statements are true.
    B. Both statements are false.
    C. The first statement is true, and the second statement is false.
    D. The first statement is false, and the second statement is true.

72. The overall, or global, prognosis may be different from the prognoses for individual teeth because periodontal disease is site specific and may affect some teeth in the dentition more severely than others.
    A. Both the statement and the reason are correct and related.
    B. Both the statement and the reason are correct but NOT related.
    C. The statement is correct, but the reason is NOT.
    D. The statement is NOT correct, but the reason is correct.
    E. NEITHER the statement NOR the reason is correct.

73. Periodontal maintenance is BEST defined as
    A. disease detection.
    B. home care reinforcement.
    C. scaling, root planning, and polishing at appropriate intervals.
    D. periodic assessment and preventive treatment for early detection and treatment of recurrent disease.

74. Successful periodontal therapy, including maintenance, is likely to result in slowing the rate of tooth loss to approximately
    A. 1 tooth over 10 years.
    B. 10 teeth over 10 years.
    C. 1 tooth in the first year after treatment.
    D. 10 teeth in the first year after treatment.

75. There is a high dropout rate for maintenance patients because they often do not understand that periodontal therapy is not complete after phase I therapy.
    A. Both the statement and the reason are correct and related.
    B. Both the statement and the reason are correct but NOT related.
    C. The statement is correct, but the reason is NOT.
    D. The statement is NOT correct, but the reason is correct.
    E. NEITHER the statement NOR the reason is correct.

76. Recurrent periodontal disease may be linked to all of the following factors EXCEPT one. Which one is the EXCEPTION?
    A. Systemic conditions
    B. Poor plaque biofilm control
    C. Incomplete calculus removal
    D. Presence of faulty restorations
    E. Appropriate recall compliance

77. A patient presents with periodontal probing depths of 3 to 4 mm and attachment loss of 1 to 2 mm. This patient would be classified as having _____ periodontitis.
    A. advanced
    B. severe
    C. moderate
    D. early

78. The use of prophylactic antibiotic coverage for dental procedures is recommended for which of the following conditions?
    A. Atrial septal defect
    B. Cardiac pacemaker
    C. Prosthetic heart valve
    D. Ventricular septal defect
    E. Functional heath murmur

79. For each numbered description listed below, select the MOST closely linked term or procedure from the list provided.

Description	Term or Procedure
_____ 1. Disruption or removal of plaque biofilm	A. Root planning
_____ 2. Instrumentation of the crown and root of teeth to remove plaque, calculus, and stains	B. Polishing
_____ 3. Definitive removal of cementum or surface dentin that is rough or is impregnated with calculus, toxins, or microorganisms	C. Maintenance

Description	Term or Procedure
_____ 4. Preventive procedure to remove local irritants from the gingiva, including calculus removal	D. Periodontal debridement
_____ 5. Application of agents to remove stains and plaque biofilm from teeth	E. Plaque control
_____ 6. Scaling and root planing and disruption or removal of plaque biofilm with minimal tooth structure removal	F. Endotoxins
_____ 7. Lipopolysaccharides found in the cell wall of gram-negative bacteria that trigger a strong inflammatory response	G. Prophylaxis
_____ 8. Periodic assessment and prophylactic treatment to permit detection and treatment of disease	H. Scaling

80. From the following list, select three items that will decrease the relative risk of root caries after periodontal surgery.
    A. Increased age
    B. Daily topical fluoride
    C. High retention of teeth
    D. High intake of sugary foods
    E. Nutritional counseling and diet modification

81. Clinical response to nonsurgical therapy can be measured with a periodontal probe. Measurement of clinical attachment is computed by measuring the periodontal probe depths and then subtracting the distance to the cementoenamel junction (CEJ).
    A. Both statements are true.
    B. Both statements are false.
    C. The first statement is true, and the second statement is false.
    D. The first statement is false, and the second statement is true.

82. All of the following chemical agents are used to treat sensitivity EXCEPT one. Which one is the EXCEPTION?
    A. Fluoride
    B. Silver nitrate
    C. Zinc chloride
    D. Chlorhexidine
    E. Sodium citrate

83. Informed consent is a process that allows the patient full understanding of the disease process, treatment options, and probable outcomes. This consent must always be in writing and signed by the patient.
   A. Both statements are true.
   B. Both statements are false.
   C. The first statement is true, and the second statement is false.
   D. The first statement is false, and the second statement is true.

84. Continuous or intermittent closure of the jaws under vertical pressure is termed
   A. spasm.
   B. trismus.
   C. bruxism.
   D. myalgia.
   E. clenching.

85. A less common form of aggressive periodontal disease, referred to as *necrotizing ulcerative gingivitis* (NUG), features specific, identifiable bacterial species. Symptoms of NUG include sudden onset, pain, pseudomembranous film on the papillae, and very bad breath.
   A. Both statements are true.
   B. Both statements are false.
   C. The first statement is true, and the second statement is false.
   D. The first statement is false, and the second statement is true.

86. The dental hygienist should refrain from treating patients with primary herpetic gingivostomatitis because it is a viral infection characterized by pain in the gingiva, fever, malaise, and vesicle formation.
   A. Both the statement and the reason are correct and related.
   B. Both the statement and the reason are correct but NOT related.
   C. The statement is correct, but the reason is NOT.
   D. The statement is NOT correct, but the reason is correct.
   E. NEITHER the statement NOR the reason is correct.

87. The relationship of the accumulation of plaque biofilm and the development of gingivitis is well documented. The dental hygienist is responsible for treating and preventing recurrence of the condition.
   A. Both statements are true.
   B. Both statements are false.
   C. The first statement is true, and the second statement is false.
   D. The first statement is false, and the second statement is true.

88. At the 4-week reevaluation appointment of multiple sessions of nonsurgical therapy, the dental hygienist identifies that three specific areas of the periodontium have not responded to phase I therapy. The BEST course of action is to
   A. refer the patient to the periodontist.
   B. place a local delivery antimicrobial agent.
   C. retreat the area and reassess at the next appointment.
   D. assume that there is an underlying systemic condition inhibiting healing.

89. For each of the descriptions listed, select the MOST closely linked process from the list provided.

Description	Process
____ 1. Wedge-shaped lesions located apical to the cementoenamel junction	A. Erosion
____ 2. Loss of enamel and dentin from the chemical action of dietary and gastric acids	B. Attrition
____ 3. Wear from tooth-to-tooth functional contact	C. Fenestration
____ 4. Tooth wear as a result of excessive forces exerted by a foreign object	D. Abfraction
____ 5. Window in the bone covering the facial surface of a root	E. Dehiscence
____ 6. Denuded area of bone on the root surface	F. Abrasion

90. Which characteristic is MOST indicative of an endodontic abscess?
   A. Constant pain
   B. Tooth vitality
   C. Localized pain
   D. Apical radiolucency

91. The presence of calculus is almost always associated with bacterial plaque biofilm because calculus is the plaque biofilm mineralized by salivary calcium and phosphate salts.
   A. Both the statement and the reason are correct and related.
   B. Both the statement and the reason are correct but NOT related.
   C. The statement is correct, but the reason is NOT.
   D. The statement is NOT correct, but the reason is correct.
   E. NEITHER the statement NOR the reason is correct.

92. Which of the following scaling instruments is primarily designed to remove heavy, supragingival calculus?
   A. Sickle scalers
   B. Universal curettes
   C. Ultrasonic scalers
   D. Extended shank curettes
   E. Area-specific curettes

93. The removal of plaque biofilm may be accomplished with power-driven scalers at a level comparable with that of hand instrumentation. There is no antimicrobial effect to the periodontal pocket from ultrasonic instrumentation.
    A. Both statements are true.
    B. Both statements are false.
    C. The first statement is true, and the second statement is false.
    D. The first statement is false, and the second statement is true.

94. Match each numbered organism to the period in which it appears within undisturbed plaque biofilm.

Organism	Time Period
____ 1. Vibrios and spirochetes	A. Days 1–2
____ 2. *Streptococcus mutans* and *Streptococcus sanguis*	B. Days 4–7
____ 3. Filamentous rods and fusobacteria	C. Days 7–14

95. *Coaggregation* is defined as the ability of
    A. current bacterial strains to multiply.
    B. bacteria in biofilms to communicate.
    C. biofilm to calcify and become calculus.
    D. new bacterial strains to attach to existing bacteria.

96. For each numbered PDL fiber group listed, select the MOST closely linked major function from the list provided.

PDL Fiber Group	Major Function
____ 1. Alveolar crest	A. Transfers occlusal pressure to tension on bone; largest periodontal fiber group
____ 2. Horizontal	B. Suspends tooth and protects bone between the roots of multirooted teeth
____ 3. Oblique	C. Retains tooth in socket; opposes lateral forces; most coronal of PDL fibers
____ 4. Apical	D. Attaches root surface to alveolar bone in perpendicular fashion
____ 5. Interradicular	E. Suspends tooth; only present in fully erupted teeth

97. Phase II periodontal therapy involves surgery, which is the intentional cutting of soft tissue to control disease or change the size and shape of tissues. The MAJOR benefit and indication for periodontal surgery is elimination of periodontal pockets.
    A. Both statements are true.
    B. Both statements are false.
    C. The first statement is true, and the second statement is false.
    D. The first statement is false, and the second statement is true.

98. Pockets with the junctional epithelium coronal to the alveolar crest are termed
    A. suprabony defects.
    B. biologic width defects.
    C. intrabony (infrabony) defects.

99. Which procedure is NOT an indication for periodontal surgery?
    A. Root access
    B. Repair of clefts
    C. Pocket reduction or elimination
    D. Correction of mucogingival defects

100. Oral irrigation is an adjunctive method for the arrest and control of gingival infections. Professional oral irrigation is more effective in control of oral biofilm and inflammation than daily home oral irrigation.
    A. Both statements are true.
    B. Both statements are false.
    C. The first statement is true, and the second statement is false.
    D. The first statement is false, and the second statement is true.

101. Which of the following procedures is defined as the removal of alveolar bone with the supporting periodontal ligament fibers?
    A. Osteoplasty
    B. Osteoectomy
    C. Gingivectomy
    D. Gingivoplasty

102. Osseous defects are classified by the number of walls of the remaining supporting alveolar bone. A one-wall defect would have the best prognosis.
    A. Both statements are true.
    B. Both statements are false.
    C. The first statement is true, and the second statement is false.
    D. The first statement is false, and the second statement is true.

103. For each numbered bone graft below, select the most closely linked definition from the list provided.

Bone Graft	Definition
____ 1. Autograft	A. Bone that comes from another person
____ 2. Alloplast	B. Bone that comes from another species
____ 3. Allograft	C. Bone that comes from the patient's own body
____ 4. Xenograft	D. Synthetic bone

104. Which of the following cells is the FIRST to arrive at an acutely inflamed site?
    A. Plasma
    B. Fibroblast
    C. Neutrophil
    D. Macrophage

105. Aggressive periodontitis and refractory periodontitis exhibit the same clinical symptoms. Aggressive periodontitis is recognized by its rapid cycles of disease progression and can be maintained or controlled through regular periodontal maintenance appointments.
    A. Both statements are true.
    B. Both statements are false.
    C. The first statement is true, and the second statement is false.
    D. The first statement is false, and the second statement is true.

106. Osseointegration is defined as
    A. inflammation in and around the area of a dental implant.
    B. an osseous defect in bone that surrounds one or more teeth.
    C. growth and bonding of bone tissue directly to the implant surface.
    D. the technical term for the appliance that secures the abutment to the implant.

107. Slight periodontitis is associated with clinical attachment loss of 2 to 3 mm. Slight periodontitis may present with edematous, erythematous tissue as well as radiographic bone loss of 10% or less.
    A. Both statements are true.
    B. Both statements are false.
    C. The first statement is true, and the second statement is false.
    D. The first statement is false, and the second statement is true.

108. The role of the dental hygienist in dealing with emergency conditions is focused on
    A. treatment and referral.
    B. recognition and referral.
    C. treatment of the emergent condition.
    D. recognition and treatment of the emergent condition.

109. The col is the depression between the buccal and lingual papillae of two adjacent teeth. It is made of nonkeratinized tissue and conforms to the interproximal contact area.
    A. Both statements are true.
    B. Both statements are false.
    C. The first statement is true, and the second statement is false.
    D. The first statement is false, and the second statement is true.

110. Periodontitis is a risk factor for all of the following systemic diseases EXCEPT one. Which one is the EXCEPTION?
    A. Cardiovascular disease
    B. Bacterial pneumonia
    C. Tuberculosis
    D. Diabetes mellitus

1. The therapeutic end point of periodontal debridement is

ANS: A
Restoration of gingival health (A), including pocket depth reduction and improvement or maintenance of clinical attachment level, is considered the therapeutic end point of periodontal debridement. The therapeutic endpoint is determined at the periodontal reevaluation appointment, usually 4 to 6 weeks after treatment. Creating nonretentive root surfaces (B) and removing detectable biofilm and calculus (C) are related to the clinical end point, that is, the tooth surface's preparedness for healing, which is determined immediately after the procedure. The use of chemotherapeutic agents (D) is considered an adjunct therapy in the prevention and control of oral diseases.

2. When performing periodontal debridement procedures on multirooted tooth surfaces, it is recommended that each root be instrumented as a separate tooth. The use of longer-shanked, miniature-bladed, area-specific curettes is helpful in accessing these surfaces.

ANS: A
Both statements are true (A). A systematic approach is necessary for successful debridement of multirooted tooth surfaces. Treating each root as a separate tooth assists in completing the meticulous task. The use of miniature blades allows for better adaptation to root surfaces and less tissue distension. The longer-shanked instruments provide better adaptation into deep pockets and along the long root surfaces. The use of area-specific curettes facilitates adaptation to root surfaces because of the specific bends of the instruments. Choices B, C, and D do not correctly reflect the statements.

3. Frequent periodontal debridement of subgingival root surfaces for the purpose of removing biofilm is important for the treatment of periodontal disease because most subgingival biofilm is not easily reached during patient self-care.

ANS: A
Both the statement and the reason are correct and related (A). The progress or arrest of periodontal disease is related to the presence of biofilm and calculus in the pocket. To maintain a subgingival environment that supports oral health and healing, biofilm must be kept at a minimum. It is difficult for patients to clean the subgingival environment well by using the toothbrush, floss, and rinses. Frequent periodontal debridement appointments assist in

eliminating biofilm in areas the patient is unable to clean. Choices B, C, and D do not correctly reflect the statement.

4. Each of the following is a common response to successful periodontal debridement EXCEPT one. Which one is the EXCEPTION?

ANS: C
Formation of new alveolar bone (C), new cementum, or new periodontal ligament (PDL) is not considered a common response to periodontal debridement. Common responses to successful periodontal debridement include reduction of probing depths (A); reduction of tissue swelling (B), or edema; and formation of a long junctional epithelium (D).

5. The "gross scale" technique of removing only the large deposits of supragingival calculus at the first appointment is no longer recommended because of the potential problems from incomplete calculus removal.

ANS: A
Both the statement and the reason are correct and related (A). Removing only the coronal calculus while allowing the subgingival pathogenic microflora beneath soft tissue to remain is an approach that was abandoned many years ago because of several potential problems. Tissue shrinkage at the gingival margin allows for the proliferation of microorganisms in the subgingival environment, with the risk for periodontal abscess formation. The tightened tissue makes subgingival instrumentation more difficult at subsequent appointments, and the roughened calculus left by partial removal facilitates bacterial recolonization. The patient loses motivation for further treatment when viewing the tissue, which appears healed. Choices B, C, and D do not correctly reflect the statements.

6. Which of the following instruments is designed for removal of fine deposit in a deep, narrow pocket on the distal root surface of tooth #27?

ANS: D
The micro-miniature 13/14 Gracey curette (D) is designed for removal of fine calculus on distal tooth surfaces in areas with difficult access. It has a 20% thinner blade than a miniature Gracey curette and is 3 mm longer than the lower shank of a standard Gracey curette, and the working-end is half the length of a standard Gracey curette. The 15/16 Gracey curette (A) is intended to be used on posterior mesial

surfaces. The intended use of the 6/7 anterior sickle scaler (B) is removal of supragingival calculus on anterior teeth. The 3/7 Hirschfeld periodontal file (C) is intended to be used on the facial and lingual surfaces of posterior teeth.

7. Chronic periodontitis may be either localized or generalized. The disease progresses continuously over time.

ANS: C
The first statement is true, and the second statement is false (C). It is true that chronic periodontitis is classified as localized (< 30% of involved sites) or generalized (> 30% of involved sites). The second statement is false because the disease progresses intermittently in response to local factors such as biofilm, with episodic bursts of activity that cause loss of attachment. The disease progression slows or ceases when immune response or therapy enhances host resistance. Choices A, B, and D do not correctly reflect the statements.

8. Phase I of periodontal therapy, or the etiologic phase, includes each of the following procedures EXCEPT one. Which one is the EXCEPTION?

ANS: D
Endodontic therapy (D) is part of phase II of periodontal therapy, which is the surgical phase, and includes procedures intended to reduce the effects of the disease. Phase I describes procedures designed to control or eliminate the etiologic factors of the disease process and includes biofilm control (A), occlusal therapy (B), patient education (C), periodontal debridement (E), and correction of contributing restorative and prosthetic factors.

9. The severity of periodontal disease is most accurately measured over time by

ANS: D
Clinical attachment loss (D) best describes the severity of periodontal disease because it describes the attachment loss from the cementoenamel junction, which, as a fixed reference point, provides a good indication of the amount of periodontal ligament destroyed and bone loss. Caries rate (A) is related to the caries disease process, not to periodontal therapy. Probing depths (B) assist in identifying risk for disease, oral self-care concerns, and instrumentation needs. Probing depths, combined with gingival recession measurements, provide a more complete assessment of the loss of supporting structures than probing depths alone. Gingival bleeding (C) is considered a risk predictor and is associated with persistent inflammation.

10. Which of the following is NOT an underlying objective of periodontal maintenance?

ANS: D
Although a reduction in intervals between periodontal maintenance visits (D) may occur as a result, it is not a goal related to the overall objective or a requirement for maintaining periodontal health. The overall objective of periodontal maintenance is to prevent the development of new or recurrent periodontal disease through a combination of daily personal hygiene and professional care. Control of inflammation (A), maintenance of alveolar bone height (B), preservation of clinical attachment levels (C), and evaluation and reinforcement of patient oral hygiene (E) are important criteria and strategies for maintaining periodontal health and are considered four of the five underlying objectives. The fifth underlying objective is maintenance of optimal oral health.

11. Probing depth is usually equal to clinical attachment loss. Periodontal surgery is most successful when treating periodontal pockets with probing depths of 5 to 9 mm.

ANS: D
The first statement is false, and the second statement is true (D). Probing depth is the measurement from the gingival margin to the base of the pocket. Clinical attachment loss is measured from the cementoenamel junction (CEJ) to the base of the pocket. If the gingival margin is located coronal to the CEJ, then the probing depth is greater than the loss of attachment. If the gingival margin is located apical to the CEJ, then the probing depth is less than the loss of attachment. Periodontal surgery is most successful when treating periodontal pockets with probing depths of 5 to 9 mm. Research has shown that nonsurgical debridement of pockets 4 mm or less is generally adequate in controlling periodontal disease. Pocket depths greater than 9 mm are generally associated with extreme loss of attachment, which negatively affects long-term prognosis for maintaining the teeth. Choices A, B, and C do not correctly reflect the statements.

12. Periodontal surgery is not indicated for patients under 30 years old who present with pocket depths exceeding 5 mm and loss of half of their supporting bone because they likely have a slowly progressing form of periodontal disease.

ANS: D
Neither the statement nor the reason is correct (D). Periodontal surgery is strongly indicated for patients under 30 years of age presenting with pocket depths exceeding 5 mm and loss of half their supporting

bone because it is likely they have an aggressive form of periodontal disease. Patients older than 60 years presenting with the same conditions are more likely to have a slow-progressing form of periodontal disease, and the need for periodontal surgery may be less critical. Choices A, B, and C do not correctly reflect the statements.

13. Which of the following is the preferred form of excisional surgery for the treatment of drug-induced gingival enlargement?

ANS: B
Gingivectomy (B) is an excisional surgery commonly used for treatment of drug-induced gingival enlargement. Ostectomy (A), periodontal flap surgery (C), and guided tissue regeneration (D) are not considered excisional surgical procedures.

14. The goal of periodontal flap procedures is

ANS: A
Periodontal flap procedures are intended to provide access to the root surface (A) to facilitate removal of biofilm by patients and professional debridement procedures, including scaling and root planing. Periodontal flap procedures are used when pocket reduction by apical repositioning (D) is not necessary and preserving gingival tissue is a goal. Guided tissue regeneration (B) is a separate procedure to promote healing by selected cell repopulation. Periodontal flap procedures may be used in conjunction with osseous surgical procedures (C) but are not osseous surgical procedures.

15. Which of the following is a contraindication to osseous recontouring?

ANS: B
Bone defects too deep to allow for removal of osseous walls (B) do not provide conditions for successful recontouring procedures. Interproximal bone that is apical to facial or lingual bone, or reverse alveolar bony architecture (A); thick bony ledges that interfere with gingival flap procedures (C); and infrabony pockets (D) that extend apically below the osseous crest are all changes in bone architecture and benefit from recontouring procedures.

16. The surgical procedure which only involves removal of bony ledges or nonsupporting bone is called

ANS: B
During osteoplasty (B) only bony ledges or nonsupporting bone is removed. During ostectomy (A), the bone removed also contains supporting periodontal

ligament fibers. Apicoectomy (C) is surgery that removes the apex of the tooth for access to the root canal for endodontic treatment. Gingivectomy (D) is a type of excisional surgery that removes excess gingival tissue.

17. The type of periodontal bone grafting created from synthetic bone minerals is a/an

ANS: B
Alloplasts (B) are periodontal grafts that use a variety of synthetic bone materials, whereas allografts (A) are created from the bone of another person. Autografts (C) use donor bone from the same patient, and xenografts (D) are created from the bone of another species, usually bovine or porcine.

18. Lasers are considered an adjunct therapy for removal of soft tissue within the periodontal pocket. The Er:YAG laser has been shown to be safe for use around implants.

ANS: A
Both statements are true (A). Lasers have been used in periodontics for removal of soft tissue within the periodontal pocket. The 2.94-micrometer (μm) wavelength of the Er:YAG laser has been proven to be safe and effective for use around implants. Choices B, C, and D do not correctly reflect the statements.

19. Evaluating mobility is a critical tool in assessment of implant success. Probing is a less useful assessment tool in evaluating implant success.

ANS: A
Both statements are true (A). Assessment of mobility is important, as healthy implants do not exhibit clinical signs of mobility because of the rigid bone-to-implant interface. Probing is less reliable because the lack of a true connective tissue attachment into the implant surface makes it easier for probes to penetrate the attachment, especially in the presence of inflammation. Choices B, C, and D do not correctly reflect the statements.

20. Professionally placed controlled-release local drug delivery is indicated for deep pockets and nonresponsive sites because it routinely provides superior results in reducing pocket depths and attachment levels compared with periodontal debridement.

ANS: C
The statement is correct, but the reason is NOT. Adjunct therapies such as professionally placed controlled-release local drug delivery are recommended for patients with severe and

unresponsive periodontal diseases to maximize the therapeutic opportunity. The reason for this statement, however, is NOT correct. Studies of controlled-release drug delivery agents placed locally after nonsurgical periodontal debridement procedures have shown very limited reduction of periodontal pockets and clinical attachment levels. Choices A, B, and D do not correctly reflect the statement and the reason.

21. Which of the following regions of the dentition has the narrowest width of attached gingiva?

ANS: E
The mandibular premolars (E) have the least amount of attached gingiva, with an average of 1.8 millimeters (mm). Maxillary molars and incisors (A, B) have an average width of 3.5 to 4.5 mm. Mandibular molars (C) have an average width of 3.3 to 3.9 mm. Maxillary premolars (D) have an average width of 1.9 mm.

22. Which of the following types of tissue makes up the outer layer of gingival tissue?

ANS: E
Stratified squamous epithelial (E) tissue forms the outer layer of gingival tissue. It covers connective tissue. Epithelial tissue serves as a barrier to protect the underlying connective tissue and is attached to connective tissue by basal cells. The different layers of keratinized stratified squamous epithelium include the stratum basal, stratum spinosum, stratum granulosum, and stratum corneum. Cuboidal cell epithelial (A) tissue is a single layer of epithelium that lines most glands. Connective tissue provides shape and structure and the nervous and vascular supply. There are several types of connective tissue: dense, regular (B) and irregular (C), areolar, adipose, and compact. Simple squamous epithelial (D) tissue comprises the endothelium of the heart, blood vessels, and lymph nodes.

23. For each numbered term listed, select the most closely associated description.

ANS: 1D; 2F; 3A; 4G; 5C; 6B; 7H; 8E
The interdental gingiva or the interdental papilla is the gingival tissue between two teeth, consisting of two papillae: the facial papilla and the lingual papilla (1D). The mucogingival junction is the point at which the attached gingival meets the alveolar mucosa (2F). The gingival margin is the coronal border of the gingiva (3A). The sulcus is the unattached area between the free gingiva and the epithelial junction on the tooth (4G). The alveolar or lining mucosa is located below the mucogingival junction (5C). The free gingival groove demarcates the border of the free gingiva and the attached gingiva (6B).

The shallow depression between the two interdental papillae is known as the *col* (7H). Periodontal ligament fibers suspend the tooth in the socket (8E).

24. Crevicular fluid increases its flows in the gingival sulcus during gingival health. It decreases in flow in the presence of plaque biofilm and inflammation.

ANS: B
Both statements are false (B). There are very small amounts of crevicular fluid found in the sulcus during gingival health. As plaque biofilm accumulates and inflammation develops, the flow of gingival crevicular fluid increases. Choices A, C, and D do not correctly reflect the statements.

25. Each of the following is a function of the periodontal ligament EXCEPT one. Which one is the EXCEPTION?

ANS: B
Formation of secondary dentin (B) is the action of odontoblasts and is not a function of the PDL. The periodontal ligament has many functions in addition to supporting the tooth in alveolar bone (A) by attaching to cementum. It transmits sensations of touch and pressure (C), provides nutrients to cementum and bone via the blood supply to the periodontium (D), and provides regeneration (E) and resorption for cementum and bone. Other functions of the PDL include acting as a shock absorber and converting pressure into tension to strengthen alveolar bone.

26. Order the steps (from first to last) in the spread of inflammation seen with vertical bone loss. Match each letter with its appropriate number.

ANS: 1B, 2C, 3A
Oral biofilm initiates the inflammatory process so that the oral structures closest to the biofilm are affected first. Biofilm accumulates at the gingival margin, and the inflammatory reaction spreads from the outermost structures to the more internal structures. In vertical bone loss, the inflammation first occurs in the gingival connective tissue (1B), then moves into the PDL space (2C), and finally spreads into alveolar bone (3A).

27. There is a greater prevalence and severity of periodontal disease among the female population in the United States than among the male population. A person in his or her 60s is at greater risk for periodontal disease than an individual in his or her 40s.

ANS: D
The first statement is false, and the second statement is true (D). The first statement is false. Men in the United States have a greater prevalence (number

of cases) of periodontal disease compared with females. This is believed to occur because females use health care services in greater numbers and with greater frequency compared with males. The second statement is true. Periodontal disease is a multifactorial cumulative disease; as people age, they are at greater risk for developing periodontal disease. Risk factors associated with aging, for example, decreased dexterity, medications, systemic illnesses, stress, and smoking, all contribute to increasing prevalence in the older population. Choices A, B, and C do not correctly reflect the statements.

28. Which of the following are local contributing factors for periodontal disease? (Select all that apply.)

ANS: C, D, E
Although all are factors that contribute to periodontal disease, only biofilm growth (C), faulty restorations (D), and tooth concavities (E) are considered local factors because of the localized destruction caused by plaque retention. Smoking (A) is considered an environmental factor in the progression of periodontal diseases. Medications (B) are considered systemic factors that may cause periodontal disease to progress.

29. For each numbered component of the immune system listed, select the function that most closely matches it from the list provided. Not all functions will be used.

ANS: 1D; 2A; 3G; 4B; 5F; 6C
B-lymphocytes (1D) are responsible for humoral immunity. They are white blood cells that produce plasma cells, which produce antibodies or immunoglobulins and memory B-lymphocytes. The antibodies destroy antigens and activate complement. Memory B-cells will quickly produce antibodies on future contact with the same antigens, greatly speeding up the body's response to the pathogen and conferring continuing immunity. PMNs or neutrophils (2A) are the first white blood cells to arrive at site of injury. These short-lived granular cells begin the process of phagocytosis; release cytokines and lysosomes, which destroy the pathogen; and recruit other inflammatory cells to the site. T-lymphocytes (3G) are responsible for cellular immunity. There are many types of T-lymphocytes or T-cells, with CD4 helper T-cells providing a critical link between cellular and humoral immunity. T-cells secrete cytokines and other inflammatory mediators that increase the inflammatory response and recruit other phagocytic cells and cytotoxic T-cells to the site. Immunoglobulins (4B) are a class of large molecule proteins produced by B-lymphocytes. Some immunoglobulins will become antibodies, but

other functions include neutralizing bacterial toxins, activating complement system, chemotaxis, and opsonization, or coating bacteria for phagocytosis. The macrophage (5F) is a large phagocytic granular white blood cell that arrives soon after the neutrophil in response to inflammatory mediators. The macrophage ingests and digests microorganisms, releases cytokines, prostaglandins, and lysosomes and is the critical link between humoral immunity and cellular immunity. The complement system (6C) is a series of plasma proteins that starts chemotaxis, activates lysis of the cell membrane and phagocytosis, and recruits additional phagocytic cells to the area of injury.

30. All the following describe the plaque biofilm overgrowth phase of early gingivitis EXCEPT one. Which one is the EXCEPTION?

ANS: B
Osteoclasts are activated (B) during the tissue destruction phase, which occurs in periodontitis, not gingivitis. During plaque biofilm overgrowth, pathogens enter connective tissue by way of the epithelium; invaded epithelial cells release cytokines (A), PMNs are recruited by cytokines (C), macrophages are recruited to connective tissue (D), and PMNs destroy healthy gingival connective tissue (E).

31. Which systemic risk factor for periodontitis is characterized by a gradual onset, an inadequate supply of insulin, or the inability to use produced insulin effectively?

ANS: D
Type 2 diabetes (D) results from insulin resistance and insulin secretory defect and is characterized by a gradual onset, unlike the abrupt onset of type 1 diabetes. Many of those individuals with type 2 diabetes can control it with diet and exercise. If blood glucose levels are not well-controlled, the individual is at risk for the development of periodontitis in addition to a number of other complications. Leukemia (A) is a cancer involving abnormal white blood cells. Osteoporosis (B) is decreased bone density with an increased risk of fracture. It is most often seen in postmenopausal women, sedentary individuals, and persons on long-term steroid therapy. In type 1 diabetes mellitus (C), the pancreas does not produce insulin at all, and this type of diabetes must be controlled with insulin, although diet and exercise also help. Gestational diabetes (E) occurs during pregnancy and is often a precursor to development of type 2 diabetes mellitus later in life.

32. A person with uncontrolled type 2 diabetes mellitus is at greater risk for periodontal disease compared with a person with controlled type 1 diabetes mellitus because the uncontrolled diabetic has an impaired host response, disruption in collagen formation, and higher glucose levels in the gingival crevicular fluid.

ANS: A
Both the statement and the reason are correct and related (A). A person with uncontrolled diabetes is at greater risk of periodontal disease compared with a person whose blood glucose levels are controlled, whether that individual has type 1 or type 2 DM. The high plasma glucose levels lead to increased glucose in the gingival crevicular fluid. The increased glucose levels feeds oral biofilm, reduces polymorphonuclear neutrophil function, disrupts chemotaxis, increases prostaglandin and interleukin levels, and affects collagen production. Choices B, C, D, and E do not accurately reflect the statement and reason.

33. Smoking affects the periodontium in all the following ways EXCEPT one. Which one is the EXCEPTION?

ANS: D
Smoking does not affect the accumulation of plaque (D). Conversely, smoking may result in increased bone loss (A) and tissue fibrosis (B), decreased bleeding response (C), and decreased inflammatory response (E).

34. Your patient presents with gingival redness, inflammation, bleeding, sensitivity, and tenderness. There is visible plaque biofilm at the gingival margin. There is no bone loss indicated on dental images. This individual most likely has

ANS: E
The descriptors listed are classic signs and symptoms of gingivitis associated with dental plaque biofilm (E). Chronic periodontitis (A) is directly related to the presence of plaque biofilm and calculus deposits. The gingiva may be pale pink, red, or purple, with inflammation and bleeding on probing (bleeding may be spontaneous) and an increase in crevicular fluid. There is loss of attachment, and dental images indicate bone loss. Healthy tissue (B) does not exhibit any of those signs and symptoms. Aggressive periodontitis (C) presents as rapid loss of attachment and bone. Gingival tissues may or may not be inflamed, ulcerative, and red. Gingivitis associated with an allergic reaction (D) is present with little or no plaque biofilm. The gingiva appears erythematous (fiery red) and may be ulcerative.

35. Rapid periodontal destruction, including bone loss, tissue necrosis, severe pain, tissue sloughing, spontaneous bleeding, and fiery red erythematous tissue, all describe which of the following conditions?

ANS: D
Rapid periodontal destruction, including bone loss, tissue necrosis, severe pain, tissue sloughing, spontaneous bleeding, and fiery red erythematous tissue are all classic signs and symptoms of necrotizing ulcerative periodontitis (NUP) (D). In primary herpetic gingivostomatitis (A), the patient has severe pain, vesicular ulcers, gingival inflammation, low-grade fever, headache, swollen lymph nodes, and a sore throat. In gingivitis induced by malnutrition (B), patients with ascorbic acid deficiency present with fiery red erythematous, inflamed, ulcerative, and bleeding tissue. Necrotizing ulcerative gingivitis (NUG) (C) exhibits the same signs and symptoms as NUP, but there is no bone loss in NUG.

36. For each numbered inherited disease with risk of periodontal disease listed, select the most closely linked description from the list provided.

ANS: 1C; 2E; 3A: 4B; 5F; 6D; 7G.
Leukocyte adhesion deficiency is an inherited immunodeficiency disease with recurrent bacterial infections and impaired wound healing. Neutrophil adhesion defects cause periodontal bone and tooth loss beginning at tooth eruption (1C). Papillon-Lefévre syndrome (2E) is an inherited disease exhibited by hyperkeratosis of the palms of hands and the soles of feet (palmoplantar keratoderma). Periodontal defects are severe, including bone and tooth loss of all primary teeth by age 5 years and all permanent teeth by age 15 years. Cohen syndrome (3A) is an inherited disease in which individuals exhibit developmental delay, a small head, intellectual disability, hyperelasticity of skin, and weak muscle tone. They may have a short philtrum, a vaulted palate, and prominent maxillary central incisors. They are also susceptible to periodontal disease. Chediak-Higashi syndrome (4B) is an inherited immune disorder exhibited by pale-colored hair, eyes, and skin. Neutrophil chemotaxis is compromised, and periodontitis is aggressive. Patients exhibit severe tooth loss in both dentitions and are at high risk for fatal bacterial infection. Extractions are recommended to decrease infections. Down syndrome (5F), or Trisomy 21, is a birth defect caused by an additional chromosome 21. People with this disorder have mild to moderate intellectual disability. Onset of severe aggressive periodontitis at an early age is common. These individuals often have generalized heavy plaque, deep pocketing, and gingival inflammation.

Familial and cyclic neutropenia (6D) are disorders that affect the bone marrow and neutrophil levels. Persons with cyclic neutropenia may exhibit severe bone and tooth loss, in which deciduous teeth and permanent teeth exfoliate as soon as they erupt. Glycogen storage disease (7G) interferes with the storage of carbohydrates as glycogen. It causes neutropenia, which may result in tooth loss at a young age.

37. Periodontal disease is associated with coronary heart disease, diabetes mellitus, preeclampsia, hospital-acquired pneumonia, and some types of cancer. Association indicates causation.

ANS: C
The first statement is true, and the second statement is false (C). Although a relationship has been established between periodontal disease and coronary heart disease, diabetes mellitus, preeclampsia, hospital-acquired pneumonia, and some types of cancer, correlation does not always mean causation. Choices A, B, and D do not correctly reflect the statements.

38. Which of the following nutrients is MOST critical for wound healing and collagen formation in the periodontium?

ANS: D
Vitamin C (D) is critical for collagen formation and wound healing in the periodontium. Calcium (A) and vitamin D (C) are vital for formation of strong bones and teeth. Protein (B) is needed for cellular components, antibodies, collagen, and enzymes. Antioxidants (E) help reverse cellular damage caused by free radicals.

39. Order the five phases of therapy in the periodontal treatment plan. Match each letter with its proper sequence number.

ANS: 1E, 2C, 3A, 4B, 5D
The first phase in a periodontal treatment plan is the assessment and preliminary (1E) therapy phase, which includes data collection and referral for emergency care. Next is nonsurgical periodontal (2C) therapy, or phase I therapy, which includes nonsurgical care, dental hygiene care, and patient education. If the nonsurgical periodontal therapy is not successful, the surgical (3A) therapy phase, or phase II therapy, which includes periodontal surgery and implantation, is implemented. During the restorative (4B) therapy phase, or phase III therapy, dental restorations are performed. Finally, the periodontal maintenance (5D) phase, or phase IV therapy, focuses on maintenance of periodontal health.

40. Periodontal debridement is beneficial for each of the following conditions EXCEPT one. Which one is the EXCEPTION?

ANS: A
Periodontal debridement is not beneficial for treatment of allergic gingivitis (A), which has an immunologic, rather than oral biofilm, etiology. Periodontal debridement is a recommended part of the treatment plan for all of the other gingival and periodontal diseases: chronic periodontitis (B), aggressive periodontitis (C), dental plaque–induced gingivitis (D), and NUP (E). Although referral to a periodontist and periodontal surgery may be indicated for patients with chronic periodontitis (B), aggressive periodontitis (C) and NUP (E), these individuals will usually undergo periodontal debridement as the first step of their treatment prior to surgery.

41. Most cases of halitosis originate in the oral cavity. Pyridine has been identified as the leading cause of halitosis.

ANS: C
The first statement is true, and the second statement is false (C). Most cases of halitosis originate in the oral cavity. Although pyridine is a causative agent of halitosis (oral malodor), the volatile sulfur compounds (mainly hydrogen sulfide and methylmercaptan) are the main causative agents. Oral malodor occurs when sulfur containing amino acids are broken down by anaerobic bacteria and form a noxious gas. Choices A, B, and D do not correctly reflect the statements.

42. Tetracyclines are bacteriocidal. They are broad-spectrum antibiotics that affect gram-positive and gram-negative bacteria.

ANS: D
The first statement is false, and the second statement is true (D). Tetracyclines are bacteriostatic, not bacteriocidal, slowing, rather than killing, the harmful bacteria. Tetracyclines are broad-spectrum antibiotics that affect gram-positive and gram-negative bacteria; they slow bacterial growth and proliferation to allow the host's immune response to respond. Choices A, B, and C do not correctly reflect the statements.

43. The reestablishment of junctional epithelium after periodontal debridement occurs within

ANS: A
The junctional epithelium reestablishes within 1 to 2 weeks after periodontal debridement (A). Gain in clinical attachment level takes 4 to 6 weeks (B). Connective tissue healing will continue at 6 to

8 weeks (C). For the complete reestablishment of junctional epithelium, 24 to 48 hours (D) and 48 to 64 hours (E) are insufficient lengths of time.

44. All the following are characteristics of chronic periodontitis EXCEPT one. Which one is the EXCEPTION?

ANS: D
In chronic periodontitis, the amount of dental biofilm is usually proportionate to the amount of tissue destruction (D). Periodontal disease is transmissible among family members (A), prevalence and severity increases with age (B), and it is the most common form of periodontitis (C).

45. A patient who has previously had nonsurgical periodontal surgery returns for the 4-month periodontal maintenance appointment. The patient presents with visible plaque, increased pocket depth and clinical attachment loss, inflammation with exudate, and bleeding on probing in the maxillary right molar region. There is also some evidence of increased bone loss on dental images. All other areas have remained stable. Which of the following is the BEST course of action?

ANS: E
The best course of action is to perform localized nonsurgical periodontal therapy (E) in the problem area. When the patient's oral home care is insufficient, treatment should begin with nonsurgical periodontal therapy. If the oral hygiene is good, then periodontal surgery (A) may be the best option. Involvement would be more generalized if there were a systemic reason for the problem (B). Increasing the number of periodontal maintenance visits (C) would not benefit the patient until the problem with the upper right area has been corrected, and decreasing the frequency of these visits (D) also would not provide any benefit to a patient who is experiencing problems. Periodontal pathogens are the most likely cause of the problem in the upper right region, and debridement is the most effective treatment.

46. The maintenance interval schedule for the first year after the placement of an implant is

ANS: B
For the first year after implant placement, the patient should be placed on a 3-month maintenance interval schedule (B). After 1 year, the patient should be seen every 3 to 6 months, depending on individual needs. Maintenance intervals of 1 month (A), 4 months (C), and 6 months (D) are not recommended for the first year after implant placement.

47. Which gram-negative, nonmotile pathogen is found in small numbers in the healthy periodontium and in large numbers in recurrent disease sites with deep periodontal pockets?

ANS: C
P. gingivalis (C) is a gram-negative, nonmotile pathogen found in small numbers in the healthy periodontium and large numbers in recurrent disease sites and deep periodontal pockets. It inhibits leukocyte migration and induces an elevated host response. *T. forsythia* (A) is a gram-negative, nonmotile, spindle-shaped rod and is a risk factor for periodontitis. *T. forsythia* is commonly found in the epithelial cells of periodontal pockets and is associated with clinical attachment loss in adolescents. *T. denticola* (B) is a motile, gram-negative spirochete that has been associated with periodontal disease. *A. actinomycetemcomitans* (D) is a gram-negative, nonmotile rod associated with aggressive periodontitis.

48. Dentinal sensitivity can only be managed with the use of fluoride toothpaste because the sensitivity is more often related to root caries than exposure of root surfaces.

ANS: E
NEITHER the statement NOR the reason is correct (E). Sensitivity is most often related to exposure of root surfaces, since root caries are usually painless. Choices A, B, C, and D do not correctly reflect the statement and the reason.

49. Periodontal disease is almost always preceded by gingivitis. Gingivitis almost always leads to periodontal disease.

ANS: C
The first statement is true, and the second statement is false (C). Although gingivitis is usually the first stage of periodontal disease, it is reversible and does not always lead to periodontal disease. Choices A, B, and D do not correctly reflect the statements.

50. To determine immediate success of scaling and root planning, the clinician must rely on

ANS: A
Immediate success of periodontal debridement may be determined by tactile evaluation (A) by using a hand instrument to check for residual deposits. Visual examination (B) would not determine immediate success, since resolution of inflammation takes 1 to 2 weeks. Microscopic evaluation (C) of periodontal pathogens would not immediately indicate treatment

success because of inflammatory byproducts. Radiographic evaluation (D) would only give historic evidence of changes in bone.

51. Order the healing events after treatment for gingivitis. Match each letter with its proper sequence number.

    ANS: 1E; 2B; 3F; 4C; 5D; 6A
    Healing occurs in the following general order, although there is some overlap: Fibroblasts replace inflammatory cells (1E). Collagen is deposited (2B). Collagen becomes functionally oriented (3F). Clinical probing depth is reduced as ulcerated epithelium heals and prevents the probe tip from penetrating connective tissue (4C). Tissue color returns to normal as inflammatory vascular changes are resolved (5D). Stippling reappears as the increased flow of gingival crevicular stops, reversing epithelial edema (6A).

52. The most common form of gingivitis is plaque-induced gingivitis. The most common symptoms of the disease are pain and bleeding.

    ANS: C
    The first statement is true, and the second statement is false (C). Plaque-induced gingivitis is the most common form of gingivitis and is known to affect almost all adults by the age of 50 years. The most common symptoms are bleeding, changes in gingival contours, and redness. Pain is rarely associated with this disease. Choices A, B, and D do not correctly reflect the statements.

53. From the following list, select the three items that characterize gingivitis.

    ANS: B, D, E
    Characteristics of gingivitis include degree of inflammation (B) (slight, moderate, or severe), extent of involvement as localized or generalized (D), and the involvement of the marginal or papillary tissues (E). Bone loss (A) and clinical attachment loss (C) are associated with periodontal disease.

54. Systemic factors may modify the patient's reaction to plaque biofilm. The patient's reaction to plaque biofilm may be caused by alterations in the immune system caused by stress, endocrine-related changes, and drug-induced changes.

    ANS: A
    Both statements are true (A). Systemic factors may increase the patient's reaction to the presence of plaque biofilm. These factors may be internally produced alterations in the immune system in times of intense stress, hormone-related changes, and drug-induced

changes such as those caused by antiseizure drugs. Choices B, C, and D do not correctly reflect the statements.

55. Pregnancy gingivitis is a condition that occurs because the elevation of female hormones cause exaggerated cellular and vascular proliferation, and microvessel leakage in response to oral biofilm. Pregnancy gingivitis is an unavoidable outcome of pregnancy.

    ANS: C
    The first statement is true, and the second statement is false (C). Pregnancy gingivitis is a common condition caused by increased inflammatory response to oral biofilm with increasing hormone levels, and it is exacerbated by poor oral hygiene. This condition is manageable with good oral hygiene at home and regular dental hygiene visits, although it may not resolve completely until after delivery. Choices A, B, and D do not correctly reflect the statements.

56. From the following list, select the three items that are characteristic of the contents of the inflamed periodontal pocket.

    ANS: C, D, E
    The contents of the periodontal pocket include increased gingival crevicular fluid (C), which escapes easily from the proliferation of blood vessels in the adjacent connective tissues. Other contents include virulent bacteria (D), both in biofilm and planktonic forms, sheltered from self-cleansing efforts and oral hygiene techniques. Purulent exudate (E) is often found because of the destruction of tissue and cell death in the pocket. Osteoclastic cells (A) are found on the surface of the bone, not in the pocket, and collagen fibers (B) are in connective tissue.

57. Periodontal disease activity is

    ANS: D
    Periodontal disease has been shown to be both episodic (A, D), occurring in bursts of activity, and site specific (B, D). It often occurs associated with some teeth but not all, and progression varies greatly. Periodontal disease is not continuously active (B, E), but it occurs in phases of activity (exacerbation) and inactivity (quiescence).

58. Bleeding on probing is a sign of active periodontal disease. Bleeding sites are indicative of increasing bone loss and soft tissue destruction.

    ANS: B
    Both statements are false (B). Bleeding does indicate active inflammatory changes in tissue, but it does

not indicate that the site or sites that are bleeding are experiencing active tissue destruction. The important corollary is that sites that do NOT bleed are not undergoing active tissue destruction. Therefore, bleeding is an important indicator of inflammation but is not a marker of active disease. Choices A, C, and D do not correctly reflect the statements.

59. Chronic periodontal disease is consistent with the amount of oral biofilm found in the mouth, including the presence of subgingival calculus. Chronic periodontitis progresses at a slow rate, with short bursts of disease progression.

ANS: A

Both statements are correct (A). Chronic periodontal disease is consistent with the amount of oral biofilm and subgingival calculus found in the mouth. It progresses slowly, with bursts of disease activity. Choices B, C, and D do not correctly reflect the statements.

60. Clinical characteristics such as the rate of bone loss and age of onset are the most reliable distinguishing features between aggressive periodontal disease and chronic periodontal disease because both conditions present with a similar bacterial microflora.

ANS: A

Both the statement and the reason are correct and related (A). Both types of periodontal disease present with gram-negative, microbial complexes with loosely adherent components and motile forms. No specific organism or organisms are found 100% of the time, so assessment of the disease is based on clinical presentation. For that reason, clinical characteristics such as the rate of bone loss and age of onset are the best indicators for the diagnosis of the condition. Choices B, C, D, and E do not correctly reflect the statement or the reason.

61. After periodontal surgery, all of the following postoperative instructions should be given EXCEPT one. Which one is the EXCEPTION?

ANS: B

Smoking (B) is discouraged after periodontal surgery because it may slow wound healing. Patients who have undergone periodontal surgery are advised to eat a soft diet (A), limit physical activity (C), and use light pressure to control any bleeding from the surgical site (D) to maximize and support healing.

62. Which of the following BEST describes the progress of surgical wound healing at the 1-week postoperative visit?

ANS: B

At the 1-week postoperative visit, the clinician can expect to see the wound completely reepithelialized (B), as epithelial cells will migrate about 1 mm per day. Bone (C) and connective tissue (D) will continue to reorganize and remodel for weeks to months before healing is complete (A).

63. Which of the following is the earliest period after surgery when it is safe to probe the surgical site?

ANS: D

It takes approximately 4 weeks (D) for connective tissue to organize and heal sufficiently so that the probe tip does not damage the healing tissue. After 4 weeks, the clinician can expect to attain accurate probing depths, even though some tissue remodeling will continue to occur. Tissue damage and inaccurate probe reading result when healing tissues are probed before 4 weeks (A, B, C). Waiting 6 weeks (E) after surgery is unnecessary because probing is safe and accurate 4 weeks after surgery.

64. In the first few days after periodontal surgery, the dental hygienist is likely to see all of the following clinical signs or symptoms in the periodontal patient EXCEPT one. Which one is the EXCEPTION?

ANS: B

The dental hygienist is not likely to see new caries formation (B), even though the roots have been exposed because of the surgery. Mobility (A), root sensitivity (C), and larger spaces between teeth (D) are commonly noted as a result of the trauma of the procedure and the changes in the gingival architecture.

65. The MOST common type of implant used in clinical dentistry is the

ANS: C

The most common type of implant used today is the endosseous implant (C). The endosseous implant is a cylindrical or screw-shaped titanium implant placed into bone to integrate with bone tissue. This process, known as *osseointegration,* greatly improves the long-term survival of dental implants. Blade implants (A) were early endosseous implants but are no longer used because of the high complication or failure rate. Transosteal implants (B) and subperiosteal implants (D) sit on the surface of alveolar bone, are only placed in the mandible, and are used much less frequently compared with endosseous implants.

66. The formation of an intimate lattice between the implant surface and bone is referred to as

ANS: D
The contact between bone and the implant surface is referred to as *osseointegration* (D). The bone grows into the implant surface with only a 20- to 24-nanometer (nm) nonmineralized interface between the two in the successfully integrated implant. Ankylosis (A) is the fusion of the cementum of the tooth to alveolar bone with no intervening periodontal ligament. Ossification (B) is the formation of bone from cartilage. Mineralization (C) is the deposition of minerals such as calcium and phosphate onto a surface.

67. Plaque biofilm and calculus removal for dental implants should be performed with

ANS: A
Nonabrasive instruments (A), including plastic, nylon, titanium, graphite, or gold-plated curettes, may be used for cleaning titanium dental implants. Conventional metal tipped ultrasonic (B) instruments and conventional stainless steel (C) instruments may cause roughness and increase biofilm retention. Dental implants may also be polished (D), but using a nonabrasive paste such as zirconium silicate is least likely to cause scratches.

68. Home care for patients with implants is very important because they require the same cleaning aids as do patients with natural teeth.

ANS: C
The statement is true, but the reason is NOT (C). It is true that compliance with home care regimens is very important, but the reason is incorrect because implant patients who have previously lost teeth are prone to future breakdown. Patients with implants require specialized oral hygiene aids such as floss threaders and interproximal brushes with nylon stems. Choices A, B, D, and E do not correctly reflect the statement and the reason.

69. Maintenance visits for implant patients should occur every 3 months during the first year. After the first year, recall intervals may be extended to 4 to 6 months if the gingival health is good and home care is excellent.

ANS: A
Both statements are true (A). Implants need to be monitored postoperatively at regular 3-month intervals, after which the interval may be extended slightly for compliant patients who have excellent gingival health

and daily plaque control. Choices B, C, and D do not correctly reflect the statements.

70. Implant-supported removable prostheses should be removed at home daily by patients because the supporting abutments need to be cleaned thoroughly with soft toothbrushes, single-tufted toothbrushes, and other devices, as needed.

ANS: A
The statement and the accompanying reason are both correct and related (A). Patients with removable prostheses must remove them daily to clean them. If this cleaning is not performed, the plaque biofilm will remain and begin to become more virulent as the plaque ages and matures, increasing the risk of peri-implantitis. Choices B, C, D, and E do not correctly reflect the statement and the reason.

71. The expected outcome after treatment is termed the *overall* or *global prognosis* for the periodontal patient. Risk factors such as diabetes or tobacco use may alter the prognosis for the individual.

ANS: A
Both statements are true (A). The expected outcome after treatment is modified based on risk factors. In this example, patients with uncontrolled diabetes have altered healing responses, and smoking slows healing and may mask inflammation. Choices B, C, and D do not correctly reflect the statements.

72. The overall, or global, prognosis may be different from the prognoses for individual teeth because periodontal disease is site specific and may affect some teeth in the dentition more severely than others.

ANS: A
Both the statement and the accompanying reason are correct and related (A). The global prognosis is the expected outcome for the patient. In many cases, some teeth have poorer prognoses compared with other teeth because the periodontal conditions are more severe in those sites. Choices B, C, D, and E do not correctly reflect the statement and the reason.

73. Periodontal maintenance is BEST defined as

ANS: D
Periodontal maintenance is best defined as a periodic assessment and preventive treatment for early detection and treatment of recurrent disease (D). The goal of maintenance therapy is to assess tissues, detect problems early, provide appropriate intervention, and reinforce compliance. Although it is designed to detect disease (A), reinforce home care (B), and perform

periodontal debridement as needed (C), it is much more than each individual element of the process.

74. Successful periodontal therapy, including maintenance, is likely to result in slowing the rate of tooth loss to approximately

ANS: A
Data from long-term studies indicate that periodontal therapy and compliance with maintenance will slow the loss of teeth to approximately one tooth over 10 years (A). Choices B, C, and D do not correctly define tooth loss after successful periodontal therapy that includes maintenance.

75. There is a high dropout rate for maintenance patients because they often do not understand that periodontal therapy is not complete after phase I therapy.

ANS: A
Both the statement and the reason are correct and related (A). Patients often do not understand that maintenance is part of active therapy. Special attention should be paid to helping the patient understand at the outset of treatment that success requires a long-term commitment to regular recall appointments and excellent daily home care. Choices B, C, D, and E do not correctly reflect the statement and the reason.

76. Recurrent periodontal disease may be linked to all of the following factors EXCEPT one. Which one is the EXCEPTION?

ANS: E
Compliance to recall (E) is directly related to successful long-term outcomes, not to recurrent periodontal disease. Systemic conditions (A) may alter healing and patient response to plaque biofilm, making it a possible cause of recurrent periodontal disease. Poor plaque control (B), residual calculus (C), and faulty restorations (D) all increase retained plaque biofilm, which increases the probability of inflammation and tissue destruction.

77. A patient presents with periodontal probing depths of 3 to 4 mm and attachment loss of 1 to 2 mm. This patient would be classified as having _____ periodontitis.

ANS: D
Early (or slight) periodontitis (D) is characterized by progression of gingival inflammation into the alveolar bone crest, early bone loss resulting in attachment loss of 1 to 2 mm, and periodontal probing depths of 3 to 4 mm. Advanced or severe

periodontitis (A, B) involves severe destruction of the periodontal structures, clinical attachment loss over 5 mm, increased bone loss, increased pocket depth (usually 7 mm or greater), and increased tooth mobility. Moderate periodontitis (C) shows increased destruction of periodontal structures, clinical attachment loss up to 4 mm, moderate-to-deep pockets (5 to 7 mm), moderate bone loss, and some tooth mobility.

78. The use of prophylactic antibiotic coverage for dental procedures is recommended for which of the following conditions?

ANS: C
Prosthetic heart valves (C) are considered by the American Heart Association (AHA) to be in a high-risk category for the risk of developing the potentially fatal condition known as *infective endocarditis*, and patients with this condition should be provided antibiotic coverage for dental procedures, including scaling and root planing. Any exceptions to this rule should be at the direction of the patient's cardiologist. The AHA no longer recommends that patients with atrial septal defects (A), cardiac pacemakers (B), ventricular septal defects (D), or heart murmurs (E) be given antibiotics before dental treatment because the risk of possible adverse drug effects outweighs the small possibility of developing infective endocarditis.

79. For each numbered description, select the MOST closely linked term or procedure from the list provided.

ANS: 1E; 2H; 3A; 4G; 5B; 6D; 7F; 8C
Plaque control (1E) is the destruction or removal of plaque biofilm. Scaling (2H) is the instrumentation of the crown and root of the teeth to remove plaque, calculus, and stains. Root planing (3A) is the definitive removal of cementum or surface dentin that is rough or is impregnated with calculus, toxins, or microorganisms. Prophylaxis (4G) is a preventive procedure to remove local irritants to the gingiva, which includes calculus removal. Polishing (5B) is the application of agents to remove stains and plaque biofilm from teeth. Periodontal debridement (6D) is the process of scaling and root planing and disruption or removal of plaque biofilm with minimal tooth structure removal. Endotoxins (7F) are lipopolysaccharides found in the cell wall of gram-negative bacteria that trigger a strong immune response when the cell is lysed during phagocytosis. Maintenance (8C) describes the periodic assessment and prophylactic treatment to permit detection and treatment of disease.

80. From the following list, select three items that will decrease the relative risk of root caries after periodontal surgery.

    ### ANS: B, C, E
    Fluoride therapy (B), retaining one's teeth (C), nutritional counseling, and diet modification (E) will decrease the patient's risk for developing root caries after periodontal surgery. Root caries risk increases as individuals age (A), eat sugary foods (D), lose tissue attachment, smoke or use tobacco products, or fail to maintain good oral hygiene.

81. Clinical response to nonsurgical therapy can be measured with a periodontal probe. Measurement of clinical attachment is computed by measuring the periodontal probe depths and then subtracting the distance to the cementoenamel junction (CEJ).

    ### ANS: C
    The first statement is true, and the second statement is false (C). A periodontal probe is used to measure the clinical response to nonsurgical periodontal therapy. The accepted technique used to measure clinical attachment loss is to take the probing depth and then *add* the distance to the CEJ. The clinician would only subtract the measurement when inflammation causes the gingival margin to extend coronally to the CEJ. Choices A, B, and D do not correctly reflect the statements.

82. All of the following chemical agents are used to treat sensitivity EXCEPT one. Which one is the EXCEPTION?

    ### ANS: D
    Chlorhexidine (D) is an antibacterial agent that reduces plaque and gingivitis. It is not used to treat sensitivity. Fluoride (A), silver nitrate (B), zinc chloride (C), and sodium citrate (E) are all chemical agents used to treat dentin sensitivity.

83. Informed consent is a process that allows the patient full understanding of the disease process, treatment options, and probable outcomes. This consent must always be in writing and signed by the patient.

    ### ANS: C
    The first statement is true, and the second statement is false (C). Informed consent is a process through which the patient gains a full understanding of the disease process, treatment options, and probable outcomes. It is best if informed consent is a written document signed by the patient, but the patient and provider may engage in a verbal contract that is also a binding agreement. Choices A, B, and D do not correctly reflect the statements.

84. Continuous or intermittent closure of the jaws under vertical pressure is termed

    ### ANS: E
    Clenching (E) involves continuous or intermittent closure of the jaws under vertical pressure. Both clenching and grinding are parafunctional habits that may be destructive to the patient. Spasm (A) is the involuntary contraction of a muscle or muscles, often painful and interfering with function. Trismus (B) describes a spasm in the masticatory muscles associated with a disturbance in the trigeminal nerve. Bruxism (C) is a grinding or gnashing of teeth, usually during sleep, and may cause pain and discomfort in the jaw. Myalgia (D) describes pain in a muscle.

85. A less common form of aggressive periodontal disease, referred to as *necrotizing ulcerative gingivitis* (NUG), features specific, identifiable bacterial species. Symptoms of NUG include sudden onset, pain, pseudomembranous film on the papillae, and very bad breath.

    ### ANS: A
    Both statements are true (A). The bacteria most associated with NUG are spirochetes and fusiforms, most notably *Prevotella intermedia.* Symptoms such as sudden onset, pain, pseudomembranous film on the papillae, and very bad breath are pathognomonic of the disease. Choices B, C, and D do not correctly reflect the statements.

86. The dental hygienist should refrain from treating patients with primary herpetic gingivostomatitis because it is a viral infection characterized by pain in the gingiva, fever, malaise, and vesicle formation.

    ### ANS: B
    Both the statement and the reason are correct but NOT related (B). The dental hygienist should not treat individuals with primary herpetic gingivostomatitis, which is a viral infection characterized by gingival pain, fever, malaise, and vesicle formation. However, the statement is not related to the reason. The dental hygienist should refrain from treating primary herpetic gingivostomatitis because it is a highly infectious disease and the hygienist is at risk for developing secondary infections such as herpetic whitlow of the finger or herpetic infection of the cornea. There is also the danger that dental hygiene treatment may spread the herpetic infection to other sites on the patient. Choices A, C, D, and E do not correctly reflect the statement and the reason.

87. The relationship of the accumulation of plaque biofilm and the development of gingivitis is well documented. The dental hygienist is responsible for treating and preventing recurrence of the condition.

ANS: C
The first statement is true, and the second statement is false (C). Plaque biofilm is the causative agent of gingivitis in an otherwise healthy patient. Even in cases in which underlying systemic conditions exist, improved plaque control will improve oral health. Although it is the primary responsibility of the dental hygienist to assess the gingival condition, educate the patient, and treat the gingivitis, the patient must take an active role in therapy to prevent recurrence of the disease. Choices A, B, and D do not correctly reflect the statements.

88. At the 4-week reevaluation appointment of multiple sessions of nonsurgical therapy, the dental hygienist identifies that three specific areas of the periodontium have not responded to phase I therapy. The BEST course of action is to

ANS: C
During the reevaluation appointment, if areas of the periodontium have not healed as expected, those areas should be retreated (C). Retreatment would include scaling and root planning to remove residual calculus, reviewing and possibly modifying home care techniques, and possible use of antimicrobial agents. Referral to a periodontist (A) would be appropriate if the retreatment is unsuccessful. Placement of a local delivery antimicrobial agent (B) is recommended after retreatment as an adjunctive therapy. If the patient did not respond to retreatment, the dental hygienist could refer the patient for a medical consultation, on the assumption that there is an underlying systemic condition inhibiting healing (D); however, treatment failure is usually from failure to remove sufficient biologic irritants such as biofilm and calculus.

89. For each of the descriptions listed, select the MOST closely linked process from the list provided.

ANS: 1D; 2A; 3B; 4F; 5C; 6E
Abfraction (1D) describes wedge-shaped lesions located close to the CEJ, believed to be caused by flexing of the tooth surface from excessive occlusal forces. Erosion (2A) is the loss of enamel and dentin from the chemical action of dietary and gastric acids. Attrition (3B) is wear from tooth-to-tooth functional contact. Abrasion (4F) is tooth wear as a result of excessive forces exerted by a foreign object. Fenestration (5C) is a window in the bone covering the facial surface of a root. Dehiscence (6E) is a denuded area of bone on the root surface.

90. Which characteristic is MOST indicative of an endodontic abscess?

ANS: D
An endodontic abscess will typically have an apical radiolucency (D) in a nonvital tooth. Tooth vitality (B) and constant (A), localized (C) pain are more indicative of a periodontal abscess.

91. The presence of calculus is almost always associated with bacterial plaque biofilm because calculus is the plaque biofilm mineralized by salivary calcium and phosphate salts.

ANS: A
Both the statement and the reason are correct and related (A). Although calculus is not an etiologic agent of periodontal disease by itself, is virtually always associated with plaque biofilm, which is the etiologic agent of periodontal disease. Calculus is plaque biofilm mineralized by calcium and phosphate salts found in saliva, and its rough surface facilitates additional plaque attachment, so its removal is associated with improved periodontal health. Choices B, C, and D do not correctly reflect the statement and the reason.

92. Which of the following scaling instruments is primarily designed to remove heavy, supragingival calculus?

ANS: A
Sickle scalers (A) are primarily designed to remove heavy supragingival calculus. The sickle tip ends in a sharp point, making it difficult to adapt for scaling subgingivally into periodontal pockets. The sickle has two cutting edges on each blade that can be adapted to break off ledges of calculus. Universal curettes (B) are designed to be used in any area of the mouth but are not designed for removal of heavy calculus. The universal curette has a rounded toe that can be adapted both supragingivally and subgingivally, with two parallel cutting edges. Ultrasonic scalers (C) may be used for removal of heavy calculus with the appropriate tip; however, they are not specifically designed for this purpose. Extended shank curettes (D) have extra-long terminal shanks with a rounded toe to allow access to deep periodontal pockets, but the thin shank is not designed to remove heavy calculus. Area-specific curettes (E) have a rounded toe and a lower cutting edge that adapts to specific surfaces of specific teeth. The rounded toe allows subgingival access as well as supragingival access, but these instruments are considered finishing instruments for the removal of fine calculus.

93. The removal of plaque biofilm may be accomplished with power-driven scalers at a level comparable with

that of hand instrumentation. There is no antimicrobial effect to the periodontal pocket from ultrasonic instrumentation.

ANS: C
The first statement is true, and the second statement is false (C). Ultrasonic instrumentation is remarkably efficient at removing plaque biofilm from root surfaces. Cavitation, the inwardly collapsing bubbles of water that are produced as the stream touches the vibrating tip, appears to have an antimicrobial effect in lysing the bacterial walls and flushing debris out of the pockets. Choices A, B, and D do not correctly reflect the statements.

94. Match each numbered organism to the period in which it appears within undisturbed plaque biofilm.

ANS: 1C; 2A; 3B
Plaque develops in stages and over a period. As the length of time increases, the strains of bacteria change from mainly aerobic and facultative anaerobic, nonmotile, gram-positive cocci to motile, anaerobic, gram-negative species. Days 1 to 2 (2A) consist primarily of *S. mutans* and *S. sanguis*. During days 4 to 7 (3B), filamentous rods and fusobacteria increase, with vibrios and spirochetes (1C) appearing in large numbers during days 7 to 14. Plaque biofilm is considered mature when large numbers of vibrios and spirochetes are present.

95. *Coaggregation* is defined as the ability of

ANS: D
Coaggregation is the ability of new bacterial strains to attach to existing bacteria (D), or the direct attachment between the surface components of two species. The ability of current strains to multiply (A) is colonization. Chemical signaling (B) is the ability of bacteria in biofilms to communicate. The calcification of biofilm to become calculus (C) is mineralization.

96. For each numbered periodontal ligament (PDL) fiber group listed, select the MOST closely linked major function from the list provided.

ANS: 1C; 2D; 3A; 4E; 5B
Alveolar crest fibers (1C) retain the tooth in the socket and oppose lateral forces. These fibers are the most coronal of the PDL fibers. Horizontal fibers (2D) attach the root surface to alveolar bone, running perpendicular from cementum to bone. Oblique fibers (3A) are the largest group of periodontal fiber bundles; they transfer occlusal pressure to tension on the bone strengthening the alveolar bone

with mastication. Apical fibers (4E) are probably suspensory because they do not occur in erupting teeth. Interradicular fibers (5B) are suspensory and protect interradicular bone; they are present only in multirooted teeth.

97. Phase II periodontal therapy involves surgery, which is the intentional cutting of soft tissue to control disease or change the size and shape of tissues. The MAJOR benefit and indication for periodontal surgery is elimination of periodontal pockets.

ANS: C
The first statement is true, and the second statement is false (C). Phase II periodontal therapy involves surgery, which is the intentional cutting of soft tissue to control periodontal disease. The MAJOR benefit and indication for periodontal surgery is to gain access the root surfaces for root planing and scaling. Elimination or reduction of periodontal pockets often occurs when the pockets are accessible and effective debridement of the root surfaces can take place. Choices A, B, and D do not correctly reflect the statements.

98. Pockets with the junctional epithelium coronal to the alveolar crest are termed

ANS: A
In suprabony (A) periodontal pockets, the base of the pocket lies above the crest of alveolar bone. Suprabony pockets are most often associated with horizontal bone loss and chronic periodontitis. Biologic width (B) refers to the 1 to 2 mm of connective tissue attachment covered by epithelium between the junctional epithelium and the crest of alveolar bone. If bone loss occurs too rapidly, biologic width may be violated, creating a defect in biologic width. The base of the intrabony or infrabony (C) pocket is apical to the crest of alveolar bone; intrabony or infrabony pockets are most often associated with vertical bone loss, traumatic occlusion, and aggressive periodontal disease.

99. Which procedure is NOT an indication for periodontal surgery?

ANS: B
Procedures for repair of clefts (B) are not indications for periodontal surgery. The generally accepted indications for periodontal surgery include procedures to access root surfaces (A), procedures for pocket reduction or elimination (C), procedures for correcting mucogingival defects (D), procedures for treatment of osseous defects, and procedures to promote new attachments.

100. Oral irrigation is an adjunctive method for the arrest and control of gingival infections. Professional oral irrigation is more effective in control of oral biofilm and inflammation than daily home oral irrigation.

ANS: C

The first statement is true, and the second statement is false (C). Oral irrigation is an adjunctive method used when trying to control and arrest gingival infections. Oral irrigation is most effective when used on a daily basis as part of home care compared with professional irrigation, which occurs infrequently. The continuous daily detoxification and disruption of the oral biofilm is critical to controlling inflammation. It is important to stress to the patient that brushing and flossing are still necessary because complete plaque removal is not achieved through oral irrigation. Choices A, B, and D do not correctly reflect the statements.

101. Which of the following procedures is defined as the removal of alveolar bone with the supporting periodontal ligament fibers?

ANS: B

If the periodontal ligament fibers that support the tooth are removed with alveolar bone, it is termed an *osteoectomy* (B). If only bony ledges or nonsupporting bone are removed, the procedure is termed *osteoplasty* (A). These two procedures are often performed together. *Gingivectomy* (C) is the surgical removal of portions of the gingiva, usually for treatment of gingival overgrowth. *Gingivoplasty* (D) refers to the recontouring or shaping of the gingival tissue, often done in conjunction with gingivectomy.

102. Osseous defects are classified by the number of walls of the remaining supporting alveolar bone. A one-wall defect would have the best prognosis.

ANS: C

The first statement is true, and the second statement is false (C). Osseous defects are classified by the number of walls of the remaining supporting alveolar bone. The amount of remaining bone is important in determining whether periodontal surgery will be beneficial. A three-wall defect has three intact bony walls remaining around the tooth and has a better prognosis for periodontal surgery compared with a one-wall defect. Choices A, B, and D do not correctly reflect the statements.

103. For each numbered bone graft, select the most closely linked definition from the list provided.

ANS: 1C; 2D; 3A; 4B

Autografts (1C) are created from donor bone from the patient's own body. Alloplasts (2D) are created from a variety of synthetic bone minerals. They may be hydroxyapatite mineral or ceramics. Allografts (3A) are created from bone that comes from another person, for example, cadaver bone. Xenografts (4B) are created from bone taken from another species such as cow or pig.

104. Which of the following cells is the FIRST to arrive at an acutely inflamed site?

ANS: C

Neutrophils (C), also called *polymorphonuclear neutrophils* (PMNs), are the first cells to be attracted to acute inflammation by the process of chemotaxis. PMNs are phagocytic granulocytic cells that contain granules of lysozyme, which destroys the pathogen ingested. Plasma cells (A) are part of the body's immune response, not the inflammatory response. They are produced by B-lymphocytes and will become antibodies. Fibroblasts (B) are connective tissue cells responsible for collagen production. Mediators within macrophages result in a proliferation of fibroblasts, which produce the collagen necessary for wound healing. Macrophages (D) are phagocytic scavenger cells that can engulf and digest a wide variety of bacteria. They arrive at the site of inflammation after the neutrophils and are involved in both the inflammatory and immune responses.

105. Aggressive periodontitis and refractory periodontitis exhibit the same clinical symptoms. Aggressive periodontitis is recognized by its rapid cycles of disease progression and can be maintained or controlled through regular periodontal maintenance appointments.

ANS: C

The first statement is true, and the second statement is false (C). Clinically, the symptoms of aggressive periodontitis and refractory periodontitis are similar. The primary characteristic of both aggressive periodontitis and refractory periodontitis is that periodontal tissue does not respond to tissue therapy. Aggressive periodontitis causes rapid tissue destruction and is very difficult to maintain or control through regular periodontal maintenance appointments. Choices A, B, and D do not correctly reflect the statements.

106. Osseointegration is defined as

ANS: C

Osseointegration is the structural and functional connection between living bone and the surface of the implant (C), in which bone grows and bonds to the implant. *Peri-implantitis* is a term for inflammatory reactions that affect soft and hard tissues around the implant (A), and it may lead to loss of supporting bone and implant failure. *Osseous defects* (B) is a term that describes patterns of triangular bone loss in periodontal disease, but this term is not used in reference to implants or failure of osseointegration. The appliance that connects the abutment to the implant fixture (D) is an abutment screw.

107. Slight periodontitis is associated with clinical attachment loss of 2 to 3 mm. Slight periodontitis may present with edematous, erythematous tissue as well as radiographic bone loss of 10% or less.

ANS: A
Both statements are true (A). Individuals with slight periodontitis may have clinical attachment loss of 2 to 3 mm. They may exhibit tissues with edema and redness as well as radiographic bone loss of 10% or less. Choices B, C, and D do not correctly reflect the statements.

108. The role of the dental hygienist in dealing with emergent conditions is focused on

ANS: B
The dental hygienist's role in the management of emergencies is to recognize them (B) and make

appropriate referrals. The dental hygienist is generally not allowed to perform treatment (A, C, D).

109. The col is the depression between the buccal and lingual papillae of two adjacent teeth. It is made of nonkeratinized tissue and conforms to the interproximal contact area.

ANS: A
Both statements are true (A). The col is the depression between the buccal and lingual papillae of two adjacent teeth. The col is nonkeratinized tissue that conforms to the interproximal contact area. Choices B, C, and D do not correctly reflect the statements.

110. Periodontitis is a risk factor for all of the following systemic diseases EXCEPT one. Which one is the EXCEPTION?

ANS: C
No studies have shown any correlation between periodontal disease and tuberculosis (C). A correlation between periodontal infections and cardiovascular disease (A), bacterial pneumonia (B), and diabetes mellitus (D) has been established, but does not necessarily establish causality.

## CHAPTER 11

Using Preventive Agents

Debbie K. Arver, Christine French Beatty,
Connie E. Beatty

QUESTIONS

1. Which of the following statements describes the incorporation of chemotherapeutic agents in the control of bacterial components of plaque biofilm?
   A. Replaces brushing and flossing
   B. Supplements brushing and flossing
   C. Recommended for use by all patients
   D. No antibacterial role in plaque biofilm control

2. Which of the following fluoride compounds is NOT used in professionally administered fluoride products to prevent dental caries?
   A. Sodium fluoride (NaF)
   B. Stannous fluoride (SnF_2)
   C. Acidulated phosphate fluoride (APF)
   D. Sodium monofluorophosphate (MFP)

3. For each chemotherapeutic agent listed, select the MOST closely linked description on the agent's use from the list provided.

Chemotherapeutic Agent	Use
_____ 1. MI paste and NuvaMin	A. Added to dentifrices to control gingivitis as well as dental caries; does not usually cause staining at the low dose required for dentifrice
_____ 2. Hydrogen peroxide	B. Added to dentifrices to control formation of supramarginal calculus

Chemotherapeutic Agent	Use
_____ 3. Pyrophosphates	C. Complex of casein phosphopeptides and amorphous calcium phosphate; used to manage dental caries by enhancing remineralization, especially in patients with inadequate saliva
_____ 4. Quaternary ammonium compound	D. Broad-spectrum antimicrobial detergent formulation added to dentifrices as an antiplaque, antigingivitis, and antiinflammatory agent
_____ 5. Recaldent chewing gum	E. Only fluoride used for water fluoridation and in professionally applied fluoride treatments
_____ 6. Sodium fluoride	F. Releases oxygen for antimicrobial effect to reduce gingivitis and malodor; used in treatment of NUG
_____ 7. Sodium bicarbonate	G. Mouth rinse that binds to oral tissues; side effects include a burning sensation in the oral soft tissues and epithelial desquamation
_____ 8. Stannous fluoride	H. Amorphous calcium phosphate complex added to prophylaxis paste and professionally dispensed dentifrice to enhance remineralization
_____ 9. Triclosan	I. Used to neutralize acid after vomiting in patients with bulimia or those undergoing chemotherapy

4. Which of the following additives has been shown to control dental caries by preventing the transmission of cariogenic bacteria from mother to infant?
   A. Xylitol
   B. Sorbitol
   C. Triclosan
   D. Stannous fluoride
   E. Hydrogen peroxide

5. Which of the following over-the-counter mouthrinses has been accepted by the ADA and approved by the FDA to control and treat plaque biofilm and gingivitis?
   A. Chlorine dioxide
   B. Chlorhexidine gluconate (Peridex)
   C. Essential oils (Listerine and generic versions)
   D. Cetylpridinium chloride (CPC), Crest Pro-Health, Scope

6. All the following are effective ways to control volatile sulfur compounds (VSC)–producing organisms that cause breath malodor EXCEPT one. Which one is the EXCEPTION?
   A. Using breath mints
   B. Brushing the tongue
   C. Rinsing with Listerine
   D. Using a tongue scraper

7. Chlorhexidine has been shown to be effective as an antimicrobial to control dental caries in patients who are at high risk for caries. The recommended protocol is the same as that used to control gingivitis.
   A. Both statements are true.
   B. Both statements are false.
   C. The first statement is true, and the second statement is false.
   D. The first statement is false, and the second statement is true.

8. Which of the following is considered the major mechanism of action of fluoride in the inhibition of dental caries progression?
   A. Antimicrobial effect on acidogenic bacteria
   B. Enhancement of remineralization in the demineralization–remineralization cycle
   C. Formation of fluorapatite during the development of enamel prior to eruption
   D. Inhibition of demineralization through fluoride adsorption by enamel mineral crystals

9. Which of the following dentifrice ingredients should be avoided if a nonabrasive dentifrice is recommended?
   A. Triclosan
   B. Baking soda
   C. Stannous fluoride
   D. Carbamide peroxide

10. Which of the following actions should be performed *before* the placement of dental sealants?
    A. Application of fluoride
    B. Dental prophylaxis
    C. Caries risk assessment
    D. Oral hygiene instruction

11. Pit and fissure sealants should be used in combination with fluorides for prevention of other types of caries because they are primarily effective in preventing pit and fissure caries.
    A. Both the statement and reason are correct and related.
    B. Both the statement and reason are correct but not related.
    C. The statement is correct, but the reason is not.
    D. The statement is NOT correct, but the reason is correct.
    E. NEITHER the statement NOR the reason is correct.

12. The emphasis in toothbrushing instruction to prevent and control gingivitis and mild to moderate periodontitis should be on developing and maintaining an effective technique. The emphasis on toothbrushing to prevent and control dental caries should be on increasing the frequency and duration of brushing with fluoride toothpaste.
    A. Both statements are true.
    B. Both statements are false.
    C. The first statement is true, and the second statement is false.
    D. The first statement is false, and the second statement is true.

13. Which of the following foods naturally contains the MOST fluoride?
    A. Fish and tea
    B. Meats and eggs
    C. Milk and cheese
    D. Fruits and vegetables

14. Fluoride is stored in the body in which of the following two locations?
    A. Blood
    B. Liver
    C. Saliva
    D. Teeth
    E. Bones

15. Ingested fluoride is excreted primarily through saliva. Excretion of fluoride through saliva is the reason that water fluoridation has posteruptive caries reduction benefits in both children and adults.
    A. Both statements are true.
    B. Both statements are false.
    C. The first statement is true, and the second statement is false.
    D. The first statement is false, and the second statement is true.

16. Fluoride supplements are recommended by the FDA because research has shown them to be safe to the developing fetus. Research has demonstrated that fetal plasma fluoride levels increase as a result of prenatal fluoride supplementation, but the benefit of prenatal fluoride to the child is minimal.
    A. Both statements are true.
    B. Both statements are false.
    C. The first statement is true, and the second statement is false.
    D. The first statement is false, and the second statement is true.

17. Which of the following first aid steps should be taken FIRST if a child swallows a toxic dose of fluoride?
    A. Have the child drink milk
    B. Induce vomiting
    C. Administer cardiopulmonary resuscitation (CPR)
    D. Administer oxygen

18. When the fluoride ion replaces the hydroxyl ion in the enamel structure, which of the following is the MOST stable result?
    A. Fluorapatite
    B. Hydroxyapatite
    C. Carbonated apatite

19. Which of the following statements is MOST correct regarding the benefits of water fluoridation?
    A. The benefits of water fluoridation continue even after it is discontinued.
    B. Water fluoridation does not benefit adults because their teeth have already erupted.
    C. Partial exposure to water fluoridation provides benefits in proportion to the amount of fluoride in the water.
    D. Because of current multiple exposures to fluorides, water fluoridation is no longer considered cost effective and is not recommended by public health experts.

20. Which of the following is the MOST commonly used fluoride compound in water fluoridation?
    A. Sodium fluoride
    B. Stannous fluoride
    C. Hydrofluosilicic acid
    D. Sodium silicofluoride

21. Mild to moderate fluorosis occurs at which of the following parts per million (ppm) levels?
    A. < 1 ppm
    B. > 2 ppm
    C. > 5 ppm
    D. > 10 ppm

22. Which of the following are benefits of water fluoridation? (Select all that apply.)
    A. Greater overall oral health
    B. Reduction of childhood caries

C. Savings in dental treatment costs

D. Reduction in cases of oral cancer

E. Lower rates of coronal and root caries in adults

23. There are greater caries reduction benefits from combining several methods of self-administered topical fluoride products with water fluoridation rather than one method alone. Combining several methods of topical fluorides and water fluoridation will cause fluorosis in the adult patient.

A. Both statements are true.

B. Both statements are false.

C. The first statement is true, and the second statement is false.

D. The first statement is false, and the second statement is true.

24. School water fluoridation requires adjustment of the amount of fluoride to four to five times the optimal level that is required to fluoridate the community water supply. School water fluoridation is no longer recommended by the Centers for Disease Control and Prevention (CDC).

A. Both statements are true.

B. Both statements are false.

C. The first statement is true, and the second statement is false.

D. The first statement is false, and the second statement is true.

25. A 5-year-old child presents to the dental office in a community in which the water is not fluoridated and the natural level of fluoride in the water is 0.2 ppm. Which of the following daily dosages of sodium fluoride (NaF) supplement tablets should be prescribed for this child?

A. No supplement

B. 0.25 mg NaF

C. 0.50 mg NaF

D. 1.0 mg NaF

26. Which of the following is the LOWEST probable toxic dose (PTD) of fluoride for a child who weighs 20 kilograms?

A. 100 mg fluoride or 640 g NaF

B. 200 mg fluoride or 1280 g NaF

C. 640 mg fluoride or 100 g NaF

D. 1280 mg fluoride or 200 g NaF

27. All of the following statements are true EXCEPT one. Which one is the EXCEPTION?

A. Fluorosis can be controlled in the population by controlling the risk factors.

B. The trend in the United States is an increase in the prevalence of slight fluorosis in children.

C. The new CDC recommendation to reduce fluoride levels in water supplies indicates that some public health care professionals consider the level of fluorosis to be a public health problem.

D. The rate of fluorosis is continuing to increase because of the high level of fluoride in children's toothpaste.

28. Detergent ingredients in dentifrices help loosen debris through their foaming action. An example of a detergent is sodium lauryl sulfate.

A. Both statements are true.

B. Both statements are false.

C. The first statement is true, and the second statement is false.

D. The first statement is false, and the second statement is true.

29. A patient presents with sloughing of the oral mucosa that has been present for 1 week and wonders why his gingival tissue is peeling. Which is the MOST likely cause for the patient's condition?

A. Allergic reaction

B. Brushing too vigorously

C. Inadequate toothbrushing

D. Oral manifestation of a new systemic condition

30. Your patient has just concluded orthodontics therapy and is upset about the white areas in the former location of the brackets. Which of the following would be the BEST dentifrice recommendation for this patient?

A. Anticaries dentifrice with fluoride

B. Antiplaque dentifrice with triclosan

C. Whitening dentifrice to even out enamel coloration

D. Remineralization dentifrice with fluoride and calcium phosphate

31. All of the following are important considerations for a mouth rinse marketed for xerostomia EXCEPT one. Which one is the EXCEPTION?

A. Is nonstaining

B. Contains fluoride

C. Has lubricating properties

D. Has moisturizing qualities

32. One suitable option for an antiplaque mouth rinse recommendation is chlorhexidine. Chlorhexidine is readily available as an over-the-counter medication.

A. Both statements are true.

B. Both statements are false.

C. The first statement is true, and the second statement is false.

D. The first statement is false, and the second statement is true.

33. Which of the following characteristics represent ideal properties of an antimicrobial mouth rinse? (Select all that apply.)
    A. Substantivity
    B. No adverse reactions
    C. Promotes microbial resistance
    D. Targets pathogenic microflora

34. Which of the following products are commonly associated with staining of teeth, tongue, and tooth-colored restorations? (Select all that apply.)
    A. Listerine
    B. Chlorhexidine
    C. Stannous fluoride
    D. Crest Pro-Health

35. Sugar-free gums primarily use xylitol or sorbitol for their sweetening agents. Chewing gum may be a useful home care recommendation to stimulate saliva.
    A. Both statements are true.
    B. Both statements are false.
    C. The first statement is true, and the second statement is false.
    D. The first statement is false, and the second statement is true.

36. Which of the following situations are indications for placement of a dental sealant? (Select all that apply.)
    A. A deep occlusal fissure
    B. An incipient Class I carious lesion
    C. A deep dentinal Class I carious lesion
    D. Shallow fissures in an adult with no history of caries

37. Which of the following BEST describes the purpose of using an etchant or tooth conditioner during the sealant application process?
    A. Bonds the sealant material to the tooth
    B. Increases the surface area for the sealant material
    C. Removes debris and stain from the surface to be sealed
    D. Enhances uptake of fluoride from the sealant material

38. If a sealant was lost within the first couple of months after application, which would be the MOST likely cause of failure?
    A. Operator error
    B. Carious lesions
    C. Expired materials
    D. Patient compliance

39. Sealant material often contains filler particles. The purpose of the filler is to make the sealant more resistant to abrasion and wear.
    A. Both statements are true.
    B. Both statements are false.

C. The first statement is true, and the second statement is false.
D. The first statement is false, and the second statement is true.

40. Modern sealant products polymerize or "cure" through use of a blue light source. The disadvantage of using a light-cured system is that clinicians may experience wrist fatigue if necessary precautions are not utilized.
    A. Both statements are true.
    B. Both statements are false.
    C. The first statement is true, and the second statement is false.
    D. The first statement is false, and the second statement is true.

41. Which of the following BEST describes the purpose for the use of a sealant material with fluoride added?
    A. It increases the long-term retention of the sealant.
    B. It adds to the resistance against wear and abrasion.
    C. It acts as a long-term reservoir for fluoride in the oral cavity.
    D. It inhibits caries growth in the enamel surrounding the sealant.

42. When preparing a tooth for sealant placement, the amount of time required for the acid etchant to remain in place depends on the operator's clinical judgment. If the tooth surface presents with a white chalky or frosty appearance on drying after rinsing the etchant, it is a good clinical indicator that the etching period was insufficient and should be repeated.
    A. Both statements are true.
    B. Both statements are false.
    C. The first statement is true, and the second statement is false.
    D. The first statement is false, and the second statement is true.

43. Which of the following represents the ADA's recommendation for maintaining a dry field during sealant placement?
    A. Use of cotton rolls
    B. Use absorbent pads
    C. Use of a rubber dam
    D. Use of two operators

44. Which of the following strategies serve as effective patient management tools during sealant placement in children? (Select all that apply.)
    A. Use an assistant whenever possible.
    B. Have the parent stay in the treatment area.
    C. Keep the child distracted and calm through conversation.

D. Have all supplies and materials ready before seating the child.

E. Employ the "Tell, Show, Do" strategy to avoid any surprises.

45. Which of the following concentrations of neutral sodium fluoride is considered a professionally applied fluoride (in-office-administration) agent?
    A. 0.1%
    B. 0.5%
    C. 0.2%
    D. 2.0%

46. Which of the following formulations are considered professionally applied fluoride products and have been approved by the FDA for in-office use? (Select all that apply.)
    A. 2.0 % sodium fluoride
    B. 1.1% sodium fluoride
    C. 5% sodium fluoride varnish
    D. 8.0% stannous fluoride solution
    E. 1.23% acidulated phosphate fluoride

47. When fluoride reacts with stomach acid, the reaction product is hydrogen fluoride. The initial symptoms of chronic fluoride toxicity are nausea, gastrointestinal pain, and vomiting.
    A. Both statements are true.
    B. Both statements are false.
    C. The first statement is true, and the second statement is false.
    D. The first statement is false, and the second statement is true.

48. The purpose of converting neutral sodium fluoride into acidulated phosphate fluoride is to lower the pH of the product. Evidence-based research indicates that a pH of 4 or lower enhances fluoride uptake.
    A. Both statements are true.
    B. Both statements are false.
    C. The first statement is true, and the second statement is false.
    D. The first statement is false, and the second statement is true.

49. Which of the following items are considered antibacterial agents for dental caries? (Select all that apply.)
    A. Xylitol
    B. Chlorhexidine
    C. Dental sealants
    D. Sodium bicarbonate
    E. Carbamide peroxide

50. Topically applied fluorides are most effective for prevention of dental caries formation in the pits and fissures of teeth. Dental sealants should be the primary preventive consideration by the dental hygienist for reduction in pit and fissure caries of teeth.
    A. Both statements are true.
    B. Both statements are false.
    C. The first statement is true, and the second statement is false.
    D. The first statement is false, and the second statement is true.

51. Which of the following are the methods of classification for sealants? (Select all that apply.)
    A. Cost
    B. Color
    C. Placement site
    D. Sealant content
    E. Polymerization method

52. The dental hygienist has finished placing a pit and fissure sealant and discovers a bubble in the cured sealant material. Which of the following actions is MOST appropriate?
    A. Using a high-speed hand piece and smooth the surface
    B. Adding more sealant material and polymerizing the area
    C. Leaving the bubble; mastication will remove the imperfection
    D. Reetching, washing and drying the tooth, and applying additional material

53. Dental sealants may be filled or unfilled resins or glass ionomers that contain fluoride. Glass ionomer sealants are the sealant of choice for occlusal surfaces.
    A. Both statements are true.
    B. Both statements are false.
    C. The first statement is true, and the second statement is false.
    D. The first statement is false, and the second statement is true.

54. During the placement of dental sealants, which of the following is used as an etching agent?
    A. 25% phosphoric acid
    B. 35% phosphoric acid
    C. 10% carbamide peroxide
    D. 15% carbamide peroxide
    E. 15% hydrogen peroxide

55. Continuous use of fluoridated water from birth may result in 40% to 65% fewer carious lesions. Anterior teeth, particularly maxillary anterior teeth, receive more protection from fluoride compared with posterior teeth because of the direct contact of drinking water as it passes into the mouth and earlier eruption dates.
    A. Both statements are true.
    B. Both statements are false.

C. The first statement is true, and the second statement is false.
D. The first statement is false, and the second statement is true.

56. Fluoride is added to the surface of enamel before tooth eruption. The uptake of fluoride depends on the level of fluoride in the oral environment and the length of time of exposure.
A. Both statements are true.
B. Both statements are false.
C. The first statement is true, and the second statement is false.
D. The first statement is false, and the second statement is true.

57. Which of the following conditions can be prevented by a fixed or removable prosthodontic appliance?
A. Impaction
B. Supraeruption
C. Occlusal reduction
D. Periodontal disease

58. Which of the following preventive measures can be beneficial in the reduction of anterior disc displacement (RADD) and/or control the symptoms?
A. Oral surgery
B. Occlusal splint
C. Occlusal adjustment
D. Orthodontic treatment

59. Which of the following is a best practice for the use of an oral irrigator?
A. Flush gingival sulcular areas directly.
B. Gradually increase the intensity of the stream to high.
C. Direct the stream perpendicular to the long axis of the tooth.
D. Use in limited access areas without soft-tissue inflammation.

60. Negative outcomes for failure to remove or smooth an overhanging restoration include all the following EXCEPT one. Which one is the EXCEPTION?
A. Bony defects
B. Tissue irritation
C. Occlusal trauma
D. Food entrapment

61. Communication can be considered a preventive agent when a dental professional identifies harmful habits and encourages changes in patient behavior; therefore, the dental professional should avoid discussing a patient's recreational drug use.
A. Both the statement and the reason are correct and related.

B. Both the statement and the reason are correct but NOT related.
C. The statement is correct, but the reason is not.
D. The statement is NOT correct, but the reason is correct.
E. NEITHER the statement NOR the reason is correct.

62. Smokeless or spit tobacco education should include all the following teaching points EXCEPT one. Which one is the EXCEPTION?
A. Causes vasodilation
B. Affects leukocyte migration
C. Fosters persistence of pathogens
D. Increases severity of periodontal disease

63. Which of the following preventive measures is recommended for a patient taking medication to lower blood pressure?
A. Use iodized salt.
B. Limit fatty food.
C. Add zinc supplements.
D. Restrict sodium intake.

64. Which of the following self-care devices is most appropriate for plaque biofilm removal from proximal tooth surfaces and shallow pockets?
A. Dental floss
B. Toothpicks
C. End-tuft brushes
D. Powered toothbrush

65. Characteristics of patient-centered tobacco cessation communication include all the following EXCEPT one. Which one is the EXCEPTION?
A. Listening
B. Collaboration
C. Eliciting of information
D. Emphasis on expert authority

66. Use of a properly fitted mouth guard while an individual plays sports helps to protect against all the following conditions EXCEPT one. Which one is the EXCEPTION?
A. Bruxism
B. Clenching
C. Head injuries
D. Mouth breathing

67. Which of the following is the primary purpose of a mandibular advancement device (MAD)?
A. Eliminate bruxism
B. Increase upper airway volume
C. Replace positive airway pressure
D. Retain tongue in forward position

68. A 65-year-old patient with a history of uncontrolled high blood pressure who is currently taking medication to lower blood pressure and a diuretic presents for an emergency dental appointment. Which of the following preventive agents is safe for this patient?
    A. Sugar
    B. Oxygen
    C. Norepinephrine
    D. General anesthesia

69. A female patient reports an allergic reaction when wearing certain types of jewelry. Which of the following agents should be reduced in the fabrication of her new crown for tooth #30?
    A. Zinc
    B. Nickel
    C. Copper
    D. Chromium

70. Which of the following conditions would indicate bonded retainer failure?
    A. Occlusal wear
    B. Tooth mobility
    C. Presence of biofilms
    D. Stripping of attached gingiva

71. Education for a patient who wears an obturator should include all the following teaching points EXCEPT one. Which one is the EXCEPTION?
    A. Food takes longer to clear the oral cavity.
    B. Soft-food consumption increases caries risk.
    C. Tenacious nature of nasal fluids promotes biofilm retention.
    D. Systemic fluorides are contraindicated due to risk of choking.

1. Which of the following statements describes the incorporation of chemotherapeutic agents in the control of bacterial components of plaque biofilm?

ANS: B
Incorporation of chemotherapeutic agents in plaque biofilm control is always recommended as a supplement to brushing and flossing (B). Chemotherapeutic agents are never a replacement for brushing and flossing (A). The use of chemotherapeutic agents is recommended when regular and routine oral hygiene care is insufficient to control gingivitis, dental caries, or malodor, based on the level of risk of the patient and the effectiveness of oral hygiene. With high-risk patients, chemotherapeutic agents are recommended to control the bacterial components of biofilm (C). Patients who practice effective oral hygiene and are in a low-risk category for periodontal diseases and dental caries do not need chemotherapeutic agents to control these diseases (D).

2. Which of the following fluoride compounds is NOT used in professionally administered fluoride products to prevent dental caries?

ANS: D
MFP (D) is NOT used in professionally administered fluoride products to prevent dental caries, although it is found in many widely used dentifrices. NaF (A), or neutral fluoride, is preferred for professional applications for patients with mucositis, sensitivity, and esthetic restorations. NaF is the active agent in professionally applied fluoride varnish. SnF_2 (B) is available in professionally dispensed gels for dentinal hypersensitivity and as professional rinses, although the rinses have largely been replaced by other professional fluorides. APF (C) provides the greatest uptake when used for professional topical fluoride gel and foam applications because of the low pH.

3. For each chemotherapeutic agent listed, select the MOST closely linked description on the agent's use from the list provided.

ANS: 1H; 2F; 3B; 4G; 5C; 6E; 7I; 8A; 9D.
Calcium and phosphate in saliva (1H) are involved in the remineralization process. The addition of calcium and phosphate to oral products is designed to enhance remineralization. Two professionally dispensed products are MI paste and NuvaMin. Hydrogen peroxide (2F) is used as an oxygenating mouth rinse for antimicrobial effect to reduce gingivitis and malodor, and in the treatment of NUG.

Various soluble pyrophosphate formulas (3B) have an anticalculus effect by inhibiting crystal growth to retard calculus formation. These agents are only effective on supramarginal calculus formation because of the different natures and locations of supragingival and subgingival calculus. Quaternary ammonium compounds (4G) are mouth rinses that bind to oral tissues. Side effects include increased calculus formation, occasional burning sensation, and epithelial desquamation. The most common quaternary ammonium compound is cetylpridinium chloride, contained in Cepacol, Scope, and Crest Pro-Health mouth rinses. Its mechanism of action is the rupture of bacterial cell walls and alteration of cytoplasmic contents. Recaldent (5C) is a complex of casein phosphopeptides and amorphous calcium phosphate, derived from milk protein. Available as a chewing gum, it is used to manage dental caries by enhancing remineralization. Those patients with inadequate saliva are likely to benefit from the availability of increased calcium and phosphate. Sodium fluoride (6E) is the only fluoride used for both water fluoridation *and* in professionally applied fluoride treatments. Sodium bicarbonate (7I) is used to neutralize acid from acid reflux and after vomiting in patients with bulimia or those undergoing chemotherapy. It should be used as soon as possible after the acid attack and is especially recommended to manage dental caries in patients who have inadequate saliva. It is available as a chewing gum and dentifrices or can be used by rinsing with two teaspoons of baking soda mixed in 8 ounces of water, in which case it should not be swallowed to minimize the ingestion of excessive sodium. Stannous fluoride (8A) is added to dentifrices to control gingivitis, dental caries, and hypersensitivity. At the low dose required for dentifrices, staining is not usually a problem. Triclosan (9D) is a broad-spectrum antimicrobial detergent agent with antiplaque, antigingivitis, and antiinflammatory actions when added to dentifrices. Triclosan is the active antimicrobial agent in Colgate Total dentifrice and is approved by the U.S. Food and Drug Administration (FDA) and accepted by the American Dental Association (ADA) to treat gingivitis.

4. Which of the following additives has been shown to control dental caries by preventing the transmission of cariogenic bacteria from mother to infant?

ANS: A
Chewing xylitol (A) gum in adequate amounts by mothers of young children in the first 2 years of the children's lives prevented the vertical transmission of cariogenic bacteria from caregivers to infants. Sorbitol

(B) is a nutritive sweetener that does not promote tooth decay but has not been proven to prevent the transmission of cariogenic bacteria from mother to infant. Studies have not found this protective effect is not seen with triclosan (C), stannous fluoride (D), or hydrogen peroxide (E).

5. Which of the following over-the-counter mouthrinses has been accepted by the ADA and approved by the FDA to control and treat plaque biofilm and gingivitis?

ANS: C
Listerine and its generic versions (C) are the only ADA-accepted, over-the-counter mouth rinses used to treat plaque biofilm, gingivitis, and volatile sulfur compounds producing organisms that cause malodor. Chlorine dioxide (A) is an oxygenating agent found in mouth rinses such as Oxygene, Clo-Syst II. These agents do not have ADA or FDA endorsement, and long-term studies have not shown their beneficial effects on plaque or gingivitis reduction. Chlorhexidine gluconate (Peridex) (B) also has ADA acceptance and FDA approval for treatment of gingivitis but is only available by prescription. Quarternary ammonium compounds such as cetylpridinium chloride (CPC), the active ingredient in Crest Pro-Health (D) have been shown to be effective against plaque and gingivitis but do not have ADA or FDA endorsement for reducing the volatile sulfur compounds linked to oral malodors.

6. All the following are effective ways to control volatile sulfur compounds (VSC)–producing organisms that cause breath malodor EXCEPT one. Which one is the EXCEPTION?

ANS: A
Breath mints (A) will help to mask breath malodor but will not impact the VSCs. Research indicates that 80% to 90% of oral malodor originates from the oral cavity. Oral malodor is caused by VSCs, which are byproducts of bacterial metabolism. Use of chemotherapeutic agents such as Listerine (C) that neutralize VSCs, combined with brushing the tongue (B) or using a tongue scraper (D), is effective against malodor if it has an oral cause.

7. Chlorhexidine has been shown to be effective as an antimicrobial to control dental caries in patients who are at high risk for caries. The recommended protocol is the same as that used to control gingivitis.

ANS: C
The first statement is true, and the second statement is false (C). Chlorhexidine is used in two ways to treat dental caries. Professionally, it is used as a cavity cleanser during restorative treatment. It is also prescribed as a self-administered oral rinse of 0.12%

chlorhexidine gluconate. The protocol for the rinse for control of gingivitis is to rinse twice a day for 30 seconds with 15 milliliters (mL) of chlorhexidine for up to 6 months. In contrast, the protocol for prevention of dental caries is to rinse once a day with 15 mL for 1 minute for 1 week of each month until the bacterial load is reduced, as measured by a salivary bacterial culture. Choices A, B, and D do not accurately reflect the statements.

8. Which of the following is considered the **major** mechanism of action of fluoride in the inhibition of dental caries progression?

ANS: B
Fluorides enhance the remineralization of enamel in the continual demineralization–remineralization cycle (B), and this posteruptive remineralization is believed to be the major mechanism of action of fluoride in the inhibition of dental caries progression. Other benefits include fluoride's antimicrobial effect on acidogenic bacteria (A), the formation of fluorapatite during the development of enamel prior to eruption (C), and inhibition of demineralization through fluoride adsorption by the enamel mineral crystals (D). The salivary level of fluoride is the critical factor in these posteruptive benefits. Water fluoridation continues to have a posteruptive topical effect because it is excreted into the saliva.

9. Which of the following dentifrice ingredients should be avoided if a nonabrasive dentifrice is recommended?

ANS: B
Baking soda (B) as a dentifrice ingredient in whitening toothpastes and should be avoided if a nonabrasive dentifrice is recommended. Triclosan (A) is added to dentifrices as an antibacterial agent and is nonabrasive. Stannous fluoride (C) is added to dentifrices as an anticaries, antibacterial, and desensitizing agent, but is not an abrasive ingredient. Carbamide peroxide (D) is added to whitening toothpastes but is not abrasive.

10. Which of the following actions should be performed *before* the placement of dental sealants?

ANS: C
Risk assessment (C) is the first approach in prevention. By identifying the risk factors, preventive recommendations can be individualized to the patient's needs. Fluoride treatment (A) is recommended *after* sealant application to remineralize enamel surfaces etched during sealant preparation. Dental prophylaxis (B) is not necessary

before placement of dental sealants, although the surfaces should be cleaned in preparation for sealant application. Oral hygiene instruction (D) is part of comprehensive dental hygiene treatment but does not necessarily have to be done before pit and fissure placement.

11. Pit and fissure sealants should be used in combination with fluorides for prevention of other types of caries because they are primarily effective in preventing pit and fissure caries.

ANS: A

Both the statement and the reason are correct and related (A). Sealants are directed toward the prevention of pit and fissure caries. Fluorides have the greatest effect in the prevention of smooth surface caries. Combining both preventive measures provides a comprehensive approach for prevention of tooth decay. Choices B, C, D, and E do not accurately reflect the statements.

12. The emphasis in toothbrushing instruction to prevent and control gingivitis and mild to moderate periodontitis should be on developing and maintaining an effective technique. The emphasis on toothbrushing to prevent and control dental caries should be on increasing the frequency and duration of brushing with fluoride toothpaste.

ANS: A

Both statements are true (A). The effectiveness of toothbrushing technique is important to maximize biofilm removal to prevent and control gingivitis and periodontitis. The addition of fluoride dentifrice aids in removal of plaque biofilm and increases the resistance of the enamel to acid attack. Increasing the frequency and duration of toothbrushing increases the bioavailability of the fluoride to enhance remineralization, prevents demineralization, and increases the antimicrobial effect. Choices B, C, and D do not correctly reflect the statements.

13. Which of the following foods naturally contains the MOST fluoride?

ANS: A

Fish from the sea naturally contains 1 part per million (ppm), and black tea contains from 1 to 6 ppm of fluoride (A). Fluoride is a naturally occurring compound in water and soil, so all foods contain some fluoride, especially those grown in soil that is irrigated with fluoridated water. However, the amounts of fluoride provided in meats (B), dairy products (C), and fruits and vegetables (D) are insignificant.

14. Fluoride is stored in the body in which of the following two locations?

ANS: D, E

Excess fluoride is stored in the hard tissues of bones and the developing enamel of teeth (D, E). Ingested fluoride is absorbed from the acid pH environment of the stomach and upper intestine by blood (A) and is carried in blood plasma throughout the body as ionic fluoride. The liver (B) does not store fluoride. Excess fluoride is excreted rapidly primarily in urine but also in saliva. Saliva serves as a temporary reservoir of fluoride for continual topical benefit (C). The kidneys are responsible for excreting excess fluoride, so kidney health is important to maintain the fluoride balance in the body. Patients on kidney dialysis must use mineral-free water that has been treated with reverse osmosis to remove fluoride and other chemicals.

15. Ingested fluoride is excreted primarily through saliva. Excretion of fluoride through saliva is the reason that water fluoridation has posteruptive caries reduction benefits in both children and adults.

ANS: D

The first statement is false, and the second statement is true (D). The primary excretion of excess fluoride is in urine, not saliva. Saliva is a secondary means by which fluoride is excreted, providing topical benefits. The second statement is true. When fluoride is consumed regularly through water, food, supplements, or all of these, saliva provides continual intraoral bioavailability of fluoride for enhanced remineralization, prevention of demineralization, and an antimicrobial effect. Choices A, B, and C do not correctly reflect the statements.

16. Fluoride supplements are recommended by the FDA because research has shown them to be safe to the developing fetus. Research has demonstrated that fetal plasma fluoride levels increase as a result of prenatal fluoride supplementation, but the benefit of prenatal fluoride to the child is minimal.

ANS: D

The first statement is false, and the second statement is true (D). The FDA does not recommend fluoride supplements because the benefit to the developing fetus is minimal, not because of any safety concerns. This is because enamel formation of permanent teeth occurs after birth and the primary benefits of fluoride occur after teeth erupt following birth. There are no ill effects of optimal fluoride consumption by the mother on the development of the fetus.

17. Which of the following first aid steps should be taken FIRST if a child swallows a toxic dose of fluoride?

ANS: B
The first step in the administration of first aid if a child swallows a toxic dose of fluoride is to empty the stomach of excess fluoride by inducing vomiting (B). Any fluoride remaining in the stomach can be neutralized by having the child ingest a calcium-rich product such as a glass of milk (A) or calcium antacids, which will chemically bind with the fluoride so it will not be absorbed into the bloodstream. Symptoms depend on the amount swallowed and include increased salivation, nausea, vomiting, abdominal pain, diarrhea, cramps, cardiac arrhythmia, and coma, resulting in death if not treated. If symptoms continue, the emergency medical services (EMS) should be activated; the individual should be taken to the hospital, and the stomach may have to be pumped. CPR (C) and oxygen (D) would only be necessary if early first aid measures fail.

18. When the fluoride ion replaces the hydroxyl ion in the enamel structure, which of the following is the MOST stable result?

ANS: A
When the fluoride ion replaces the hydroxyl ion in the hydroxyapatite of enamel, the resulting fluorapatite (A) crystal becomes more stable and less soluble. Fluorapatite is very resistant to dissolution by acid. Hydroxyapatite (B) is the pure form of minerals in calcified structures such as enamel, dentin, alveolar bone, cementum, and even calculus. However, in reality, hydroxyapatite exists in dental structures as carbonated apatite (C), in which it has been contaminated by carbonate and other minerals that make the tooth structure more soluble in plaque acids.

19. Which of the following statements is MOST correct regarding the benefits of water fluoridation?

ANS: C
Even in suboptimal levels of water fluoridation, there are still benefits in proportion to the amount of fluoride in the water (C). Further, even in children who receive the secondary preeruptive benefits during tooth development, the caries reduction benefits of water fluoridation do not remain if it is discontinued because the primary action of the fluoride occurs in the posteruptive period through the salivary reservoir of fluoride (A). It was once believed that the primary action of systemic fluoride consumption was preeruptive, in which case adults would have limited benefit from water fluoridation. However, currently, the evidence for the posteruptive action of fluoride is much stronger, making fluoride beneficial to everyone (B). Although it is true that multiple exposures to fluorides are now available through food sources as well as dentifrices, rinses, and other products, the addition of fluoride to the community water supply still significantly reduces the caries incidence in the population, saves considerably more in treatment costs than the cost of implementing fluoridation, is more cost effective than any other method of caries control, and has social equity (D).

20. Which of the following is the MOST commonly used fluoride compound in water fluoridation?

ANS: D
Sodium silicofluoride (D) is the most commonly used compound in community water fluoridation, and the least expensive because it is a byproduct of fertilizer production. Three fluoride compounds are used for water fluoridation: sodium fluoride (A), sodium silicofluoride (D), and hydrofluosilicic acid (C). The type of fluoride selected by a community is determined by the type of equipment used for fluoridation, which is dependent on the size of the community (the volume of water being treated). Stannous fluoride (B) is used in professionally applied topical gels, foams, and solutions, not in community water fluoridation.

21. Mild to moderate fluorosis occurs at which of the following parts per million (ppm) levels?

ANS: B
Mild to moderate fluorosis occurs at levels of greater than 2 ppm (B). The ideal level of fluoride in community water supplies is 0.7 ppm for all geographic locations in the United States. The Environmental Protection Agency (EPA) recommends defluoridation if water supplies have a fluoride level greater than 2 ppm. At levels less than 1 ppm (A), fluorosis is rare. Levels of fluoride greater than 5 ppm (C) and 10 ppm (D) will result in severe fluorosis in most populations. The EPA mandates defluoridation if water supplies contain greater than 4 ppm of fluoride.

22. Which of the following are benefits of water fluoridation? (Select all that apply.)

ANS: A, B, C, E
There are many benefits of water fluoridation. Reduction of caries results in lower rates of tooth loss, which is a factor in periodontal health and prevention of malocclusion, resulting in improvements in overall oral health (A). Water fluoridation is strongly correlated to reduction of childhood caries (B).

Prevention of caries translates to savings in dental treatment costs for both individuals and governmental agencies (C). Water fluoridation is not related to reduction in cases of oral cancer (D). The primary action of fluoride is posteruptive, so lower rates of coronal and root caries in adults are a benefit of water fluoridation (E).

23. There are greater caries reduction benefits from combining several methods of self-administered topical fluoride products with water fluoridation rather than one method alone. Combining several methods of topical fluorides and water fluoridation will cause fluorosis in the adult patient.

ANS: C

The first statement is true, and the second statement is false (C). Fluoride has a dose–response relationship, so exposure to multiple sources of fluoride, especially in lower concentrations administered daily, increases the caries reduction benefits. High-risk patients will benefit from the combination topical fluoride products to the consumption of fluoridated water. The second statement is false. Fluorosis occurs only when fluoride is ingested in excessive amounts during the late secretion to early maturation stage of enamel formation in the course of tooth development. Once tooth development is complete, any amount of topical fluoride exposures, whether in combination with water fluoridation or not, is not a risk factor for fluorosis. Swallowing of topical fluoride products regularly by young children during tooth development has the potential to cause fluorosis, so children should be supervised when using topical fluoride products. Choices A, B, and D do not accurately reflect the statements.

24. School water fluoridation requires adjustment of the amount of fluoride to four to five times the optimal level that is required to fluoridate the community water supply. School water fluoridation is no longer recommended by the Centers for Disease Control and Prevention (CDC).

ANS: A

Both statements are true. School water fluoridation requires adjustment of the amount of fluoride to 4.5 times the optimal level of fluoride that is required to fluoridate the community water supply. This is based on the fact that children consume less water at school because they are in school only part of the day, a portion of the week, and some of the months. The second statement is true. School water fluoridation is no longer recommended by the CDC for two reasons. The increase in community water fluoridation in the United States and the increase of fluoride availability

from other sources have reduced the need for school water fluoridation. In addition, quality assurance for school water fluoridation is more difficult than community water fluoridation, which has resulted in fluoride spills into the water that produced excessive levels of fluoride in the school water supply. Choices B, C, and D do not accurately reflect the statements.

25. A 5-year-old child presents to the dental office in a community in which the water is not fluoridated and the natural level of fluoride in the water is 0.2 ppm. Which of the following daily dosages of sodium fluoride (NaF) supplement tablets should be prescribed for this child?

ANS: C

For children age 3 to 6 years, 0.50 mg NaF is recommended if the community water supply contains 0.3 ppm or less fluoride (C), 0.25 mg is recommended if it contains 0.3 to 0.6 ppm fluoride (B), and no supplementation (A) is recommended if it contains more than 0.6 ppm. 1.0 mg/day (D) would only be given in ages 6 to 16 for a water supply of less than 0.3 ppm. The ADA has recommended the dosage for fluoride supplements based on the age of the child and the amount of fluoride in the water. Use of supplements above the recommended dose may cause fluorosis. The ADA recommendations are listed below.

Fluoride Ion Level in Drinking Water (in ppm)

Age	<0.3 ppm	0.3-0.6 ppm	>0.6 ppm
Birth–6 months	None	None	None
6 months–3 years	0.25 mg/day	None	None
3–6 years	0.50 mg/day	0.25 mg/day	None
6–16 years	1.0 mg/day	0.50 mg/day	None

Supplementation is based on age and fluoride content of water.

26. Which of the following is the LOWEST probable toxic dose (PTD) of fluoride for a child who weighs 20 kilograms?

ANS: A

The PTD is the same as the estimated lethal dose. It is the dose that will cause toxic signs and symptoms and possibly death and should trigger therapeutic intervention and hospitalization. The PTD is 32 to 64 mg fluoride or 5 to 10 g (50 to 100 mg) NaF/kg body weight (1 kg=2.20 pounds) (A). At the low end of this range for a child who weighs 20 kg, the PTD would be 640 mg fluoride or 100 g NaF (32×20=640; 5×20=100). The amount contained in some self-administered products is the PTD for young children. Therefore, the ADA recommends that the amount of fluoride in these fluoride products that are kept in the home be controlled. There is a need for parent education and parental supervision with the use of these products to prevent children from consuming a toxic dose. The higher levels in choices B, C, and D do not accurately reflect the question.

27. All of the following statements are true EXCEPT one. Which one is the EXCEPTION?

ANS: D
The concern about increasing fluorosis has led to the recent development of children's dentifrices with lower or no fluoride, not high levels (D). Fluorosis can be controlled in the population by controlling the risk factors (A) such as fluoride ingestion during the development stage of enamel formation. This begins as early as 22 months for the maxillary central incisors when children cannot control swallowing during tooth brushing and continues for several years until enamel has formed on all permanent teeth. The trend over the last few decades has been an increase in fluorosis, especially in the very mild to mild categories, primarily because of children inadvertently swallowing fluoride dentifrices (B). The new CDC recommendation to lower the optimal level of fluoride in community water supplies to 0.7 ppm for all geographic areas of the United States is in response to health care professionals' concern that higher rates of fluorosis have become a public health problem (C).

28. Detergent ingredients in dentifrices help loosen debris through their foaming action. An example of a detergent is sodium lauryl sulfate.

ANS: A
Both statements are true (A). The purpose of adding a detergent agent to a dentifrice is to help loosen debris, produce a foaming action, and act as a surfactant. Sodium lauryl sulfate is the most commonly utilized detergent for dentifrices. Choices B, C, and D do not accurately reflect the statements.

29. A patient presents with sloughing of the oral mucosa that has been present for 1 week and wonders why his gingival tissue is peeling. Which is the MOST likely cause for the patient's condition?

ANS: A
Sloughing is most likely a result of an allergic reaction to a product (A), frequently a flavoring, preservative, whitening agent, mouth rinse product, or detergent agent in a dentifrice. The patient should be questioned as to whether there has been a recent change in the brand of oral care product to determine whether that is the causative agent for the condition. Studies have found that the detergent sodium lauryl sulfate may cause mucosal irritation in some individuals.

Cinnamon flavoring is another common allergen. Too vigorous brushing results in trauma, not sloughing (B). Inadequate toothbrushing results in gingival erythema and bleeding (C). Although it is possible that the sloughing is a result of an oral manifestation of a new systemic condition, this occurs less frequently than allergic reactions to products (D).

30. Your patient has just concluded orthodontics therapy and is upset about the white areas in the former location of the brackets. Which of the following would be the BEST dentifrice recommendation for this patient?

ANS: D
A remineralizing dentifrice with fluoride and calcium phosphate (D) will promote reversal of incipient carious or "white spot lesions" by enhancing the uptake of fluoride and minerals into the enamel surface. White spot demineralized lesions often result from orthodontic therapy because of compromised oral hygiene during treatment. The remineralized area is a harder, stronger fluorapatite crystalline structure within enamel that can better withstand bacterial acid attacks. An anticaries dentifrice with fluoride (A) is beneficial but is not as effective as a dentifrice specifically formulated for remineralization. The effectiveness of triclosan (B) is in relation to control of inflammation and gingivitis, not dental caries. A whitening dentifrice to even out enamel coloration (C) would not effectively treat the white spot lesions.

31. All of the following are important considerations for a mouth rinse marketed for xerostomia EXCEPT one. Which one is the EXCEPTION?

ANS: A
Stain (A) is a cosmetic concern and holds no pathologic effects; if a xerostomia mouth rinse causes staining, the stain is easily removed during a patient's routine oral prophylactic treatment. Reduction in saliva results in an increased risk for dental caries because of the important role the saliva has in remineralizing areas of demineralization, so the addition of fluoride (B) helps offset caries risk. Xerostomia mouth rinses are designed to provide artificial lubrication (C) to the oral cavity while supplementing the moisturizing qualities (D) of saliva.

32. One suitable option for an antiplaque mouth rinse recommendation is chlorhexidine. Chlorhexidine is readily available as an over-the-counter medication.

ANS: C
The first statement is true, and the second statement is false (C). Chlorhexidine is used as

an antimicrobial agent to destroy bacterial cell membranes; controlling microbial levels in patients at high risk for caries or periodontal disease. It is recommended as a prescription antiplaque agent (not available over-the-counter) for high-risk patients because it inhibits bacterial colonization and prevents pellicle formation. Its substantivity promotes bacterial suppression for several hours at a time. Choices A, B, and D do not accurately reflect the statements.

33. Which of the following characteristics represent ideal properties of an antimicrobial mouth rinse? (Select all that apply.)

ANS: A, B, D
Chemotherapeutic agents are useful as a supplement to manual plaque removal. Ideal characteristics include: substantivity, or the ability to be slowly released over time for increased (A); FDA approval, which signifies that the products have demonstrated safety with the absence of adverse reactions in multiple clinical trials (B); and inhibition of plaque formation and growth, specifically targeting pathogenic microflora and sparing the normal microflora (D). Chemotherapeutic agents should not promote microbial resistance (C), which would render the agent ineffective against pathogenic microorganisms.

34. Which of the following products are commonly associated with staining of teeth, tongue, and tooth-colored restorations? (Select all that apply.)

ANS: B, C, D
Chlorhexidine (B) is notable for brown staining of teeth, tongue, and tooth-colored restorations. Stannous fluoride (SnF2) (C) may produce an extrinsic black line stain when used for therapeutic purposes. Crest Pro-Health mouth rinse (D), with cetylpyridinium chloride (CPC), stannous fluoride, and sodium hexametaphosphate as active ingredients, has been connected with light extrinsic staining with long-term use. Listerine (A) is generally NOT associated with staining.

35. Sugar-free gums primarily use xylitol or sorbitol for their sweetening agents. Chewing gum may be a useful home care recommendation to stimulate saliva.

ANS: A
Both statements are true (A). Xylitol, sorbitol, mannitol, and erythritol are useful sweeteners for chewing gum because they are not metabolized by oral bacteria, nor can they be used to produce

acid byproducts. Chewing gum stimulates saliva that buffers acids in the mouth and enhances remineralization. Research indicates that chewing xylitol gum specifically additionally reduces the population of cariogenic bacteria. When saliva is stimulated with xylitol gum, it buffers acids secreted by the oral flora; works to flush and rinse debris from teeth; lubricates oral tissues; maintains calcium, phosphate, and other ion levels; and has antibacterial effects. Research has shown that xylitol effectively reduces caries incidence when used in sufficient quantities (6 to 10 g of xylitol gum, chewed three to five times per day). Choices B, C, and D do not accurately reflect the statements.

36. Which of the following situations are indications for placement of a dental sealant? (Select all that apply.)

ANS: A, B
Indications for dental sealants include deep pits, fissures, and shallow fossae so that bacteria, particularly *Streptococcus mutans,* cannot be harbored for growth (A). Research indicates the safety of sealing over incipient lesions as a way of arresting progression of the carious lesion (B). A deep dentinal Class I carious lesion (C) needs to have a conventional restoration, as a sealant is insufficient to stop advanced caries. Shallow fissures in an adult with no history of caries (D) are not an indication for sealants because the caries risk is extremely low in this patient.

37. Which of the following BEST describes the purpose of using an etchant or tooth conditioner during the sealant application process?

ANS: B
Etching the enamel with 35% to 37% orthophosphoric acid removes the outer 5 to 10 micrometers of enamel, creating an uneven, roughened surface. The irregularities in the surface are termed *tags*, and they increase the surface area for the sealant material (B), increasing adhesion of the sealant to the tooth and enhanced long-term retention. Etchants do not bond the sealant to the tooth (A) because sealants are retained by micromechanical retention using the enamel tags. Etchants are not the appropriate material for cleaning the surface of the tooth before sealant placement (C); most manufacturer instructions recommend using a pumice flour paste or air polishing for debris removal. The etchant does not contribute to fluoride adsorption by the tooth (D), fluoride slowly leaches from the sealant material into the surrounding enamel over time.

38. If a sealant was lost within the first couple of months after application, which would be the MOST likely cause of failure?

ANS: A
Failure to obtain sealant retention for longer than 3 to 6 months is almost always related to an error on the part of the operator or clinician (A). Inability to keep the field moisture free during the actual application of the sealant often has been the primary causative factor in retention failure. A carious lesion (B) would not contribute to failure of a sealant; instead, studies have demonstrated that many times a sealant will arrest the progression of an incipient lesion. Expired materials (C) are less likely to cause sealant failure than operator error. Patient compliance (D) may increase the difficulty of keeping a dry field during placement, but an effective operator should be able to employ effective patient management to place the sealant effectively.

39. Sealant material often contains filler particles. The purpose of the filler is to make the sealant more resistant to abrasion and wear.

ANS: A
Both statements are true (A). Filled sealant material usually contains the same or similar filler materials as composite resins: glass beads, quartz, or other particles. The filler particles themselves are slightly more resistant to abrasion and wear, and when combined in a resin-based sealant, they create a more resilient material that can withstand masticatory forces better. Choices B, C, and D do not accurately reflect the statements.

40. Modern sealant products polymerize or "cure" through use of a blue light source. The disadvantage of using a light-cured system is that clinicians may experience wrist fatigue if necessary precautions are not utilized.

ANS: C
The first statement is true, and the second statement is false (C). Light-curing or light activation of sealant material is the most commonly used curing method today. The light source emits a white light through a blue filter, which reacts with a specific catalyst within the resin to produce the polymerization reaction. Long-term consequences of optical discomfort can be avoided by utilizing a protective dark yellow/orange shield, either on the light source or as protective operator eyewear. The weight of the curing light is not heavy enough nor is it manipulated long enough to cause wrist fatigue to the clinician. Choices A, B, and D do not accurately reflect the statements.

41. Which of the following BEST describes the purpose for the use of a sealant material with fluoride added?

ANS: D
Studies currently demonstrate evidence of fluoride release into the surrounding enamel as a means of inhibiting caries growth (D). Although research has shown that fluoride-incorporated sealants have high retention rates up to 48 months following placement, after that, their long-term retention decreases dramatically, failing to add to the overall retention (A). Sealants with fluoride added do not have any additional resistance against wear and abrasion (B). Adding fluoride to the sealant material has not been shown to serve as a reservoir for continuous fluoride uptake and release into the oral cavity (C).

42. When preparing a tooth for sealant placement, the amount of time required for the acid etchant to remain in place depends on the operator's clinical judgment. If the tooth surface presents with a white chalky or frosty appearance on drying after rinsing the etchant, it is a good clinical indicator that the etching period was insufficient and should be repeated.

ANS: B
Both statements are false (B). It is imperative to follow manufacturer's directions, not operator judgment, for using the acid etchant during sealant application. Although some variance exists among products, generally the etching time is 20 to 30 seconds. A white chalky or frosty appearance after rinsing and drying indicates that sufficient time was allowed for etching and that enough enamel tags have been created on the surface to adequately retain the sealant after placement. Choices A, C, and D do not accurately reflect the statements.

43. Which of the following represents the ADA's recommendation for maintaining a dry field during sealant placement?

ANS: D
The ADA recommends the use of two operators to maintain a dry field during sealant placement, allowing one clinician to focus on moisture control (D). Cotton rolls (A) and absorbent pads (B) are effective during sealant placement, but the presence of a second operator is more effective. A rubber dam (C) is very effective in isolating and maintaining a dry area; however, many dental hygienists prefer not to use this technique because of the extra time involved in placement and the potential for patient discomfort.

44. Which of the following strategies serve as effective patient management tools during sealant placement in children? (Select all that apply.)

    ANS: A, C, D, E
    Using an assistant improves time management to enhance patient comfort and maximizes the effectiveness of moisture control to ensure long-term retention of the sealant (A). Keeping the child distracted and calm through conversation (C) is another technique for gaining cooperation with the child during the sealing process. Children have a much shorter attention span compared with adults, so being organized by having all supplies and materials ready before seating the child for a sealant procedure prior to seating is beneficial (D). Employing the "Tell, Show, Do" strategy of explaining, showing on models, and demonstrating the procedure to prevent any surprises orients children and helps calm any anxiety they might have about receiving sealants (E). Having the parent stay in the treatment area (B) is not always helpful because the child may focus attention on the parent rather than paying attention to the dental hygienist.

45. Which of the following concentrations of neutral sodium fluoride is considered a professionally applied fluoride (in-office-administration) agent?

    ANS: D
    Neutral sodium fluoride 2.0% (D) gel or foam is a professionally applied agent available by prescription and used twice annually or as caries incidence requires. Neutral sodium fluoride 0.1% (A) is used in over-the-counter dentifrices twice daily, whereas NSF 0.5% (B) is used in over-the-counter rinses twice daily. NSF 0.2% (C) is used once a week in rinses, also available over-the-counter.

46. Which of the following formulations are considered professionally applied fluoride products and have been approved by the FDA for in-office use? (Select all that apply.)

    ANS: A, C, D, E
    The four high-potency topical fluoride systems that have been approved by the FDA for in-office use are 2.0% sodium fluoride (A), 5% sodium fluoride varnish (C), 8.0% stannous fluoride (D), and 1.23% acidulated phosphate fluoride (E). The remaining choice, 1.1% sodium fluoride (B) is for home care and is available over-the-counter or in the dental office.

47. When fluoride reacts with stomach acid, the reaction product is hydrogen fluoride. The initial symptoms of chronic fluoride toxicity are nausea, gastrointestinal pain, and vomiting.

    ANS: C
    The first statement is true, and the second statement is false (C). When fluoride is swallowed, it reacts with acids present in the stomach; the reaction product is hydrogen fluoride, and this is considered *acute* fluoride toxicity, which produces initial symptoms of nausea, gastrointestinal pain, and vomiting. *Chronic* fluoride toxicity, on the other hand, occurs over a length of time when the enamel is forming and leads to hypomineralization of the enamel, or dental fluorosis. Choices A, B, and D do not accurately reflect the statements.

48. The purpose of converting neutral sodium fluoride into acidulated phosphate fluoride is to lower the pH of the product. Evidence-based research indicates that a pH of 4 or lower enhances fluoride uptake.

    ANS: A
    Both statements are true (A). The primary purpose of converting neutral sodium fluoride to acidulated phosphate fluoride is to lower the pH of the product, which increases fluoride uptake into the enamel surface. Neutral sodium fluoride has a pH of around 7, and acidulation drops the pH to 3 to 5. Evidence-based research indicates that a pH of 4 or lower enhances fluoride uptake. Choices B, C, and D do not accurately reflect the statements.

49. Which of the following items are considered antibacterial agents for dental caries? (Select all that apply.)

    ANS: A, B, D, E
    Xylitol (A) is a sweetener that looks and tastes like sucrose but has the ability to inhibit attachment and transmission of bacteria. Chlorhexidine gluconate (B) is a broad-spectrum antibacterial agent that works by disrupting the cell membranes of bacteria. Sodium bicarbonate (D) neutralizes acids produced by acidogenic bacteria and has antibacterial properties. Carbamide peroxide (E) is found in botanical-based mouth rinses as well as serving as bleaching agent for teeth. Dental sealants (C) are physical barriers that prevent plaque bacteria from entering pits and fissures but are not considered antibacterial agents.

50. Topically applied fluorides are most effective for prevention of dental caries formation in the pits and fissures of teeth. Dental sealants should be the primary

preventive consideration by the dental hygienist for reduction in pit and fissure caries of teeth.

ANS: D
The first statement is false, and the second statement is true (D). Topically applied fluorides are most effective for preventing dental caries formation on the smooth surfaces of teeth and least effective in pits and fissures. The second statement is true. Dental sealants are highly effective in reducing caries in the pits and fissures of teeth and should be a primary preventive consideration for dental hygienists. Choices A, B, and C do not accurately reflect the statements.

51. Which of the following are the methods of classification for sealants? (Select all that apply.)

ANS: B, D, E
Sealants are classified by their color, which may be clear, tinted, or opaque (B); their content, which may be filled, unfilled, or glass ionomer (D); and by their method of polymerization, which may be either autopolymerization or photopolymerization (E). Cost (A) and placement site (C) are not considered in sealant classification.

52. The dental hygienist has finished placing a pit and fissure sealant and discovers a bubble in the cured sealant material. Which of the following actions is MOST appropriate?

ANS: D
Air bubbles leave a void and do not provide effective caries prevention. The best action is to reetch the tooth (D) so that the surface feels hard and smooth and firmly bonded to the tooth. Air bubbles should not be present. Smoothing the area (A) could expose the void and leave an unprotected enamel surface, and adding more sealant material (B) could interfere with occlusion. Leaving the bubble and expecting mastication to fix the problem (C) is not a good solution, since most sealants today are filled and are resistant to occlusal wear.

53. Dental sealants may be filled or unfilled resins or glass ionomers that contain fluoride. Glass ionomer sealants are the sealant of choice for occlusal surfaces.

ANS: C
The first statement is true, and the second statement is false (C). Both filled and unfilled resins and glass ionomers may be used for dental sealants. The second statement is false. Glass ionomer materials are susceptible to wear and loss and are not the best choice for the high rates of wear that occur on occlusal surfaces, even though they contain slow-release

fluoride, which enhances the caries resistance of the tooth. Choices A, B, and D do not accurately reflect the statements.

54. During the placement of dental sealants, which of the following is used as an etching agent?

ANS: B
Once isolated, cleaned and dried, the enamel surface is etched with a solution of 35% to 50% phosphoric acid (B). Carbamide and hydrogen peroxide solutions (C, D, E) are used for bleaching, whereas 25% phosphoric acid (A) is not the standard concentration used in dentistry.

55. Continuous use of fluoridated water from birth may result in 40% to 65% fewer carious lesions. Anterior teeth, particularly maxillary anterior teeth, receive more protection from fluoride compared with posterior teeth because of the direct contact of drinking water as it passes into the mouth and earlier eruption dates.

ANS: A
Both statements are true (A). Continuous use of fluoridated water from birth may result in 40% to 65% fewer carious lesions, with many more individuals being caries free when fluoride is in the water. Anterior teeth, particularly maxillary anterior teeth, receive more protection from fluoride compared with posterior teeth because of the direct contact of drinking water as it passes into the mouth. Choices B, C, and D do not accurately reflect the statements.

56. Fluoride is added to the surface of enamel before tooth eruption. The uptake of fluoride depends on the level of fluoride in the oral environment and the length of time of exposure.

ANS: D
The first statement is false, and the second statement is true (D). Fluoride is added to the surface of the enamel *after* tooth eruption. The second statement is true. The uptake of fluoride depends on the level of fluoride in the oral environment and the length of time of exposure. Choices A, B, and C do not accurately reflect the statements.

57. Which of the following conditions can be prevented by a fixed or removable prosthodontic appliance?

ANS: B
Tooth replacement with a fixed or removable prosthodontic appliance can prevent the occurrence of supraerupted teeth (B) in the opposing arch. Placement of a prosthodontic appliance will not prevent tooth impaction (A). Occlusal reduction (C) is a therapeutic

procedure that aids in occlusal adjustments. Periodontal disease (D) is caused by biofilm and prevention occurs through biofilm reduction and removal.

58. Which of the following preventive measures can be beneficial in the reduction of anterior disc displacement (RADD) and/or control the symptoms?

ANS: B
Occlusal splint (B) therapy can be beneficial in the treatment or prevention of RADD and restoring normal jaw function such as chewing and talking. Oral surgery (A) is a treatment choice rather than a preventive control measure. Occlusal adjustment (C) and orthodontic treatment (D) are not beneficial in the treatment or prevention of RADD.

59. Which of the following is a best practice for the use of an oral irrigator?

ANS: C
When an oral irrigator is being used, the stream of water should be directed perpendicular to the long axis of the tooth (C), just above the interproximal papilla. The irrigating stream should not be aimed directly into the gingival sulcus (A). The stream intensity should remain on low (B). The irrigator is useful in limited access areas with soft-tissue inflammation present (D).

60. Negative outcomes for failure to remove or smooth an overhanging restoration include all the following EXCEPT one. Which one is the EXCEPTION?

ANS: C
Overhanging restorations cause interproximal problems that do not include occlusal trauma (C). Removal of an overhanging restoration is recommended because it can cause negative outcomes such as bony defects (A), tissue irritation (B), and food and plaque entrapment (D), which in turn contributes to periodontal disease advancement.

61. Communication can be considered a preventive agent when a dental professional identifies harmful habits and encourages changes in patient behavior; therefore, the dental professional should avoid discussing a patient's recreational drug use.

ANS: C
The statement is correct, but the reason is not (C). Communication can be considered a preventive agent when a dental professional identifies harmful habits and encourages changes in patient behavior; therefore, the dental professional should discuss all conditions and observations, including drug use, related to the patient and behaviors. Choices A, B, D, and E do not accurately define the statement.

62. Smokeless or spit tobacco education should include all the following teaching points EXCEPT one. Which one is the EXCEPTION?

ANS: A
The use of smokeless or spit tobacco causes vasoconstriction (A) of blood vessels (not vasodilation), which may compromise periodontal wound healing and repair. Patients should also be advised that use of smokeless or spit tobacco affects leukocyte migration (B) and fosters persistence of pathogens (C), which can result in increases in the severity of periodontal disease (D).

63. Which of the following preventive measures is recommended for a patient taking medication to lower blood pressure?

ANS: D
Restriction of dietary sodium intake (D) is effective in lowering the mean blood pressure. Although iodine is necessary for metabolic needs, the use of iodized or plain salt (A) should be restricted in individuals with high blood pressure. Consumption of fatty foods (B) is a concern for patients with high cholesterol (HDL). Zinc supplements (C) can adversely affect HDL levels and should not be advocated for indiscriminate use.

64. Which of the following self-care devices is most appropriate for plaque biofilm removal from proximal tooth surfaces and shallow pockets?

ANS: A
Plaque biofilm removal from proximal tooth surfaces and shallow pockets is best accomplished with dental floss (A). Before recommending interdental self-care devices such as toothpicks (B) or end-tuft brushes (C), the dental hygienist should consider the contour and consistency of the gingival tissues, gingival attachment levels, and size of the embrasures. Powered toothbrushes (D) are not effective in cleaning proximal tooth surfaces thoroughly.

65. Characteristics of patient-centered tobacco cessation communication include all the following EXCEPT one. Which one is the EXCEPTION?

ANS: D
Emphasis on the patient's autonomy, rather than the expert authority (D), places the responsibility for change on the patient. Characteristics of patient-centered communication includes listening (A), collaboration (B) that honors the patient's experience

and perspectives, and the drawing out or eliciting of information (C) to learn about the patient's beliefs, values, and motivation levels.

66. Use of a properly fitted mouth guard while an individual plays sports helps to protect against all the following conditions EXCEPT one. Which one is the EXCEPTION?

ANS: D
Use of a properly fitted mouth guard while an individual is playing sports is not designed to prevent mouth breathing (D). A properly fitted mouth guard can prevent bruxism (A), clenching (B), and head injuries (C).

67. Which of the following is the primary purpose of a mandibular advancement device (MAD)?

ANS: B
The primary purpose of a mandibular advancement device (MAD) is to increase upper airway volume (B) for patients with sleep-related breathing disorders. Although use of MADs may eliminate or reduce bruxism (A) and may be used to replace cumbersome positive airway pressure (C) mechanisms, these are not the primary purposes of the oral device. Specific tongue-retaining devices (TRDs) are used to retain the tongue in a forward position (D), thus opening the airway.

68. A 65-year-old patient with a history of uncontrolled high blood pressure who is currently taking medication to lower blood pressure and a diuretic presents for an emergency dental appointment. Which of the following preventive agents is safe for this patient?

ANS: B
Oxygen (B) is the appropriate preventive agent for this patient, as it will lower the blood pressure. This is designed to prevent hypoxia, which can cause an increase in blood pressure. Sugar (A) may be appropriate for a patient in a hypoglycemic emergency. Norepinephrine (C) is not available for use as a

vasoconstrictor in the United States. Some patients with severe hypertension may be excluded from safe use of general anesthesia (D) as per the American Society of Anesthesiologists (ASA).

69. A female patient reports an allergic reaction when wearing certain types of jewelry. Which of the following agents should be reduced in the fabrication of her new crown for tooth #30?

ANS: B
As a preventive measure, the fabrication of the new crown should include the reduction of nickel (B) as part of its composition because nickel has the highest incidence of allergic response. Zinc (A), copper (C), and chromium (D) are more biocompatible with oral tissues and less likely to cause an allergic response.

70. Which of the following conditions would indicate bonded retainer failure?

ANS: B
Bonded retainers are designed to stabilize teeth and to control orthodontic alignment; therefore tooth mobility (B) would be a sign of retainer failure. Occlusal wear (A), the presence of biofilms (C), and the stripping of attached gingiva (D) are not signs of retainer failure.

71. Education for a patient who wears an obturator should include all the following teaching points EXCEPT one. Which one is the EXCEPTION?

ANS: D
Due to the increased risk of caries development, topical and systemic fluorides (D), along with dental sealants and use of therapeutic doses of xylitol-containing products are indicated. Caregivers and patients who wear obturators to cover palatal defects should be educated about the longer time needed to clear the mouth of foods (A), the relationships between soft-food consumption (B) and biofilm retention, and the tenacious nature of nasal fluids (C) with an increased risk of caries development.

## CHAPTER 12

Providing Supportive Treatment Services

Debra K. Arver, Leslie Koberna

QUESTIONS

1. From the following list, select the three materials that are considered rigid dental impression materials:
   A. Alginate
   B. Agar hydrocolloid
   C. Impression plaster
   D. Zinc oxide–eugenol (ZOE)
   E. Impression compound

2. Model plaster, dental stone, and high-strength dental stone all have the same crystal size and porosity. These three materials are all made of the same chemical, calcium sulfate hemihydrate ($CaSO_4$—$\frac{1}{2}H_2O$).
   A. Both statements are true.
   B. Both statements are false.
   C. The first statement is true, and the second statement is false.
   D. The first statement is false, and the second statement is true.

3. Select the three properties that are associated with agar from the following list.
   A. Flexible
   B. Irreversible
   C. Dimensionally stable
   D. Extracted from seaweed
   E. Complex manipulation

4. The wettability of solids by liquids, for example, the wetting of tooth enamel by pit and fissure sealants, is important in dentistry. A material that is hydrophilic shows a contact angle of 90 degrees or greater.
   A. Both statements are true.
   B. Both statements are false.
   C. The first statement is true, and the second statement is false.
   D. The first statement is false, and the second statement is true.

5. Which of the following restorative dental materials has the LOWEST compressive strength?
   A. Porcelain
   B. Glass ionomer
   C. Dental amalgam
   D. Hybrid composites

6. Which of the following dental cements inhibits the polymerization of a composite restorative material and should NOT be placed under the restoration?
   A. Zinc phosphate
   B. Calcium hydroxide
   C. Zinc polycarboxylate
   D. ZOE

7. Which of the following MOST likely caused the incisal wear to the teeth of the patient shown?

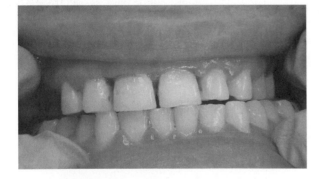

   A. Shear stress
   B. Tensile stress
   C. Reached proportional limit
   D. Lack of compressive strength

8. Select the two materials that will act as retarders for the setting of model plaster, dental stone, or high-strength stone from the following list.
   A. Borax
   B. Saliva
   C. Set gypsum particles
   D. 2% potassium sulfate
   E. Slurry water from the model trimmer

9. Which of the following waxes is classified as a pattern wax?
   A. Boxing
   B. Sticky
   C. Beading
   D. Baseplate

10. Which of the following materials with small particle sizes is intended to remove softer materials that adhere to enamel or restorative material substrates?
    A. Finishing abrasives
    B. Polishing abrasives
    C. Cleansing abrasives
    D. Aluminum oxide abrasive

11. Which of the following compositions is used as a home whitening product?
    A. 22% carbamide peroxide
    B. 30% to 35% hydrogen peroxide
    C. 35% hydrogen peroxide with silica
    D. 30% calcium, phosphate, and fluoride ions

12. Which of the following are uses of ZOE? (Select all that apply.)
    A. Base
    B. Periodontal pack
    C. Temporary cement
    D. Impression material
    E. Permanent restoration

13. Cements are created by combining different powders and liquids. For each numbered resulting cement listed, select the MOST closely linked powder–liquid components from the list provided:

Resulting Cement	Powder/Liquid
____ 1. ZOE	A. Powdered glass and polyacrylic acid
____ 2. Zinc phosphate	B. Zinc oxide and poly-acrylic acid
____ 3. Zinc polycarboxylate	C. Zinc-oxide and phos-phoric acid
____ 4. Glass ionomer	D. Zinc-oxide and eugenol
____ 5. Resin cement	E. Resin and glass materials

14. Which of the following is the term for the uptake of water by a hydrocolloid?
    A. Hysteresis
    B. Syneresis
    C. Imbibition
    D. Viscosity

15. The layer of debris that remains on the tooth after a tooth is prepared or cut for a restoration is known as a/an
    A. adherend.
    B. resin tag.
    C. enamel tag.
    D. smear layer.
    E. hybrid layer.

16. Order the steps involved in the polymerization of composite materials. Match each letter with its proper sequence number.
    1. _____ A. A free radical is formed.
    2. _____ B. Remaining free radicals combine.
    3. _____ C. A free radical reacts with a monomer, forming a new bond.
    4. _____ D. Additional monomers are added to the chain.
    5. _____ E. An initiator breaks down the double bond.

17. Which of the following characteristics apply to composite resin materials? (Select all that apply.)
    A. Used as cement
    B. Sets through condensation polymerization
    C. Expands when polymerization takes place
    D. Macrofilled composites are used most often
    E. Polymerization through heat, light, or chemical activation

18. Before a denture is made, a denture try-in is performed. The denture try-in simulates the proper bite, vertical dimension, and esthetics of the final denture.
    A. Both statements are true.
    B. Both statement s are false.
    C. The first statement is true, and the second statement is false.
    D. The first statement is false, and the second statement is true.

19. Failure of bonding of dental materials is known as *cohesive failure*. An example of cohesive failure would be an orthodontic bracket that breaks off, removing part of the tooth to which it was bonded.
    A. Both statements are true.
    B. Both statements are false.
    C. The first statement is true, and the second statement is false.
    D. The first statement is false, and the second statement is true.

20. Which of the following restorative materials releases and absorbs fluoride and is used to prevent recurrent decay?
    A. Porcelain
    B. Amalgam
    C. Glass ionomer
    D. Methyl methacrylate

21. Which composite would be the BEST choice for an occlusal restoration?
    A. Hybrid
    B. Macrofilled
    C. Microfilled

22. Which of the following are the benefits of adding high amounts of copper to an amalgam alloy? (Select all that apply.)
    A. High strength
    B. Early strength
    C. Corrosion resistant
    D. Increased expansion
    E. Increased longevity of restoration

23. All of the following practices apply when mixing alginate impression materials EXCEPT one. Which one is the EXCEPTION?
    A. Adding powder into liquid
    B. Using a clean bowl and spatula
    C. Powder-to-liquid ratio of 1:2
    D. Mixing ingredients until homogeneous
    E. Fluffing the alginate powder before dispensing

24. When filling the impression tray with alginate, begin loading the tray from the anterior portion of the tray. When inserting the impression tray in the patient's mouth, bring anterior teeth into position in the tray and then posterior teeth.
    A. Both statements are true.
    B. Both statements are false.
    C. The first statement is true, and the second statement is false.
    D. The first statement is false, and the second statement is true.

25. A Class V restoration is found in/on the
    A. occlusal pits and fissures.
    B. incisal angle of an anterior tooth.
    C. proximal surfaces of anterior teeth.
    D. proximal surfaces of a posterior tooth.
    E. gingival third of the facial or lingual tooth surface.

26. It is important to pour up alginate impressions within 30 minutes of taking the impression, because hysteresis occurs with alginate impressions.
    A. Both the statement and the reason are correct and related.
    B. Both the statement and the reason are correct but NOT related.
    C. The statement is correct, but the reason is NOT.
    D. The statement is NOT correct, but the reason is correct.
    E. NEITHER the statement NOR the reason is correct.

27. An athletic mouth guard protects teeth as it absorbs energy and then returns to its original shape and can be used again. This property is known as
    A. toughness.
    B. resilience.
    C. malleability.
    D. ultimate strength.

28. The property that causes gradual dimensional change of a dental material under load or stress is
    A. creep.
    B. fatigue.
    C. proportional limit.
    D. elastic deformation.
    E. stress concentration.

29. Which term BEST describes the intensity of a color?
    A. Hue
    B. Value
    C. Chroma
    D. Translucency

30. Light-cure sealant materials cannot be activated by natural light. The manufacturer's instructions must be followed to avoid overcuring the sealant material.
    A. Both statements are true.
    B. Both statements are false.
    C. The first statement is true, and the second statement is false.
    D. The first statement is false, and the second statement is true.

31. Percolation is a concern with composite restorations because the coefficient of thermal expansion (CTE) is higher in enamel than it is in composites.
    A. Both the statement and the reason are correct and related
    B. Both the statement and the reason are correct but NOT related.
    C. The statement is correct, but the reason is NOT.
    D. The statement is NOT correct, but the reason is correct.
    E. NEITHER the statement NOR the reason is correct.

32. The particle shape of the alloy determines the amount of mercury needed to wet the surface of the amalgam alloy particles. The purpose of mercury is to increase the strength of an amalgam.
    A. Both statements are true.
    B. Both statements are false.
    C. The first statement is true, and the second statement is false.
    D. The first statement is false, and the second statement is true.

33. A portion of the tooth surface has a glossy opaque appearance, exhibits smoothness on tactile exploration, and produces a dull sound when tapped. Which of the following is the MOST likely finding?
    A. Enamel
    B. Porcelain
    C. Composite
    D. Glass ionomer

34. All of the following are benefits of sharpening dental hygiene instruments EXCEPT one. Which one is the EXCEPTION?
    A. Patient comfort
    B. Burnished calculus
    C. Reduced clinician fatigue
    D. Improved calculus removal
    E. Increased tactile sensitivity

35. A study model is a positive reproduction of the structure it represents. The impression is a negative reproduction of the structure on which it is taken.
    A. Both statements are true.
    B. Both statements are false.
    C. The first statement is true, and the second statement is false.
    D. The first statement is false, and the second statement is true.

36. The primary indication for polishing enamel is to
    A. remove stains.
    B. create smooth surface.
    C. encourage home care.
    D. prevent plaque adherence.

37. Which two of the following factors will produce the MOST abrasion to the tooth surface?
    A. Small particle size and regular shape
    B. Large particle size and irregular shape
    C. Abrasive material not as hard as the material that is being polished
    D. High speed of application of the abrasive material with heavy pressure
    E. Low speed of application of the abrasive material with moderate pressure

38. The dental professional is encouraged to selectively rubber cup polish because the polishing agents could remove the fluoride-rich layer of enamel.
    A. Both the statement and the reason are correct and related.
    B. Both the statement and the reason are correct but NOT related.
    C. The statement is correct, but the reason is NOT.
    D. The statement is NOT correct, but the reason is correct.
    E. NEITHER the statement NOR the reason is correct.

39. Professional products are used to polish the restorations at every prophylaxis appointment because these products will not abrade the restorations.
    A. Both the statement and the reason are correct and related.
    B. Both the statement and the reason are correct but NOT related.
    C. The statement is correct, but the reason is NOT.
    D. The statement is NOT correct, but the reason is correct.
    E. NEITHER the statement NOR the reason is correct.

40. Which of the following is an indication for removal of overhanging restorative margins or for margination?
    A. Open margins
    B. Small overhang
    C. Presence of caries
    D. Difficult to access
    E. Damaged restoration

41. The fastest method for removing stain from natural dentition is to use
    A. hand scaling.
    B. air polishing.
    C. an ultrasonic scaler.
    D. rubber cup prophy.

42. Which of the following would be the MOST effective in tooth whitening if all were applied for the same length of time, under the same conditions?
    A. Carbamide peroxide 10%
    B. Hydrogen peroxide 10%

C. Carbamide peroxide 20%
D. Hydrogen peroxide 14%
E. Hydrogen peroxide 5%

43. Your patient is scheduled for placement of crowns on teeth #9 and #10 and desires teeth whitening. When should the patient make the appointment for the crowns?
    A. During whitening
    B. 2 weeks after whitening
    C. 2 weeks before whitening
    D. It does not matter when the crowns are placed

44. All of the following are acceptable home-care instructions for night guards EXCEPT one. Which one is the EXCEPTION?
    A. Air-dry.
    B. Do not expose to heat.
    C. Replace when it becomes worn.
    D. Soak in alcohol-containing mouthwash.
    E. Brush night guard with mild soap and water.

45. Causes of root sensitivity may include scaling and root planing, leaking restorations, root exposure, and caries. Occlusion of open dentinal tubules is the solution for all of these causes of root sensitivity.
    A. Both statements are true.
    B. Both statements are false.
    C. The first statement is true, and the second statement is false.
    D. The first statement is false, and the second statement is true.

Answers and Rationales

1. From the following list, select the three materials that are considered rigid dental impression materials:

   ANS: C, D, E
   Impression plaster (C), ZOE (D), and impression compound (E) are examples of rigid materials. A rigid impression material is one that sets within a specific period into a rigid form at the time of removal from the mouth. These materials have limited uses, since they are inflexible and fracture easily. Examples of flexible or elastomeric impression materials include agar hydrocolloid (B) and alginate (A). The flexibility of these materials at the time of removal from the mouth allows impression of undercut areas.

2. Model plaster, dental stone, and high-strength dental stone all have the same crystal size and porosity. These three materials are all made of the same chemical, calcium sulfate hemihydrate ($CaSO_4$—$\frac{1}{2}H_2O$).

   ANS: D
   The first statement is false, and the second is true (D). Model plaster has very porous crystals with wide variety in shape, requiring the most water when mixing. Dental stone has uniform crystals that are less porous than plaster. High-strength stone has very dense, uniform crystals that require the least amount of water for mixing. However, the second statement is true, as all three materials are made of calcium sulfate hemihydrates. Choices A, B, and C do not accurately reflect the statements.

3. Select the three properties that are associated with agar from the following list.

   ANS: A, D, E
   Agar is a flexible (A) impression material extracted from seaweed (D) and used as the active ingredient in a flexible reversible material controlled by temperature. It requires complex manipulation (E) such as three temperature-controlled water baths and water-cooled impression trays. It is reversible, not irreversible (B), and is not stable stored in air (D).

4. The wettability of solids by liquids, for example, the wetting of tooth enamel by pit and fissure sealants, is important in dentistry. A material that is hydrophilic shows a contact angle of 90 degrees or greater.

   ANS: C
   The first statement is true, and the second statement is false (C). The wettability of solids by liquids is important in dentistry. Examples include the wetting of denture base acrylics by saliva, the wetting of tooth enamel by pit and fissure sealants, the wetting of elastomeric impressions by water mixes of gypsum materials, and the wetting of wax patterns by dental investments. However, the second statement is false. The wettability of a solid by a liquid can be observed by the shape of a drop of liquid on the solid surface. If a low contact angle occurs (less than 90 degrees), the solid is readily wetted by the liquid and is hydrophilic, or water loving. If the contact angle is greater than 90 degrees, this indicates poor wetting, or a hydrophobic, material. Choices A, B, and D do not accurately reflect the statements.

5. Which of the following restorative dental materials has the LOWEST compressive strength?

   ANS: B
   Glass ionomers (B) have the lowest compressive strength and are not indicated for restorations on which heavy stress is generated. Compressive strength is the strength of a material to resist fracture under a load. Amalgam (C) has the highest compressive strength, followed by porcelain (A) and hybrid composites (D).

6. Which of the following dental cements inhibits the polymerization of a composite restorative material and should NOT be placed under the restoration?

   ANS: D
   Cements that contain eugenol such as ZOE (D) should not be used when composites are to be placed because the eugenol inhibits the polymerization process of composite materials. Zinc phosphate cements are powders of zinc oxide liquid made from phosphoric acid and water which fluoride is sometimes added. Zinc phosphate (A) cement does not inhibit the polymerization of a composite restorative material and is safe to use under these restorations. Calcium hydroxide (B) is used for pulp capping and as a protective barrier beneath composite restorations and does not interfere with the polymerization of these materials. Zinc polycarboxylate (C) cement is used for permanent luting of dental restorations. It contains zinc oxide powder and aqueous polyacrylic acid, binds chemically to the tooth surface, and has antibacterial qualities. Polycarboxylate cement does not interfere with the bonding of composites.

7. Which of the following MOST likely caused the incisal wear to the teeth of the patient shown?

ANS: A
Shear stress (A) is the most likely cause of the incisal wear to the patient's teeth, occurring when one portion of the material is forced to slide by another portion as in grinding of the incisal edges of the teeth against each other. Tensile stress (B) occurs when a material is pulled apart. Proportional limit (C) is the minimum stress at which the ratio of stress to strain of a material is no longer constant. Compressive strength (D) is the stress required to rupture a material when it is pressed together and the forces applied are opposite but toward each other.

8. Select the two materials that will act as retarders for the setting of model plaster, dental stone, or high-strength stone from the following list.

ANS: A, B
Borax (A) and saliva (B) left in the impression will retard or slow the setting reaction and may lengthen the setting time of some gypsum products to several hours present if in sufficient quantities. The rate of the gypsum reaction may be altered by chemicals that slow down (retarders) or speed up (accelerators) the setting reaction. Set gypsum particles (C), 2% potassium sulfate (D), and slurry water from the model trimmer (E), which contains particles of dehydrate, are all accelerators of the setting time.

9. Which of the following waxes is classified as a pattern wax?

ANS: D
Pattern waxes include baseplate wax (D), casting waxes, and inlay wax and are used to fabricate a restoration. Utility waxes include boxing wax (A), sticky wax (B), and beading wax (C).

10. Which of the following materials with small particle sizes is intended to remove softer materials that adhere to enamel or restorative material substrates?

ANS: C
Cleansing abrasives (C) are generally soft materials with small particle sizes and are intended to remove softer materials that adhere to enamel or restorative material substrates. Finishing abrasives (A) are generally hard, coarse abrasives used to provide the contours on restorations and gross irregularities on the surface. Polishing abrasives (B) have finer and softer particles than finishing abrasives and are used to smooth surfaces that have been roughened by finishing abrasives. Aluminum oxide abrasive (D) is an abrasive

manufactured from impure aluminum oxide and produced in various particle sizes to clean metals and carve porcelain.

11. Which of the following compositions is used as a home whitening product?

ANS: A
Home whitening products typically contain 10% to 22% carbamide peroxide (A) or 1.5% to 1.6% hydrogen peroxide. In-office whitening agents commonly contain 30% to 35% hydrogen peroxide (B) and 35% hydrogen peroxide with silica (C). Another in-office system uses 30% calcium, phosphate, and fluoride ions (D) to promote remineralization during treatment.

12. Which of the following are uses of ZOE? (Select all that apply.)

ANS: A, B, C, D
ZOE is used as a base (A) to provide thermal insulation to protect the pulp and as a periodontal pack (B) to protect surgical sites. Other uses include use as temporary cement (C) and as an inelastic impression material (D) for removable dentures. ZOE is not strong enough to be used as a permanent restoration (E).

13. Cements are created by combining different powders and liquids. For each numbered resulting cement listed, select the MOST closely linked powder–liquid components from the list provided:

ANS: 1D; 2C; 3B; 4A, 5E
Zinc oxide mixed with eugenol (1D) makes ZOE cement. Zinc oxide mixed with phosphoric acid makes zinc phosphate cement (2C). Zinc oxide mixed with polyacrylic acid makes zinc polycarboxylate (3B). Powdered glass mixed with polyacrylic acid (4A) is glass ionomer. Resin cements (5E) are made of glass materials and resin.

14. Which of the following is the term for the uptake of water by a hydrocolloid?

ANS: C
Imbibition (C) is the term for the uptake of water by a hydrocolloid, or the act of absorbing moisture. Syneresis (B) is the characteristic of gels to contract and squeeze out liquid that accumulates on the surface. Imbibition and syneresis are properties that make it important to pour up an impression quickly to avoid distortion. Hysteresis (A) is the property of a material to have two different temperatures for melting and solidifying. Viscosity (D) is the ability of a liquid material to flow, which is important to achieve good wetting properties.

the object will no longer return to its original shape. Stress concentration (E) occurs when there is a crack or a defect in the material. When force is applied, the material will fracture at the point of the crack or defect, exemplified in cutting glass. A glass cutter is used to cut the glass, the glass is tapped, and the glass fractures on the line where it was cut.

29. Which term BEST describes the intensity of a color?

    ANS: C
    Chroma (C) is the intensity or strength of a color; teeth are rather pale in color. Hue (A) is the dominant color of the wavelength detected; teeth are seen in the yellow and brown range. Value (B) describes how light (white) or dark (black) the color is. Teeth have values in the light scale of value. Translucency (D) is the quality of partially transmitting and partially scattering light; teeth are naturally translucent.

30. Light-cure sealant materials cannot be activated by natural light. The manufacturer's instructions must be followed to avoid overcuring the sealant material.

    ANS: C
    The first statement is true, and the second statement is false (C). A curing light, not natural light, is required to initiate polymerization of the sealant resin matrix. The sealant material can be undercured but cannot be overcured. Choices A, B, and D do not accurately reflect the statements.

31. Percolation is a concern with composite restorations because the coefficient of thermal expansion (CTE) is higher in enamel than it is in composites.

    ANS: C
    The statement is correct but the reason is NOT (C). Percolation is the opening and closing of the gap at the restoration–tooth interface caused by expansion and contraction of the tooth and material during temperature changes. The reason is incorrect. The CTE is the degree to which a material expands and contracts. The CTE for composites is higher (26–40) than that for enamel (11). When there is a large difference between the CTE and the restorative material, the percolation will be greater. Although composite has a larger CTE than tooth structure, bonding it to the tooth structure helps prevent percolation. Choices A, B, D, and E do not accurately reflect the statement and the reason.

32. The particle shape of the alloy determines the amount of mercury needed to wet the surface of the amalgam alloy particles. The purpose of mercury is to increase the strength of an amalgam.

    ANS: C
    The first statement is true, and the second statement is false (C). The particle shape of alloy does affect the amount of mercury needed to wet the surface of the amalgam alloy particles. Spherical-shaped alloy requires less mercury to wet the surface than lathe-cut alloy. The second statement is incorrect. The purpose of mercury is to wet the alloy particles, causing the mass to undergo change and harden. Choices A, B, and D do not accurately reflect the statements.

33. A portion of the tooth surface has a glossy opaque appearance, exhibits smoothness on tactile exploration, and produces a dull sound when tapped. Which of the following is the MOST likely finding?

    ANS: C
    Findings of a glossy, opaque tooth surface, smoothness upon tactile exploration, and producing a dull sound when tapped are indicative of a composite resin restoration (C). Enamel (A) is translucent, with a glossy surface, is smooth upon tactile exploration, and produces a sharp sound. Porcelain (B) may be opaque, is smooth on tactile exploration, and produces a sharp sound. Glass ionomer (D) is opaque, rough on tactile exploration, and produces a dull sound.

34. All of the following are benefits of sharpening dental hygiene instruments EXCEPT one. Which one is the EXCEPTION?

    ANS: B
    Burnished calculus (B) is NOT desirable because of difficulty of removal. Patient comfort (A), reduced clinician fatigue (C), improved calculus removal (D), and increased tactile sensitivity (E) are all benefits of keeping dental hygiene instruments sharpened.

35. A study model is a positive reproduction of the structure it represents. The impression is a negative reproduction of the structure on which it is taken.

    ANS: A
    Both statements are true (A). A study model, cast, and die are all examples of positive reproduction of the structures they represent or are exact replicas of those structures. The impression is a negative reproduction, or a reversed representation, of the structure on which it is taken. Choices B, C, and D do not accurately reflect the statements.

36. The primary indication for polishing enamel is to

    ANS: A
    The primary indication for polishing is to remove stain (A). Although the creation of a smooth surface

(B) helps prevents plaque adhesion (D), these can easily be accomplished with other methods. Polishing only removes plaque temporarily and does not encourage patients to take responsibility for their own home care (C).

37. Which two of the following factors will produce the MOST abrasion to the tooth surface?

ANS: B, D

Abrasion on the tooth surface is increased using large particles of irregular shapes (B) and when abrasive material is applied at high speed and with heavy pressure (D). Other factors that increase abrasions are using an abrasive material that is harder than the material being polished (C), and lack of lubrication. Abrasive agents with small particle size and regular shape (A) that are applied using low speed with moderate pressure (E) and with lubrication reduces abrasion to the tooth surface.

38. The dental professional is encouraged to selectively rubber cup polish because the polishing agents could remove the fluoride-rich layer of enamel.

ANS: A

Both the statement and the reason are correct and related (A). Evidence-based practice indicates that selective polishing causes the least damage to the tooth surface. The abrasives in most prophylaxis pastes can remove the fluoride-rich layer of enamel as well as the softer cementum and dentin surfaces. Choices B, C, D, and E do not correctly reflect the statement or the reason.

39. Professional products are used to polish the restorations at every prophylaxis appointment because these products will not abrade the restorations.

ANS: E

NEITHER the statement NOR the reason is correct (E). Only restorations with visible scratches should be polished. Even polishing with fine prophylaxis paste may abrade amalgam, porcelain, composite, glass ionomer, titanium, and gold restorations. Pastes designated for restorative materials are more abrasive than dental material and should not be used at every prophylaxis appointment. Choices A, B, C, and D do not accurately reflect the statement and the reason.

40. Which of the following is an indication for removal of overhanging restorative margins or for margination?

ANS: B

Margination should only be performed when restorations overhang or the flash is small (B) and

removal will not compromise the restoration. If the restoration has open margins (A), has caries (C), is difficult to access (D), or is damaged (E), margination should not be attempted. The dental professional should only perform margination if it is within the scope of practice for that professional.

41. The fastest method for removing stain from natural dentition is to use

ANS: B

Air polishing (B) is a faster method for stain removal than hand scaling (A), ultrasonic scaling (C), or rubber cup prophy paste (D) and creates less operator fatigue. Air polishing is recommended for the removal of difficult stains such as those caused by tobacco and chlorhexidine use.

42. Which of the following would be the MOST effective in tooth whitening if all were applied for the same length of time, under the same conditions?

ANS: D

Hydrogen peroxide 14% (D) would be the most effective tooth whitening agent if applied for the same length of time under the same conditions as the other choices because it is the highest concentration of available bleaching agent. Carbamide peroxide breaks down to hydrogen peroxide. Carbamide peroxide 10% (A) will be broken down to the equivalent of 3.3% hydrogen peroxide. Hydrogen peroxide 10% (B) is less concentrated than hydrogen peroxide 14%. Carbamide peroxide 20% (C) breaks down to hydrogen peroxide 7.3%. Hydrogen peroxide 5% (E) is less concentrated than hydrogen peroxide 14%.

43. Your patient is scheduled for placement of crowns on teeth #9 and #10 and desires teeth whitening. When should the patient make the appointment for the crowns?

ANS: B

The patient should wait at least 2 weeks after his or her teeth have been whitened (B) to have the crowns fabricated to match the new tooth color. It takes 2 weeks for the color of teeth to stabilize after whitening. The tooth surface has also been weakened and takes 2 weeks to regain strength after whitening. Whitening should not be done concurrently with restoration (A). Whitening may be done after the restoration (C), but since the color of the existing restorations will not lighten with bleaching, the best match occurs if bleaching is done before the restoration.

44. All of the following are acceptable home-care instructions for night guards EXCEPT one. Which one is the EXCEPTION?

    ANS: D
    Night guards should not be soaked in alcohol-containing mouthwash (D). Alcohol mouth rinses, denture cleaners, and bleach will damage the mouth guard, and should not be used. Care for a night guard includes letting it air-dry after cleaning (A), keeping it away from heat (B), replacing it when it becomes worn (C), brushing with mild soap and water (E), and storing in a perforated container.

45. Causes of root sensitivity may include scaling and root planing, leaking restorations, root exposure, and caries. Occlusion of open dentinal tubules is the solution for all of these causes of root sensitivity.

    ANS: C
    The first statement is true, and the second statement is false (C). Root sensitivity may be caused by scaling and root planing, leaking restorations, root exposure, caries, toothbrush abrasion, and erosion. However, the second statement is false. Coverage or occlusion of open dentinal tubules may help resolve dentinal hypersensitivity caused by scaling and root planing and root exposure, but leaky restorations and caries must be treated with definitive restoration. Choices A, B, and D do not correctly reflect the statements.

## CHAPTER 13

Professional Responsibility

Joanna Campbell, Elizabeth O. Carr, Ashley Martin Hale, Jodi L. Olmsted, Laura J. Webb

QUESTIONS

1. Select the four most important items to disclose to a patient while gaining informed consent.
   A. Treatment options
   B. Risks and benefits of treatment
   C. Discussion of patient's bill of rights
   D. Expected prognosis or treatment outcomes
   E. Diagnosis or description of patient's problem

2. All of the following are examples of correct principles of informed consent EXCEPT one. Which one is the EXCEPTION?
   A. Allow time for questions
   B. Provide information to the patient as often as needed
   C. Assess the financial concerns that the patient may have
   D. Assess the patient's ability to provide informed consent
   E. Use simplified terminology to allow the patient to understand

3. Which law (enacted in 1992) gives individuals the right to know why they were denied for credit and the name of the credit bureau that supplied the information?
   A. The Truth in Lending Act
   B. The Fair Credit Reporting Act
   C. The Fair Debt Collection Practice Act

4. Select the four elements that must be present to qualify an action as negligent.
   A. Injury
   B. Deceit
   C. Causation
   D. Duty of care
   E. Breach of legal duty

5. All of the following exemplify legal competence EXCEPT one. Which one is the EXCEPTION?
   A. Persons over the age of 18 years
   B. Mature children not requiring supervision
   C. Mentally competent individuals over a certain age
   D. Appointed legal guardians of mentally incompetent individuals

6. The Hazard Communications Standard is also called the "Employer Right to Know" standard. It requires employee access to hazardous materials information.
   A. Both statements are true.
   B. Both statements are false.
   C. The first statement is true, and the second statement is false.
   D. The first statement is false, and the second statement is true.

7. The Occupational Safety and Health Administration (OSHA) is the government agency charged with creating the expertise, information, and tools that people and communities need to protect their health. OSHA objectives include health promotion, prevention of disease, injury and disability, and preparedness for new health threats. The Centers for Disease Control and Prevention (CDC) is the government agency charged with assurance of safe and healthful working conditions for working men and women by setting and enforcing standards and by providing training, outreach, education, and assistance.
   A. Both statements are true.
   B. Both statements are false.
   C. The first statement is true, and the second statement is false.
   D. The first statement is false, and the second statement is true.

8. Match the regulation with its purpose.

Regulation	Purpose
1. Hazardous Materials Standard (HAZMAT)	A. A regulation that prescribes safeguards to protect workers against health hazards related to occupationally acquired pathogens
2. Bloodborne Pathogens Standard	B. Implemented as part of the Social Security Act, this federal act set standards for coding health information and transmission of health information; patient, provider, employer, and payer identification; to protect security of patient data; and to protect the privacy of health information
3. Freedom of Information Act	C. A regulation that provides that any person has the right to request access to federal agency records or information
4. Health Insurance Portability and Privacy Act (HIPAA)	D. Standard that applies to industries where injuries and illnesses from workplace exposure to hazardous materials are likely to occur; concerned with the distribution of material safety data sheets (MSDS) from the manufacturer to the employer

9. OSHA bloodborne pathogen training and education on the hazards of body fluid and protective measures used to minimize occupation exposures is required at all of the following times EXCEPT one. Which one is the EXCEPTION?
   A. Annually
   B. Every 6 months
   C. Upon start of employment
   D. When a new task is introduced

10. All of the following statements regarding OSHA's HAZMAT are correct EXCEPT one. Which one is the EXCEPTION?
    A. A formal training program in Hazard Communication is not required.
    B. Every office is mandated to possess a *Hazard Communication Manual*.
    C. Employees are informed about harmful chemicals and products in the workplace.
    D. MSDS are a component of the *Hazard Communication Manual*.

11. *Universal precautions* is the term for procedures developed to avoid contact with blood and blood-contaminated, potentially infectious body fluids. Engineering controls is the expanded concept that all bodily fluids except sweat are potentially infectious.
    A. Both statements are true.
    B. Both statements are false.

C. The first statement is true, and the second statement is false.
D. The first statement is false, and the second statement is true.

12. Enforcing practice codes, establishing standards, and enforcing sanctions against incompetent practitioners, to protect the health and safety of the public, are the purposes of
A. licensure.
B. malpractice.
C. credentialing.
D. statute of limitations.

13. The dental hygienist may legally perform the duties or functions allowed in that particular state. If the individual is trained and licensed in another state where the practice act is more expansive, it is also permissible to perform those expanded functions in both states.
A. Both statements are true.
B. Both statements are false.
C. The first statement is true, and the second statement is false.
D. The first statement is false, and the second statement is true.

14. The concept "Do No Harm" is known as
A. justice.
B. veracity.
C. beneficence.
D. nonmaleficence.

15. Which term is also known as the principle of truthfulness?
A. Justice
B. Veracity
C. Beneficence
D. Nonmaleficence

16. Promising patients treatment outcomes that might not be achievable is known as
A. defamation.
B. standard of care.
C. breach of contract.
D. contributory negligence.

17. Defamation is a false communication that harms a person's reputation. It may be either slander (written communication) or libel (verbal communication).
A. Both statements are true.
B. Both statements are false.
C. The first statement is true, and the second statement is false.
D. The first statement is false, and the second statement is true.

18. The dental treatment record is a comprehensive, ongoing file of assessment findings, treatment

services rendered, outcomes, notations, and patient contacts. Entries in the dental record should be signed and dated.
A. Both statements are true.
B. Both statements are false.
C. The first statement is true, and the second statement is false.
D. The first statement is false, and the second statement is true.

19. Select the factors that minimize the risk of litigation for a dental care provider. (Select all that apply.)
A. Risk management
B. Using experimental materials
C. Following the standard of care
D. Comprehensive dental treatment record
E. Clear communication with the patient regarding care and treatment

20. A dental hygienist does not move the ultrasonic cords out of the way, and the patient accidently trips, falls, and is harmed when leaving the treatment area. The hygienist is guilty of
A. deceit.
B. assault.
C. battery.
D. negligence.

21. Administering a fluoride treatment without obtaining the patient's consent is considered
A. defamation.
B. a negligent act.
C. technical battery.
D. breach of confidentiality.

22. The patient has an artificial heart valve requiring prophylactic premedication before the dental hygiene appointment and does not take the medication because of an upset stomach. The dental hygienist fails to ask if the patient has taken the premedication, and the patient develops infective endocarditis. The dental hygienist is guilty of
A. a criminal act.
B. technical battery.
C. breach of contract.
D. contributory negligence.

23. To avoid charges of patient abandonment, a dental office is required to do all of the following actions EXCEPT one. Which one is the EXCEPTION?
A. Notifying the patient verbally
B. Suggesting that the patient seek other providers
C. Using objective language in written notification
D. Providing written notification of termination and the reasons
E. Stating that the patient's records will be forwarded to new provider

24. Match each legal term below with the MOST likely corresponding type of law.

    1. Contract law   A. Violation of a societal rule
    2. Tort law   B. Civil wrong
    3. Criminal law   C. Legally binding agreement

25. Scopes of practice for care vary by state. Licensed dental hygienists are not permitted to perform any procedure that can be legally delegated to a nonlicensed provider such as a dental assistant.
    A. Both statements are true.
    B. Both statements are false.
    C. The first statement is true, and the second statement is false.
    D. The first statement is false, and the second statement is true.

26. The dental hygienist accidentally uses latex gloves on a patient with a latex allergy, and the patient has a severe allergic reaction. Which action has the dental hygienist committed? (Select all that apply.)
    A. Civil offense
    B. Intentional tort
    C. Criminal offense
    D. Unintentional tort

27. Providing written evaluation of the extent of achievement of patient-centered goals is considered a legal risk management strategy. Failure to evaluate the outcome of care may be grounds for negligence.
    A. Both statements are true.
    B. Both statements are false.
    C. The first statement is true, and the second statement is false.
    D. The first statement is false, and the second statement is true.

28. The founding principle of all health care professions is
    A. veracity.
    B. autonomy.
    C. beneficence.
    D. confidentiality.
    E. nonmaleficence.

29. Teaching careful oral hygiene self-care is an example of promoting good. "Doing good" for patients describes the principle of veracity.
    A. Both statements are true.
    B. Both statements are false.
    C. The first statement is true, and the second statement is false.
    D. The first statement is false, and the second statement is true.

30. The dental hygienist may refuse to provide a service requested by the patient if that service is in conflict with the standards of patient care. Although this decision conflicts with patient's autonomy, it is within the dental hygienist's autonomy and ethical responsibility.
    A. Both statements are true.
    B. Both statements are false.
    C. The first statement is true, and the second statement is false.
    D. The first statement is false, and the second statement is true.

31. Placing the welfare of a child suspected of child abuse over the autonomy of the parent is an example implementing the duty of *prima facie*. The welfare of the child is a stronger duty than preserving the parent's right to autonomy.
    A. Both statements are true.
    B. Both statements are false.
    C. The first statement is true, and the second statement is false.
    D. The first statement is false, and the second statement is true.

32. Practicing dental hygiene without a license is considered
    A. malpractice.
    B. a civil offense.
    C. a criminal offense.
    D. an intentional tort.
    E. an unintentional tort.

33. If the husband of a patient contacts the dental office to request information regarding his wife's health history so that he can accurately fill out insurance forms, it is permissible to share that information with the husband because the couple is married. Sharing patient information with family is a violation of confidentiality.
    A. Both statements are true.
    B. Both statements are false.
    C. The first statement is true, and the second statement is false.
    D. The first statement is false, and the second statement is true.

34. Compensatory damages are damages which are added when gross carelessness or negligence causes injury. Compensatory damages are usually covered by liability insurance.
    A. Both statements are true.
    B. Both statements are false.
    C. The first statement is true, and the second statement is false.
    D. The first statement is false, and the second statement is true.

35. When a dental hygiene malpractice suit is a civil action, the level of proof required is called a *preponderance of evidence*. A preponderance of evidence requires that the jury or judge must be 51% certain of guilt or innocence.
    A. Both statements are true.
    B. Both statements are false.
    C. The first statement is true, and the second statement is false.
    D. The first statement is false, and the second statement is true.

36. Advising the patient of the benefits, risks, and expected outcomes of their proposed treatment plan, prior to obtaining the informed consent, promotes which of the following ethical principles?
    A. Autonomy
    B. Nonmaleficence
    C. Beneficence
    D. Confidentiality

37. The dentist proposes a full mouth series of radiographs as part of a patient's treatment plan. The patient questions the dental hygienist about the need for and the safety of radiography. The hygienist educates the patient about dental radiography and answers all of the patient's questions honestly. Which ethical principle is the hygienist upholding?
    A. Justice
    B. Fidelity
    C. Veracity
    D. Accountability
    E. Responsibility

38. Which gesture or expression demonstrates respect for a patient's cultural background in the dental hygiene process of care?
    A. Acknowledging good oral hygiene with a thumbs-up gesture
    B. Using head movement signs for "yes" and "no" rather than speaking
    C. Greeting the patient with a handshake at the beginning of the appointment
    D. Obtaining permission before touching the patient during extraoral and intraoral examinations

39. The OSHA protects the dental professional by
    A. ensuring a safe and healthy workplace.
    B. allowing unpaid leave for medical reasons.
    C. mandating licensure for dentists and dental hygienists.
    D. protecting health care workers from age discrimination.

40. All of the following are functions of a state dental board EXCEPT one. Which one is the EXCEPTION?
    A. Promotion of professional ethical standards
    B. Prosecuting excessive fees for dental services
    C. Protection of the public from incompetent and fraudulent practitioners
    D. Administration of dental and dental hygiene practice acts and regulating the dental profession
    E. Investigation of complaints about professional misconduct and taking appropriate disciplinary action

41. Which is the BEST description of a Dental Practice Act?
    A. Statute
    B. Licensure
    C. Certification
    D. Accreditation

42. Which type of supervision requires prior diagnosis of the patient's condition, authorization of a procedure by a dentist, and the presence of a supervising dentist on the premises?
    A. Direct
    B. Indirect
    C. General

43. Which federal act protects health insurance coverage for workers and their families when they change or lose their jobs?
    A. Ryan White Care Act
    B. Americans with Disabilities Act (ADA)
    C. HIPAA

44. Which of the following terms is applied to providing a level of care that a reasonably prudent practitioner would exercise practicing under the rules and regulations of the state practice act?
    A. Universality
    B. Access to care
    C. Standard of care
    D. Health care disparity

45. Patients must be informed of proposed treatment, risks, options, and nature of the disease or problem before the health care professional can proceed with treatment. Informed consent is mandated by the HIPAA.
    A. Both statements are true.
    B. Both statements are false.
    C. The first statement is true, and the second statement is false.
    D. The first statement is false, and the second statement is true.

46. Which of the following BEST defines professional ethics?
    A. Adhering to state rules and regulations
    B. Complying with insurance carrier's policies
    C. Following office guidelines for treating patients
    D. Conforming to a system of moral principles and standards

47. It is the responsibility of the professional to obtain informed consent before providing treatment. If care is modified, it is not necessary to obtain informed consent again.
    A. Both statements are true.
    B. Both statements are false.
    C. The first statement is true, and the second is false.
    D. The second statement is true, and the first is false.

48. Discussing a patient's medical history with a co-worker violates which ethical principle?
    A. Beneficence
    B. Societal trust
    C. Professionalism
    D. Confidentiality

49. The dental hygienist who participates in life-long learning, attends continuing education courses, and stays current with advances in the field of dentistry and dental hygiene is upholding which ethical principle?
    A. Fidelity
    B. Autonomy
    C. Beneficence
    D. Societal trust
    E. Nonmaleficence

50. Reciprocity is when a state grants licensure, usually without further testing, to an individual who is already licensed in another state. Individuals must apply for reciprocity in another state within the first 10 years after becoming first licensed.
    A. Both statements are true.
    B. Both statements are false.
    C. The first statement is true, and the second is false.
    D. The second statement is true, and the first is false.

51. Which of the following terms refers to time restrictions during which legal proceedings may be initiated?
    A. Standard of care
    B. State practice act
    C. Informed consent
    D. Statute of limitations

52. All of the following are addressed in the Patient's Bill of Rights EXCEPT one. Which one is the EXCEPTION?
    A. The right to immediate care in the event of an emergency
    B. The right of privacy with regard to consultation and treatment
    C. The right to be responsible for associated fees for proposed services
    D. The right to receive information concerning any aspect of treatment or condition

53. The primary purpose of reporting suspected cases of child abuse is to protect the child from further abuse. Dental hygienists are required to report known or suspected cases of child abuse.
    A. Both statements are true.
    B. Both statements are false.
    C. The first statement is true, and the second is false.
    D. The first statement is false, and the second is true.

54. Malpractice is defined as
    A. deceit.
    B. abandonment.
    C. informed refusal.
    D. professional negligence or misconduct.

55. Misdemeanors and felonies are examples of civil law and involve crimes against persons or property. Civil offenses only result in monetary damages or compensation.
    A. Both statements are true.
    B. Both statements are false.
    C. The first statement is true, and the second is false.
    D. The first statement is false, and the second is true.

56. Which patient requires a signed informed refusal after being educated by the health care provider about the possible consequences of refusal? (Select all that apply.)
    A. A patient who refuses radiography
    B. A patient who declines esthetic restorations
    C. A patient who does not want his or her teeth probed
    D. A patient who declines an oral cancer screening
    E. A patient who refuses biopsy of a suspicious lesion

57. Which of the following BEST defines jurisprudence?
    A. It is the study or science of the law.
    B. It is a written law passed by a legislative body.
    C. It addresses the ethics of medical and biologic research.
    D. It is the branch of knowledge that deals with moral principles.

58. An act of omission is a form of malpractice in which the practitioner commits an act that causes harm or injury to the patient. An act of commission is a form of malpractice in which the practitioner fails to act properly to prevent harm.
    A. Both statements are true.
    B. Both statements are false.
    C. The first statement is true, and the second is false.
    D. The first statement is false, and the second is true.

59. The American Dental Hygienists' Association (ADHA) Code of Ethics
    A. regulates the practice of dental hygiene.
    B. resolves conflicts among dental professionals.

C. defines the scope of legal misconduct and liability.

D. outlines the responsibilities and obligations of the dental hygienist.

60. If a dental hygienist falsifies information on the dental hygiene license renewal application, the state board may do which actions? (Select all that apply.)
    A. Deny the renewal
    B. Revoke the license
    C. Suspend the license
    D. Put the hygienist on probation
    E. Notify the public health department

61. A dental hygienist tries to reschedule a patient's appointment with another hygienist because she does not like to treat "old people." What is the hygienist guilty of?
    A. Paternalism
    B. Harassment
    C. Malpractice
    D. Discrimination

62. Which of the following protects individuals with disabilities from employment discrimination?
    A. The Americans with Disabilities Act (ADA)
    B. The Occupational Health and Safety Act (OSHA)
    C. The Family and Medical Leave Act (FMLA)
    D. The Health Information Portability and Accountability Act (HIPAA)

63. A patient has a toothache and schedules an appointment with a dentist. By making the appointment the patient gives consent for the dentist to make a diagnosis and offer treatment. This scenario exemplifies
    A. disclosure.
    B. implied consent.
    C. informed consent.
    D. informed refusal.

64. Being accountable for one's own actions is assuming
    A. veracity.
    B. autonomy.
    C. responsibility.
    D. nonmaleficence.

65. A dental hygienist accidently mounts a radiograph backward, and the dentist does not notice this error. The dentist extracts tooth #30 instead of tooth #19. This is an example of
    A. a statute.
    B. technical battery.
    C. an intentional tort.
    D. an unintentional tort.

66. Which of the following defines an ethical dilemma?
    A. A lack of reasonable and prudent care results in harm.
    B. A situation in which two or more moral principles are in conflict.
    C. A relationship between the patient and the health care professional based on responsibility.
    D. A civil wrong that occurs when an individual does not intend the results of the action.

67. A complete dental chart should include the patient's identification data, consent forms, updated medical and dental histories, clinical assessment and diagnosis, treatment notes, radiographs, and copies of any correspondence with dental specialists or medical practitioners. Failure to keep accurate and complete patient records is considered malpractice.
    A. Both statements are true.
    B. Both statements are false.
    C. The first statement is true, and the second is false.
    D. The first statement is false, and the second is true.

68. Failure to refer a patient who has aggressive periodontal disease and severe bone loss represents which concept?
    A. Veracity
    B. Autonomy
    C. Negligence
    D. Informed consent

69. Who owns a patient's chart and radiographs?
    A. State
    B. Patient
    C. Dentist
    D. Insurance carrier

70. Which of the following would be appropriate for correction of an error recorded in the treatment notes by the dental hygienist?
    A. Draw single line through the error; enter correct information in red ink
    B. Draw single line through the error; enter correct information in black ink
    C. Cover error with correction fluid; write correct information over the original entry
    D. Completely cross out error; enter correct information in black ink

71. Which agency or group should a dental hygienist contact regarding a sexual harassment complaint?
    A. American Dental Hygienists' Association (ADHA)
    B. Equal Employment Opportunity Commission (EEOC)
    C. Healthcare Integrity and Protection Data Bank (HIPDB)
    D. Occupational Health and Safety Administration (OSHA)

72. The dental state practice act regulates the practice of dentistry and specifies the legal requirements for licensure because its primary purpose is to protect the public from incompetent health care providers.
    A. Both the statement and the reason are correct and related.
    B. Both the statement and the reason are correct but NOT related.
    C. The statement is correct, but the reason is NOT.
    D. The statement is NOT correct, but the reason is correct.
    E. NEITHER the statement NOR the reason is correct.

73. Which of the following terms refers to an effort to understand the language, culture, and behavior of diverse individuals and groups?
    A. Access to care
    B. Health literacy
    C. Cultural diversity
    D. Cultural sensitivity

74. Which of the following policies will NOT reduce the risk of malpractice allegations?
    A. Keeping accurate and complete records
    B. Obtaining informed consent from all patients
    C. Maintaining current licensure and certification
    D. Routinely performing full radiographic series on every adult patient

75. Which party or entity establishes the rules and regulations that determine the scope of practice for a dental hygienist?
    A. State governor
    B. State Board of Dentistry
    C. Council on Dental Accreditation
    D. American Dental Hygienists' Association (ADHA)

76. All of the following are examples of professional misconduct EXCEPT one. Which one is the EXCEPTION?
    A. Discussing a patient's history of drug abuse with a co-worker
    B. Failing to follow established OSHA guidelines during dental hygiene care
    C. Submitting a pit and fissure sealant as a composite restoration to Medicaid
    D. Releasing the patient's protected health information to the patient's insurance company

77. Good communication with the patient is the best defense against malpractice claims because patients are less likely to initiate a lawsuit when they have a clear understanding of proposed treatment plans and any potential treatment complications.
    A. Both the statement and the reason are correct and related.

B. Both the statement and the reason are correct but NOT related.
    C. The statement is correct, but the reason is NOT.
    D. The statement is NOT correct, but the reason is correct.
    E. NEITHER the statement NOR the reason is correct.

78. The dental hygienist may perform an action that is unethical yet is still legal. However, it is not possible to perform an action that is illegal and is still ethical.
    A. Both statements are true.
    B. Both statements are false.
    C. The first statement is true, and the second is false.
    D. The first statement is false, and the second is true.

79. Which of the following is an example of an intentional tort?
    A. Assault
    B. Malpractice
    C. Abandonment
    D. Informed refusal

80. Which of the following BEST describes the ethical principle of nonmaleficence?
    A. Truthfulness
    B. Act of doing good
    C. Avoidance of harm
    D. Act of self-determination

81. Patient autonomy allows the patient to make decisions about the treatment received. If a patient chooses a treatment option that is consistent with standards of care, but not what the dental professional recommends, the professional does not have to provide the treatment.
    A. Both statements are true.
    B. Both statements are false.
    C. The first statement is true, and the second statement is false.
    D. The first statement is false, and the second statement is true.

82. Which of the following statements represents an example of when it is legal to require a pregnant applicant to undergo medical evaluation?
    A. The applicant has been identified as having a high-risk pregnancy.
    B. There are childcare concerns with the applicant's current children.
    C. Others interviewing for the position are required to complete a medical screening.
    D. An employer wishes to prove that pregnant applicant is able to perform duties efficiently.

83. A dental hygienist finds an area on the lateral border of the tongue that is suspicious for oral cancer. The hygienist tells the patient about it and suggests a treatment which she is not qualified to perform and

which could potentially cause harm to the patient. This violates which ethical principle?
A. Justice
B. Fidelity
C. Autonomy
D. Nonmaleficence

84. The patient refuses to take the prescribed prophylactic premedication required before dental hygienist treatment. The dental hygienist's decision not to treat the patient exemplifies
A. abandonment.
B. ethical dilemma.
C. injury causation.
D. professional obligation.
E. contributory negligence.

85. Which of the following BEST represents the most valid way to make evidence-based treatment decisions?
A. Reading a magazine and trying a new procedure suggested in an article
B. Applying information the previous patient told you during his or her appointment
C. Gathering information from a peer-reviewed journal and using clinical judgment
D. Asking a fellow dental hygienist for his or her opinion concerning a treatment option

86. When a patient allows the lead apron to be put in place before radiographic examination, it is considered an expressed contract. When the patient signs the paperwork presented during a sedation consultation, it is considered an implied contract.
A. Both statements are true.
B. Both statements are false.
C. The first statement is true, and the second statement is false.
D. The first statement is false, and the second statement is true.

87. Which of the following is the BEST example of a dental professional practicing nonmaleficence?
A. Providing dental services regardless of age, race, and economic status
B. Attendance at the required number of continuing education courses per year
C. Diagnosing the correct classification of carious lesions found during an examination
D. Explaining the treatment plan thoroughly and allowing the patient to ask questions

88. If a state's dental practice act prohibits a dental hygienist from using local anesthesia on patients, which branch of the government will enforce that statute against the hygienist if he or she decides to provide anesthetic services illegally to a patient?
A. Judicial
B. Executive
C. Municipal
D. Legislative

89. The primary purpose of the American Dental Hygienists' Association (ADHA) Code of Ethics is to guide decision making and encourage professional growth. The standards within this code are also defined by law.
A. Both statements are true.
B. Both statements are false.
C. The first statement is true, and the second statement is false.
D. The first statement is false, and the second statement is true.

90. All of the following scenarios allow the dental professional to release confidential patient information EXCEPT one. Which one is the EXCEPTION?
A. Suspected child abuse
B. Subpoena in criminal prosecution
C. The noncustodial parent of a minor child
D. Infection with reportable public health disease

91. Which of the following statements BEST represents an example of due process?
A. Dental health care providers can only be charged with civil suits.
B. A dental license cannot be suspended without proper notice.
C. Ability to initiate a lawsuit is lost after a state-specified amount of time.
D. Laws may not be enforced against a hygienist solely on the basis of race.

92. A patient can request copies of the dental records at any time. If the account balance is not paid in full, the dental office is not obligated to provide the dental records to the patient.
A. Both statements are true.
B. Both statements are false.
C. The first statement is true, and the second statement is false.
D. The first statement is false, and the second statement is true.

93. During an employment interview, an applicant can be asked about all of the following EXCEPT one. Which one is the EXCEPTION?
A. Employment history
B. Criminal convictions
C. Authorization to work
D. Garnishment of wages

94. Which type of contract is created when a patient signs a consent form?
    A. Implied
    B. Apparent
    C. Expressed

95. All of the following examples represent contractual duties of dental professionals to their patients EXCEPT one. Which one is the EXCEPTION?
    A. Using standard techniques, medications, and products
    B. Completing procedures in the predetermined amount of time
    C. Providing adequate postoperative instructions following a dental extraction
    D. Providing referral for conditions that exceed the scope of the general dentist's practice

96. A noncompliant patient may be dismissed before the treatment already started has been completed. If the office dismisses a patient in active treatment without proper notification, the office may be charged with abandonment.
    A. Both statements are true.
    B. Both statements are false.
    C. The first statement is true, and the second statement is false.
    D. The first statement is false, and the second statement is true.

97. Which of the following is NOT a permissible reason to terminate a dental hygienist's employment under the at-will employment relationship?
    A. The hygienist consistently has cancellations and cannot maintain a full schedule.
    B. The dentist dismisses one hygienist and hires another hygienist from a different ethnicity to maintain diversity.
    C. The hygienist calls in sick more than 2 to 3 days per month because of a child's illness.
    D. The dental practice does not have enough dentists to allow the current number of hygienists to practice.

98. All of the following aspects of malpractice must be proven for the patient to initiate a lawsuit EXCEPT one. Which one is the EXCEPTION?
    A. The patient has incurred an injury.
    B. The dental professional has a contractual relationship with the patient.
    C. A verbal accusation was voiced by the patient that a wrongful act had been committed.
    D. Harm inflicted on the patient was a result of actions committed by the dental professional.

99. Which of the following statements BEST represents the purpose of a dental practice act?
    A. Prevention of harm to the public
    B. Protection for the dental hygienist
    C. Control of fee schedules for dental services
    D. Maintenance of dental records for patients

100. Which regulatory body grants a dental hygiene license after successful completion of board examinations?
    A. American Dental Association
    B. State Board of Dental Examiners
    C. American Dental Hygienists' Association (ADHA)
    D. Joint Commission on National Dental Examinations

101. Which of the following ethical values should a hygienist uphold if he or she finds a suspicious lesion during the intraoral examination?
    A. Justice
    B. Veracity
    C. Autonomy
    D. Nonmaleficence

102. A 12-month employment contract is an example of term employment. A hygienist hired as a term employee cannot be terminated without just cause.
    A. Both statements are true.
    B. Both statements are false.
    C. The first statement is true, and the second statement is false.
    D. The first statement is false, and the second statement is true.

103. All of the following are examples of individual risk management within a dental practice EXCEPT one. Which one is the EXCEPTION?
    A. Compliance with all statutes
    B. Maintaining dental licenses and certifications
    C. Being knowledgeable about the state's dental practice act
    D. Verbally telling patients about credentials obtained

104. Which of the following scenarios represents the BEST example of "quid pro quo" sexual harassment?
    A. The dental hygienist sends inappropriate emails to all employees.
    B. The dentist makes derogatory sexual remarks to all employees throughout the day.
    C. The dentist orders that female employees dress provocatively on Fridays.
    D. The dental hygienist submits to a dentist's sexual advances to receive a salary increase.

105. Dental records are the ongoing documentation of all occurrences and encounters with the dental patient. It is not necessary for each entry to be signed as long as a date is included.
    A. Both statements are true.
    B. Both statements are false.
    C. The first statement is true, and the second statement is false.
    D. The first statement is false, and the second statement is true.

106. Direct supervision requires that the dentist remain in the treatment room while the hygienist is performing procedures. General supervision allows the dental hygienist to perform procedures that have been authorized by the dentist, but the dentist need not be present in the facility.
    A. Both statements are true.
    B. Both statements are false.
    C. The first statement is true, and the second statement is false.
    D. The first statement is false, and the second statement is true.

107. Under which of the following circumstances is the release of protected health information allowed without violation of the HIPAA? (Select all that apply.)
    A. To provide payment
    B. For family convenience
    C. For provision of treatment
    D. To allow facility operations
    E. To governmental agencies

108. The Pregnancy Discrimination Act is an amendment to the
    A. Civil Rights Act.
    B. Family Medical Leave Act.
    C. Americans with Disabilities Act.
    D. Equal Employment Opportunity Act.

109. Which of the following BEST represents an assault?
    A. The use of another's name for purposes of financial gain
    B. An action that places someone in fear of bodily harm
    C. Communicating an untrue statement about another person
    D. Intentional infliction of offensive or harmful bodily contact

Answers and Rationales

1. Select the four most important items to disclose to a patient while gaining informed consent.

    ANS: A, B, D, E
    The most important information to give a patient while obtaining informed consent is: diagnosis of patient's problem (E); treatment options (A); risks and benefits of all proposed treatment (B); and expected prognosis or treatment outcomes (D). The Patient's Bill of Rights (C) is required to be disclosed before the patient is assessed.

2. All of the following are examples of correct principles of informed consent EXCEPT one. Which one is the EXCEPTION?

    ANS: C
    Financial concerns are important, but they should be discussed with the client prior to treatment, not during the informed consent process (C). The patient must have time to ask questions to have enough information to make a rational choice and give informed consent (A). Informed consent should be an ongoing process in which the hygienist continues to inform the patient regarding the terms of care (B). The patient must be legally competent to give consent, and in the case of a minor, consent must be given by a parent or guardian (D). The clinician needs to use simplified terminology to allow the patient to be knowledgeable and understand the treatment planned to give informed consent (E).

3. Which law (enacted in 1992) gives individuals the right to know why they were denied for credit and the name of the credit bureau that supplied the information?

    ANS: B
    The Fair Credit Reporting Act (B) was enacted in 1992 and gives individuals the right to know why they were denied for credit and the name of the credit bureau that supplied the information. The Truth in Lending Act of 1968 (A) was designed to protect consumers in their dealings with lenders and creditors. The Fair Debt Collection Practice Act was enacted in 1978 (C) as a statute to the Consumer Credit Protection Act, and it eliminates abusive practices in debt collection, promotes fair debt collection, and provides consumers with an avenue for disputing and obtaining validation of debt information.

4. Select the four elements that must be present to qualify an action as negligent.

    ANS: A, C, D, E
    Negligence is the failure of one owing a duty to another or failure to do what a reasonable and prudent person would do under the circumstances. For an action to be considered negligent, injury or harm to the patient results (A), causation of the injury from the dental hygienist is present (C), a duty of care must exist (D), and a breach of or failure to exercise a legal duty must occur (E). Deceit (B) is considered an intentional tort.

5. All of the following exemplify legal competence EXCEPT one. Which one is the EXCEPTION?

    ANS: B
    Mature children under the age of 18 years are not considered legally competent (B). Mentally competent persons over the age of 18 years are considered legally competent (A, C). Appointed legal guardians of mentally incompetent individuals (D) are considered legally competent to give consent for their wards.

6. The Hazard Communications Standard is also called the "Employer Right to Know" standard. It requires employee access to hazardous materials information.

    ANS: D
    The first statement is false, and the second statement is true (D). The first statement is false because the Hazard Communications Standard is also called the "Employee Right to Know" standard, not the "Employer Right to Know" standard. The second statement is true because the standard mandates that employees have access to hazardous materials information. Choices A, B, and C do not correctly reflect the statements.

7. The Occupational Safety and Health Administration (OSHA) is the government agency charged with creating the expertise, information, and tools that people and communities need to protect their health. OSHA objectives include health promotion, prevention of disease, injury and disability, and preparedness for new health threats. The Centers for Disease Control and Prevention (CDC) is the government agency charged with assurance of safe and healthful working conditions for working men and women by setting and enforcing standards and by providing training, outreach, education, and assistance.

    ANS: B
    Both statements are false (B). The OSHA's purpose is to assure safe and healthful working conditions for employees, enforce standards, and provide training,

outreach, education, and assistance. The CDC creates the expertise, information, and tools that people and communities need to protect their health through health promotion; prevention of disease, injury, and disability; and preparedness for new health threats. Choices A, C, and D do not accurately reflect the statements.

8. Match the regulation with its purpose.

   ANS: 1D, 2A, 3C, 4B.
   HAZMAT is a standard that applies to industries where injuries and illnesses from workplace exposure to hazardous materials are likely to occur. HAZMAT is concerned with the distribution of MSDS from the manufacturer to the employer (1D). The Bloodborne Pathogens Standard is an OSHA regulation that prescribes safeguards to protect workers against health hazards related to bloodborne pathogens (2A). The Freedom of Information Act states that any person has the right to request access to federal agency records or information (3C). The HIPAA was implemented as part of the Social Security Act. This federal act sets standards for coding health information and transmission of health information; patient, provider, employer, and payer identification; to protect security of patient data; and to protect the privacy of health information (4B).

9. OSHA bloodborne pathogen training and education on the hazards of body fluid and protective measures used to minimize occupation exposures is required at all of the following times EXCEPT one. Which one is the EXCEPTION?

   ANS: B
   OSHA bloodborne pathogen training is not required every 6 months. OSHA mandates training and education on the hazards of body fluid and protective measures used to minimize occupation exposures training annually (A), upon start of employment (C), and when new job tasks are introduced (D), specifically those that have potential for occupational exposure.

10. All of the following statements regarding OSHA's HAZMAT are correct EXCEPT one. Which one is the EXCEPTION?

    ANS: A
    A formal education program in Hazard Communication is required and staff training should occur (1) when a new employee is hired, (2) when a new chemical product is introduced to the office, and (3) once a year for all continuing employees (A). The HAZMAT standard mandates that each office possess a *Hazardous Communication Manual* (B). This standard requires that each employee is informed about harmful

chemicals and products in workplace (C). MSDS are a component of the *Hazard Communication Manual*, and must be updated whenever new MSDS information is published (D).

11. *Universal precautions* is the term for procedures developed to avoid contact with blood and blood-contaminated, potentially infectious body fluids. Engineering controls is the expanded concept that all bodily fluids except sweat are potentially infectious.

    ANS: B
    Both statements are false (B). Universal Precautions are a set of infection control and safety procedures intended to protect against bloodborne disease transmission with the concept of treating blood and blood-contaminated body fluids as if they are infectious. Standard Precautions expanded the concept by treating all body fluids except sweat as infectious. Engineering controls are devices or equipment that reduce or eliminate a hazard. Choices A, C, and D do not accurately reflect the statement.

12. Enforcing practice codes, establishing standards, and enforcing sanctions against incompetent practitioners, to protect the health and safety of the public, are the purposes of

    ANS: A
    Licensure is designed to enforce practice codes, establish standards, and sanction incompetent practitioners, all for the purpose of protecting the health and safety of the public (A). Malpractice is an act or failure to act that was the proximate cause of an injury to a patient and was below the standard of care (B). Credentialing establishes the qualifications of licensed professionals, organizational members, or organizations by assessing their background and legitimacy (C). The statute of limitations is the length of time an aggrieved person has to enter suit against another for an alleged injury (D).

13. The dental hygienist may legally perform the duties or functions allowed in that particular state. If the individual is trained and licensed in another state where the practice act is more expansive, it is also permissible to perform those expanded functions in both states.

    ANS: C
    The first statement is true, and the second statement is false (C). The first statement is true because the exact duties and services that may be performed by the dental hygienist in a particular state are based on customary parameters of practice and the state dental practice act. The second statement is false because

only duties allowed by state statute may be performed as per legal mandates in said state, whether or not the clinician is permitted to perform other functions in another area. Choices A, B, and D do not accurately reflect the statement.

14. The concept "Do No Harm" is known as

ANS: D
Nonmaleficence is the ethical principle which states that above all, a health care professional should do no harm (D). Justice is the ethical and legal principle of providing individuals or groups with what is owed, due, or deserved as a duty (A). Veracity is the ethical principle of being honest and telling the truth (B). Beneficence is the ethical principle of "doing good" or benefiting the patient by removing harm (C).

15. Which term is also known as the principle of truthfulness?

ANS: B
Veracity is the ethical principle of being honest and telling the truth (B). Justice is the ethical and legal principle of providing individuals or groups with what is owed, due, or deserved as a duty (A). Beneficence is the ethical principle of "doing good" or benefiting the patient by removing harm (C). Nonmaleficence is the ethical principle which states that above all, a health care professional should do no harm (D).

16. Promising patients treatment outcomes that might not be achievable is known as

ANS: C
Breach of contract is defined as the failure to uphold the terms of an implied or expressed contract, and health care providers should be careful not to make statements that patients may interpret as a guarantee of an outcome or result (C). Defamation is an untrue communication that injures an individual's reputation (A). The standard of care is using accepted drugs, materials, and techniques recognized by the profession in practice (B). Contributory negligence is an action or lack of action that contributes to the harm or injury of an individual and negatively affects his or her health status (D).

17. Defamation is a false communication that harms a person's reputation. It may be either slander (written communication) or libel (verbal communication).

ANS: C
The first statement is true, and the second statement is false (C). Defamation is defined as untrue communication that injures an individual's reputation. Libel is written defamation and slander is verbal defamation. Choices A, B, and D do not correctly reflect the statements.

18. The dental treatment record is a comprehensive, ongoing file of assessment findings, treatment services rendered, outcomes, notations, and patient contacts. Entries in the dental record should be signed and dated.

ANS: A
Both statements are true (A). The dental treatment record is a comprehensive, ongoing file of assessment findings, treatment services rendered, outcomes, notations, and patient contacts. All entries made in the dental treatment record should be signed and dated. Choices B, C, and D do not correctly reflect the statements.

19. Select the factors that minimize the risk of litigation for a dental care provider. (Select all that apply.)

ANS: A, C, D, E
A risk management program identifies potential risks in the delivery of care; once risks are identified, they can be minimized or eliminated (A). Following the standard of care ensures that the clinician is providing care to the professionally accepted level (C). A comprehensive dental treatment record may help defend against such charges as breach of contract, negligence, or lack of informed consent and indicates that the practitioner has met all obligations and caused no harm (D). Clear communication allows the practitioner to clearly explain the care that will occur and answer any questions the patient has, which reduces the potential for lawsuits (E). Using experimental materials or treatments increases the risk of litigation for failure to follow the standard of care (B).

20. A dental hygienist does not move the ultrasonic cords out of the way, and the patient accidently trips, falls, and is harmed when leaving the treatment area. The hygienist is guilty of

ANS: D
The hygienist is guilty of negligence, as the patient was harmed because of a breach of duty such as failure to move the cords out of the patient's path (D). Deceit occurs when a practitioner intentionally misrepresents a situation to a patient (A). Assault occurs when a person intends to cause apprehension in another person without touching them (B). Battery is unpermitted, harmful, or offensive physical contact (C).

21. Administering a fluoride treatment without obtaining the patient's consent is considered

ANS: C
Technical battery occurs when, during the course of treatment, a practitioner exceeds the consent given by the patient, for example, giving a treatment without the patient's consent (C). Defamation is communication that can harm a person's reputation (A). A negligent

act is the failure of one owing a duty to another to do what a reasonable person would have ordinarily done under the circumstances (B). Breach of confidentiality occurs when the practitioner violates the confidential relationship between the practitioner and patient (D).

22. The patient has an artificial heart valve requiring prophylactic premedication before the dental hygiene appointment and does not take the medication because of an upset stomach. The dental hygienist fails to ask if the patient has taken the premedication, and the patient develops infective endocarditis. The dental hygienist is guilty of

ANS: D
Contributory negligence is an action or lack of action (the hygienist did not ask about the premedication) that contributes to the harm or injury of an individual (D). A criminal act (A) is an act that harms society that has the punishment prescribed by criminal or penal codes. Technical battery (B) is when a practitioner exceeds what the patient has authorized, for example, performing a treatment without consent. Breach of contract is not completing a promised or required act or breaking a contract, agreement, promise, or legal duty by failing to perform a promised or required duty (C).

23. To avoid charges of patient abandonment, a dental office is required to do all of the following actions EXCEPT one. Which one is the EXCEPTION?

ANS: A
Notifying the patient verbally (A) that he or she will no longer be treated in the practice is insufficient to prevent charges of abandonment. Following a legally defensible protocol such as suggesting the patient seek another dental care provider (B) in written notification using objective language in the notice of termination (C) is important. Other preventive actions include providing the reasons in the written notification of termination (D) and stating in the notification that the patient's records will be forwarded to new provider (E). It is advisable to provide a permission slip for transfer of records.

24. Match each legal term below with the MOST likely corresponding type of law.

ANS: 1C, 2B, 3A
Contract law (1C) represents the type of law where parties enter into a legally binding agreement. Tort law (2B) is also called *civil law*; it pertains to a civil wrong in which one person or the person's property is harmed as a result of negligence or intentional acts. Criminal law (3A) is a body of law established for the purpose of preventing harm to society, and violation of these laws is codified into criminal or penal codes.

25. Scopes of practice for care vary by state. Licensed dental hygienists are not permitted to perform any procedure that can be legally delegated to a nonlicensed provider such as a dental assistant.

ANS: C
The first statement is true, and the second statement is false (C). The scopes of practice are established by each state (United States) or province (Canada), although they do have common elements. The second statement is false. Licensure allows the dental hygienists to perform any procedures that can be legally delegated to a nonlicensed provider such as a dental assistant because of the higher regulatory and educational requirement required by licensure. Choices A, B, and D do not correctly reflect the statements.

26. The dental hygienist accidentally uses latex gloves on a patient with a latex allergy, and the patient has a severe allergic reaction. Which action has the dental hygienist committed? (Select all that apply.)

ANS: A, D
The action the dental hygienist committed is a civil offense (A) because it is a wrongful act against a person that violates the person, privacy, property, or contractual rights. The dental hygienist also committed an unintentional tort (D), which was not intended to cause harm, but harm or injury did occur. An intentional tort (B) is a deliberate and purposeful act with probability of harmful consequences. A criminal offense (C) is a violation of societal rule outlined by statutory law. An example of a criminal offense is practicing dental hygiene without a license.

27. Providing written evaluation of the extent of achievement of patient-centered goals is considered a legal risk management strategy. Failure to evaluate the outcome of care may be grounds for negligence.

ANS: A
Both statements are true (A). Written evaluations in the patient's permanent record discussing the extent to which patient goals are achieved are considered a legal risk management strategy. Choices B, C, and D do not correctly reflect the statements.

28. The founding principle of all health care professions is

ANS: E
The principle of nonmaleficence (E) is considered the founding principle of all health care professions, and the first obligation to the patient is "Do no harm". Veracity (A) relates to being honest and telling the truth and is the basis of the trust between the patient and the health care provider. The principle of

autonomy (B) is the self-determination and ability of a person to be self-governing and self-directing. The principle of beneficence (C) requires that an existing harm be removed. Confidentiality (D) relates to the responsibility of health care providers to keep the information provided by patients receiving health care private.

29. Teaching careful oral hygiene self-care is an example of promoting good. "Doing good" for patients describes the principle of veracity.

    ANS: C
    The first statement is true, and the second statement is false (C). The first statement is true because teaching careful oral hygiene self-care is considered promoting good. The principle of beneficence, not veracity, focuses on "doing good" for patients, so the second statement is false. Veracity is the basis of the trust between the patient and the health care provider and relates to being honest and telling truth. Choices A, B, and D do not correctly reflect the statements.

30. The dental hygienist may refuse to provide a service requested by the patient if that service is in conflict with the standards of patient care. Although this decision conflicts with patient's autonomy, it is within the dental hygienist's autonomy and ethical responsibility.

    ANS: A
    Both statements are true (A). Dental hygienists have a duty to present all treatment options and to respect patients' decisions regarding actions that affect their bodies. When a patient selects services which are within the standards of patient care, the dental hygienist may ethically act on that choice. However, if a patient selects treatment in conflict with the standards of patient care, the dental hygienist also has the autonomy to refuse to provide unethical care. Choices B, C, and D do not correctly reflect the statements.

31. Placing the welfare of a child suspected of child abuse over the autonomy of the parent is an example implementing the duty of *prima facie*. The welfare of the child is a stronger duty than preserving the parent's right to autonomy.

    ANS: A
    Both statements are true (A). *Prima facie* means "at first glance" and refers to duties that must be performed before any other considerations. A guideline for resolving conflicting acts is to consider the act with the stronger "right." The stronger duty (*prima facie*) in this case is the good or welfare of the

child, not the parent's right of autonomy. Choices B, C, and D do not correctly reflect the statement and the reason.

32. Practicing dental hygiene without a license is considered

    ANS: C
    Practicing without a license is considered a criminal offense because it is a violation of a societal rule outlined in statutory law (C). Malpractice (A) is the performance of professional services without reasonable care or skill or in violation of ethics. A civil offense is a wrongful act against a person that violates personal body, privacy, or contractual rights (B). An intentional tort (D) is a deliberate and purposeful act with probability of harmful consequences. An unintentional tort (E) causes harm, even when none was intended.

33. If the husband of a patient contacts the dental office to request information regarding his wife's health history so that he can accurately fill out insurance forms, it is permissible to share that information with the husband because the couple is married. Sharing patient information with family is a violation of confidentiality.

    ANS: D
    The first statement is false, and the second statement is true (D). Sharing a patient's history or treatment with spouses, family, or friends without the patient's expressed permission is a violation of confidentiality. Choices A, B, and C do not correctly reflect the statements.

34. Compensatory damages are damages which are added when gross carelessness or negligence causes injury. Compensatory damages are usually covered by liability insurance.

    ANS: D
    The first statement is false, and the second statement is true (D). The first statement is false, as compensatory damages are a sum of money awarded to compensate actual injury or economic loss. Punitive damages are added when gross carelessness or negligence causes injury. The second statement is true, as compensatory damages are usually covered by liability insurance. Punitive damages are not usually covered by liability insurance. Choices A, B, and C do not correctly reflect the statements.

35. When a dental hygiene malpractice suit is a civil action, the level of proof required is called a *preponderance of evidence*. A preponderance of evidence requires that the jury or judge must be 51% certain of guilt or innocence.

ANS: A

Both statements are true (A) because dental hygiene malpractice suits are usually civil actions. In civil cases, a preponderance of evidence (51% certainty of guilt or innocence) is applicable by the judge or jury. In criminal actions, the level of proof is stricter, requiring proof *beyond a reasonable doubt*, or absolute certainty of guilt or innocence. Choices B, C, and D do not correctly reflect the statements.

36. Advising the patient of the benefits, risks, and expected outcomes of their proposed treatment plan, prior to obtaining the informed consent, promotes which of the following ethical principles?

ANS: A

Autonomy is the personal liberty of action and self-determination (A). Informed consent promotes this ethical principle and respects the patient's decision. Nonmaleficence is avoidance of harm to others (B). Beneficence is the act of doing good for the benefit of others (C). Confidentiality is the duty to respect privileged information (D).

37. The dentist proposes a full mouth series of radiographs as part of a patient's treatment plan. The patient questions the dental hygienist about the need for and the safety of radiography. The hygienist educates the patient about dental radiography and answers all of the patient's questions honestly. Which ethical principle is the hygienist upholding?

ANS: C

Veracity is the duty to be truthful when information is disclosed to patients about treatment (C). Justice requires treating each other fairly (A). Fidelity is the duty to keep promises (B). Accountability means being answerable to one's own actions (D). Responsibility is the execution of duties associated with the dental hygienist's role (E).

38. Which gesture or expression demonstrates respect for a patient's cultural background in the dental hygiene process of care?

ANS: D

Obtaining the patient's permission to touch him or her before performing extraoral and intraoral examinations displays respect and responsiveness to the patient's cultural norms (D). Hand gestures such as pointing, thumbs-up, or the V-sign, may be interpreted in different ways by people of different cultures (A). Head movement signs for "yes" and "no" may have different meanings among different cultures (B). A handshake is a common introduction in some cultures, and in other cultures physical contact may be inappropriate (C).

39. The OSHA protects the dental professional by

ANS: A.

OSHA (an agency of the U.S. Government under the Department of Labor) ensures a safe and healthy work environment (A). The Family and Medical Leave Act protects job security by allowing unpaid leave for medical reasons (B). The practice and licensure of dentistry and dental hygiene is regulated by each state (C). Dentists and dental hygienists must be licensed to practice their profession legally. The Age Discrimination in Employment Act forbids age discrimination in employment (D).

40. All of the following are functions of a state dental board EXCEPT one. Which one is the EXCEPTION?

ANS: B

The regulation and prosecution of excessive fees for dental services (B) is not a function of a state dental board. Purposes of state dental boards or board of dental examiners include promotion of professional ethical standards (A), and protection of the public from incompetent and fraudulent practitioners (C). Other functions include administration of the dental and dental hygiene practice acts and regulation of the dental profession within the state (D), and investigation of complaints regarding professional misconduct and taking appropriate disciplinary action (E).

41. Which is the BEST description of a Dental Practice Act?

ANS: A

The Dental Practice Act is an example of a statute (A). A statue is a document of law that specifies legal requirements enacted by the legislative branch of a government. Licensure (B) is the process by which states grant individuals the authority to practice a particular profession or occupation. Certification (C) is a voluntary process by which an organization grants recognition to an individual who has met certain predetermined qualifications or standards. Accreditation grants public recognition, for example, to a school, institute, college program facility, or company that has met predetermined standards (D).

42. Which type of supervision requires prior diagnosis of the patient's condition, authorization of a procedure by a dentist, and the presence of a supervising dentist on the premises?

ANS: B

Indirect supervision requires prior diagnosis of the patient's condition and authorization of a procedure by a dentist, and the presence of a supervising dentist on the premises (B). Direct supervision generally requires prior diagnosis of the patient's condition and authorization of a procedure by a dentist, the presence of a supervising dentist on the premises, and dentist approval of the work performed prior to patient dismissal (A). General supervision requires that the dentist authorize the services being delivered; however, the presence of the supervising dentist in the treatment facility is not required (C).

43. Which federal act protects health insurance coverage for workers and their families when they change or lose their jobs?

    ANS: C
    The HIPAA protects health insurance coverage for workers and their families when they change or lose their jobs (C). The Ryan White Care Act provides federal funding for medical treatment for patients with acquired immunodeficiency syndrome (A). The ADA prohibits discrimination against qualified applicants and employees on basis of disability (B).

44. Which of the following terms is applied to providing a level of care that a reasonably prudent practitioner would exercise practicing under the rules and regulations of the state practice act?

    ANS: C
    Standard of care (C) is the degree of care that a reasonably prudent professional should exercise practicing within the rules and regulations of the state practice act and is the level of care that is upheld as appropriate. Universality (A) is a concept that if a situation was duplicated, the same results would occur. Access to care (B) is the ability of the patient to obtain medical care regardless of socioeconomic status. A health care disparity (D) is an unequal distribution of the availability of health care because of factors such as economics, transportations, education, or ethnicity. *Healthy People 2020* eliminated health care disparities.

45. Patients must be informed of proposed treatment, risks, options, and nature of the disease or problem before the health care professional can proceed with treatment. Informed consent is mandated by the HIPAA.

    ANS: C
    The first statement is true, and the second statement is false (C). Patients must be informed of proposed treatment, risks, options, and nature of the disease or problem before the health care professional can proceed with treatment, this is termed *informed consent*. The second statement is false. Informed consent is considered part of the standard of care for health care and is not mandated by the HIPAA. The HIPAA regulates patient privacy, and insurance

transferability of workers. Choices A, B, and D do not accurately reflect the statements.

46. Which of the following BEST defines professional ethics?

    ANS: D
    Professional ethics are upheld when the professional conforms to a system of moral principles and standards (D). Licensed professionals are legally bound to adhere to state rules and regulations (A), but following the law does not guarantee ethical behavior. Complying with insurance carrier's policies is required by law (B) but is not proof of upholding professional ethics. Following office guidelines for treating patients (C) does not ensure compliance with professional ethics.

47. It is the responsibility of the professional to obtain informed consent before providing treatment. If care is modified, it is not necessary to obtain informed consent again.

    ANS: C
    The first statement is true, and the second is false (C). It is the professional's responsibility to obtain consent; hygienists must take the time to obtain informed consent and give the patient the opportunity to ask questions. If care is modified or if additional invasive procedures need to be performed, consent should always be obtained again. Choices A, B, and D do not accurately reflect the statements.

48. Discussing a patient's medical history with a co-worker violates which ethical principle?

    ANS: D
    Confidentiality (D) is the duty to hold private any information acquired in the professional relationship. A dental hygienist should respect the privacy of patients and hold in confidence information disclosed to them. Beneficence (A) involves caring about and acting to promote the good of another. Societal trust (B) maintains a bond of trust in the relationships between professionals and their patients. Professionalism (C) is the commitment to use and advance professional knowledge and skills to serve the patient and the public good.

49. The dental hygienist who participates in life-long learning, attends continuing education courses, and stays current with advances in the field of dentistry and dental hygiene is upholding which ethical principle?

    ANS: E
    The dental hygienist who participates in life-long learning, attends continuing education courses, and stays current with advances in the field of dentistry

and dental hygiene is upholding the ethical principle of nonmaleficence (E), the professional obligation of doing no harm. Fidelity (A) is the principle of loyalty and acting in the best interests of the patient. Beneficence (B) is the act of doing good for the benefit of others. Autonomy (B) is the personal liberty of action and self-determination. By communicating relevant information openly and truthfully, a dental hygienist assists patients in making informed choices. Societal trust (D) is the ethical principle of being worthy of the trust the public has in the profession. Clinicians practicing this principle show concern for the patient over self-interest.

50. Reciprocity is when a state grants licensure, usually without further testing, to an individual who is already licensed in another state. Individuals must apply for reciprocity in another state within the first 10 years after becoming first licensed.

    ANS: C
    The first statement is true, and the second is false (C). The first statement is true as reciprocity is when a state grants licensure, usually without further testing, to an individual who is already licensed in another state. Individual states determine on a case-by-case basis if an individual meets the requirements to be granted licensure within the state. The second statement is false because the time that an individual has been licensed does not determine if they are eligible to be granted reciprocity. Choices A, B, and D do not correctly reflect the statements.

51. Which of the following terms refers to time restrictions during which legal proceedings may be initiated?

    ANS: D
    The statute of limitations (D) is a law that sets the maximum waiting period before filing a lawsuit. The periods vary by state and by type of claim. After that period, the right to initiate a lawsuit is forfeited. The state practice act (B) adopts rules and regulations for the profession. Informed consent (C) is a process by which the patient agrees to a proposed treatment plan after a complete case presentation. Standard of care (A) is the degree of care that a reasonably prudent professional should exercise practicing within the rules and regulations of the state practice act.

52. All of the following are addressed in the Patient's Bill of Rights EXCEPT one. Which one is the EXCEPTION?

    ANS: C
    The Patient's Bill of Rights does not address the associated fees for proposed services (C). The Patient's

Bill of Rights was developed to help establish the standards of care relating to patient services. Some of these rights include the right to immediate care in event of emergency (A), the right of privacy concerning consultation and treatment (B), and the right to receive information regarding treatment or condition at any time (D).

53. The primary purpose of reporting suspected cases of child abuse is to protect the child from further abuse. Dental hygienists are required to report known or suspected cases of child abuse.

    ANS: A
    Both statements are true (A). The primary purpose of reporting suspected cases of child abuse is to protect the child from further abuse. Dental hygienists are mandated by state law to report known or suspected cases of child abuse. Choices B, C, and D do not correctly reflect the statements.

54. Malpractice is defined as

    ANS: D
    Malpractice (D) is negligence or misconduct by a professional person. It is a deviation from the acceptable standards of care. Deceit (A) occurs when a practitioner intentionally misrepresents a situation to a patient. Abandonment (B) is when the professional discontinues treatment of the patient without giving reasonable notice or providing a competent replacement. Informed refusal (C) is when the patient refuses the proposed treatment.

55. Misdemeanors and felonies are examples of civil law and involve crimes against persons or property. Civil offenses only result in monetary damages or compensation.

    ANS: D
    The first statement is false, and the second is true (D). Misdemeanors and felonies are examples of criminal law and involve crimes against society. The second statement is true; civil offenses only result in monetary damages or compensation. Choices A, B, and C do not accurately reflect the statements.

56. Which patient requires a signed informed refusal after being educated by the health care provider about the possible consequences of refusal? (Select all that apply.)

    ANS: A, C, D, E
    If a patient refuses any proposed treatment with implications for his or her health, the health care provider must inform the patient about any possible consequences and obtain the patient's informed refusal. Examples of scenarios that require informed refusal include a patient who refuses radiography (A), a

patient who does not want his or her teeth probed (C), a patient who declines an oral cancer screening (D), or a patient who refuses a biopsy of a suspicious lesion (E). Declining esthetic restorations (B) would not require informed refusal because there are no long-term health implications to refusal.

57. Which of the following BEST defines jurisprudence?

ANS: A

Jurisprudence is the study of or science of law (A). A statute is a written law passed by a legislative body (B). Bioethics is the ethics of medical and biologic research (C). Ethics is the branch of knowledge that deals with moral principles (D).

58. An act of omission is a form of malpractice in which the practitioner commits an act that causes harm or injury to the patient. An act of commission is a form of malpractice in which the practitioner fails to act properly to prevent harm.

ANS: B

Both statements are false (B). An act of omission is the failure to act properly to prevent harm, for example, failure to diagnose or treat periodontal disease. An act of commission is when the practitioner commits an act that causes harm or injury to the patient, for example, breaking an instrument tip in the patient's mouth and not telling the patient. Either of these acts may constitute malpractice if the patient was harmed in either of these scenarios. Choices A, C, and D do not accurately reflect the statements.

59. The American Dental Hygienists' Association (ADHA) Code of Ethics

ANS: D

The ADHA Code of Ethics outlines the responsibilities and obligations of dental hygienists toward patients, colleagues, and society and describes professional conduct (D). The practice act of each state adopts rules and regulates the practice of dental hygiene (A). Each state defines the scope of practice for the profession (C). The professional association does not resolve conflicts among dental professionals (B); the state board of dentistry may investigate complaints and take disciplinary action, when necessary.

60. If a dental hygienist falsifies information on the dental hygiene license renewal application, the state board may do which actions? (Select all that apply.)

ANS: A, B, C, and D

The state board of dentistry has the authority to take disciplinary action, for example, deny renewal of the

license (A), revoke the license (B), suspend the license (C), or place the hygienist on probation (D). The state board of dentistry is authorized to grant and revoke licenses and monitor licensure renewal. Notification of the public health department (E) is not a responsibility of the state dental board.

61. A dental hygienist tries to reschedule a patient's appointment with another hygienist because she does not like to treat "old people." What is the hygienist guilty of?

ANS: D

Discrimination (D) is the act of treating persons differently based on factors that one cannot control, for example, age, handicapping condition, race, or gender. Discrimination violates both ethical and legal principles. Paternalism (A) is acting with good intentions for a patient, much like a father would, but without the patient's knowledge, thus violating the patient's autonomy. Harassment (B) is the act of annoying or threatening a person by word or deed. Malpractice (C) is professional services done without reasonable care or skill or in violation of ethics.

62. Which of the following protects individuals with disabilities from employment discrimination?

ANS: A

The ADA prohibits discrimination against qualified applicants and employees on basis of disability (A), and is part of the Equal Employment Opportunity Commission (EEOC). The OSHA ensures a safe and healthy work environment for employees (B). The FMLA protects job security by allowing unpaid leave for medical reasons (C). The HIPAA protects health information and protect health insurance coverage for workers and their families when they change or lose their jobs (D).

63. A patient has a toothache and schedules an appointment with a dentist. By making the appointment the patient gives consent for the dentist to make a diagnosis and offer treatment. This scenario exemplifies

ANS: B

Implied consent (B) is the granting of permission for health care without a formal agreement between the patient and the dentist. Disclosure (A) is the act of revealing or uncovering. Informed consent (C) is a process by which the patient agrees to a proposed treatment plan after a complete case presentation. Informed refusal (D) is when the patient has been informed of the consequences of not receiving treatment and chooses not to be treated.

64. Being accountable for one's own actions is assuming

ANS: C
Responsibility (C) is a moral obligation to be
accountable for your own behavior. Veracity (A) is
the duty to tell the truth when information is disclosed
to patients about treatment. Autonomy (B) is the
personal liberty of action and self-determination.
Nonmaleficence (D) is avoidance of harm to others.

65. A dental hygienist accidently mounts a radiograph
backward, and the dentist does not notice this error.
The dentist extracts tooth #30 instead of tooth #19.
This is an example of

ANS: D
This is an example of an unintentional tort (D)
because a wrongful act by the dental hygienist
resulted in injury to the patient, but the act was not
committed with intent on the part of the hygienist.
Statutes (A) are laws that are written and enacted by
federal or state legislatures. Technical battery is an
intentional tort (B) and occurs when a practitioner
exceeds the consent given by the patient. Intentional
torts (C) are committed with intent on the part of the
person.

66. Which of the following defines an ethical dilemma?

ANS: B
An ethical dilemma is a situation in which two or
more moral or ethical principles are in conflict (B).
Negligence is a lack of reasonable and prudent care
resulting in harm (A). A fiduciary relationship is
a relationship between the patient and the health
care professional based on responsibility (C). An
unintentional tort is a civil wrong that occurs when an
individual does not intend the results of the action (D).

67. A complete dental chart should include the patient's
identification data, consent forms, updated medical
and dental histories, clinical assessment and diagnosis,
treatment notes, radiographs, and copies of any
correspondence with dental specialists or medical
practitioners. Failure to keep accurate and complete
patient records is considered malpractice.

ANS: A
Both statements are true (A). The first statement is
true, as all of the items listed are necessary to include
in the dental chart. The second statement is true,
as malpractice is professional negligence. Failure
to thoroughly document and keep accurate dental
records is a deviation from acceptable standards of
care. Choices B, C, and D do not correctly reflect the
statements.

68. Failure to refer a patient who has aggressive periodontal
disease and severe bone loss violates which of the
following standards of professional responsibility?

ANS: C
Negligence (C) is conduct that falls below the
minimum standards of behavior established by law
for the protection of others against reasonable risks
of harm. Failing to refer a patient who has aggressive
periodontal disease and severe bone loss would be an
act of negligence (C). Veracity (A) is the duty to tell
the truth when information is disclosed to patients
about treatment. Autonomy (B) is the personal liberty
of action and self-determination. Informed consent (D)
is a process by which the patient agrees to a proposed
treatment plan after a complete case presentation.

69. Who owns a patient's chart and radiographs?

ANS: C
A patient's chart and radiographs are considered
the property of the individual who initiated and
created it, the dentist (C). The state (A) would only
take possession of the patient's chart if it is used as
evidence in a criminal proceeding. Although the patient
(B) pays for the radiographs and findings recorded
in the chart, the patient is paying for the professional
expertise of the dentist and the staff, not the actual
documents. The patient has the right to obtain copies
of the contents of their chart, although the dental office
has the right to charge for the copies. The insurance
company (D) may request copies of the chart, but the
chart does not belong to the insurance company.

70. Which of the following would be appropriate for
correction of an error recorded in the treatment notes
by the dental hygienist?

ANS: B
Dental charts should be recorded legibly and written
in blue or black ink. Mistakes made in the dental chart
are corrected by drawing a single line through the error,
writing the correct information immediately after, and
signing the entry (B). The original entry should still be
legible. Red ink is not used for legal documents such as
dental charts, only blue or black ink is acceptable (A).
The mistake should never be obliterated or covered up,
as this can indicate improper altering of a chart (C, D).

71. Which agency or group should a dental hygienist
contact regarding a sexual harassment complaint?

ANS: B
The EEOC (B) is the federal agency that investigates
claims of employment discrimination and sexual
harassment. The ADHA (A) is the professional

association of dental hygienists and outlines codes of behaviors and ethics for the profession. The ADHA has no regulatory authority over complaints. The HIPDB (C) was created to combat fraud and abuse in health insurance and health care delivery. This database contains information regarding civil judgments, criminal convictions, or action by federal or state licensing agencies against a health care provider, supplier, or practitioner related to the delivery of a health care item or service. The OSHA (D) ensures a safe and healthy work environment.

72. The dental state practice act regulates the practice of dentistry and specifies the legal requirements for licensure because its primary purpose is to protect the public from incompetent health care providers.

ANS: A
Both the statement and the reason are correct and related (A). Each state practice act has established rules and regulations for the practice of dentistry and specifies the legal requirements for licensure. The primary purpose of the state practice act is to protect the public from incompetent dental health care providers. Choices B, C, D, and E do not correctly reflect the statement and the reason.

73. Which of the following terms refers to an effort to understand the language, culture, and behavior of diverse individuals and groups?

ANS: D
Cultural sensitivity (D) refers to an effort to understand the language, culture, and behavior of diverse individuals and groups. The culturally sensitive delivery of dental hygiene care can make a positive difference in oral health outcomes. Access to care (A) describes the ability to obtain health care regardless of socioeconomic status, age, or ethnicity. Health literacy (B) is a set of cognitive and social skills that determine the ability of a patient to obtain, understand, or respond to health messages and be motivated to make health decisions that promote and maintain good health. Cultural diversity (C) is the blending and integration of many different populations.

74. Which of the following policies will NOT reduce the risk of malpractice allegations?

ANS: D
Radiography should only be performed (D) when there is a clear indication, not according to a routine. Accurate and complete documentation of dental records (A) is critical to protect the health care provider against allegations of wrongdoing. Obtaining

informed consent from all patients (B) is crucial to avoiding miscommunications. Maintaining current licensure and any required certifications (C) are essential in proving competency as a part of individual risk management.

75. Which party or entity establishes the rules and regulations that determine the scope of practice for a dental hygienist?

ANS: B
Each state grants authority to a Board of Dentistry (B) (also called *Board of Dental Examiners*, *State Dental Board*, and *State Dental Commission*) to adopt rules and regulations for dental hygienists and other dental professions. These rules and regulations are referred to as the state dental practice act. The state governor (A) often appoints individuals to dental boards. The Council on Dental Accreditation (C) establishes, maintains, and applies standards to dental and dental related educational programs. The ADHA (D) is the professional organization that represents the interests of dental hygienists and promotes the highest standards of education and practice in the profession.

76. All of the following are examples of professional misconduct EXCEPT one. Which one is the EXCEPTION?

ANS: D
Releasing the patient's protected health information to the patient's insurance company (D) is not an example of professional misconduct and is permitted under HIPAA rules for the purposes of payment. Discussing a patient's history of drug abuse with a co-worker (A) violates the confidentiality of the patient. Failing to follow established OSHA guidelines during dental hygiene care (B) is a safety issue that places the patient and clinician at risk. Submitting a pit and fissure sealant as a composite restoration to Medicaid (C) is falsification of records and is professional misconduct.

77. Good communication with the patient is the best defense against malpractice claims because patients are less likely to initiate a lawsuit when they have a clear understanding of proposed treatment plans and any potential treatment complications.

ANS: A
Open communication and shared decision making between the patient and the health care professional are key to minimizing the potential risk of any legal allegations of wrongdoing (A). Choices B, C, D, and E do not correctly reflect the statement and the reason.

78. The dental hygienist may perform an action that is unethical yet is still legal. However, it is not possible to perform an action that is illegal and is still ethical.

ANS: A
Both statements are true (A). Statutory law regulates the practice of dental hygiene, providing a general outline of the requirements, provisions, and limitations of the practice of dental hygiene. These laws are the minimum level of regulation of the dental hygiene program. Ethical codes address the essential characteristics of a true profession, in areas of professional integrity, dedication, and behavior that serves as role models for others in the profession. Ethical behavior will always uphold the law; however, behavior may fall within the law and not be considered ethical. Choices B, C, and D do not correctly reflect the statements.

79. Which of the following is an example of an intentional tort?

ANS: A
Assault (A), which is any action that places one in fear of bodily harm, is an example of an intentional tort. An intentional tort is a wrongful act that results in injury to one person by another. The defendant must have intended to cause harm or injury. Malpractice (B) is a wrongful act of a professional person and an example of an unintentional tort. Abandonment (C) is when the professional discontinues treatment of the patient without giving reasonable notice or providing a competent replacement. Informed refusal (D) is when the patient refuses the proposed treatment.

80. Which of the following BEST describes the ethical principle of nonmaleficence?

ANS: C
Nonmaleficence (C) is the avoidance of harm to others. Truthfulness (A) describes the core value of veracity. Beneficence (B) is the act of doing good. Autonomy (D) is the act of self-determination.

81. Patient autonomy allows the patient to make decisions about the treatment received. If a patient chooses a treatment option that is consistent with standards of care, but not what the dental professional recommends, the professional does not have to provide the treatment.

ANS: C
The first statement is true, as the principle of autonomy does allow the patient to make decisions about treatment. The second statement is false (C) because as long as the patient chooses an option consistent with standards of care, the dental professional has an obligation to provide the treatment. Choices A, B, and D do not correctly reflect the statements.

82. Which of the following statements represents an example of when it is legal to require a pregnant applicant to undergo medical evaluation?

ANS: C
An employer can require a pregnant applicant to undergo medical evaluation if all others applicants are also required to do so (C). Identification of an applicant as having a high-risk pregnancy (A), childcare concerns with an applicant's existing children (B), or the need to prove that the pregnant applicant is able to perform efficient duties (D) are not legal reasons to require a pregnant patient to undergo medical evaluation.

83. A dental hygienist finds an area on the lateral border of the tongue that is suspicious for oral cancer. The hygienist tells the patient about it and suggests a treatment which she is not qualified to perform and which could potentially cause harm to the patient. This violates which ethical principle?

ANS: D
The principle of nonmaleficence (D) states that the health care provider must do no intentional harm to the patient. Treating a patient with fairness and equality is the definition of justice (A). Keeping an implied or explicit promise is the principle of fidelity (B). Allowing the patient to accept or reject treatment is defined as patient autonomy (C).

84. The patient refuses to take the prescribed prophylactic premedication required before dental hygienist treatment. The dental hygienist's decision not to treat the patient exemplifies

ANS: B
The dental hygienist is faced with an ethical dilemma (B). An ethical dilemma is defined as a situation in which two ethical principles are in conflict. In this situation, the patient is exercising the right of autonomy in refusing to take the premedication. The dental hygienist is ethically obligated to cause no harm, so performing dental hygiene treatment under these circumstances would violate the ethical principle of nonmaleficence. The dental hygienist faces an ethical dilemma in having to choose between the two principles. Abandonment (A) is discontinuation of an established patient–provider relationship. Injury causation (C) occurs when a patient's injury is caused by the dental hygienist's breach of duty. Professional obligation (D) is the

obligation to help regulate the profession of dental hygiene. Contributory negligence (E) is an action or lack of action that contributes to the harm or injury of an individual and negatively affects his or her health status.

85. Which of the following BEST represents the most valid way to make evidence-based treatment decisions?

ANS: C
The most valid way to make an evidence-based treatment decision is to gather information from peer-reviewed journals and use clinical judgment (C). Reading a magazine and trying a new procedure suggested in an article (A), applying information from a previous patient (B), and asking a fellow dental hygienist for his or her opinion (D) are all useful in making treatment decisions but are not based on scientific evidence.

86. When a patient allows the lead apron to be put in place before radiographic examination, it is considered an expressed contract. When the patient signs the paperwork presented during a sedation consultation, it is considered an implied contract.

ANS: B
Both statements are false (B). An expressed contract is created through oral or written communication, and an implied contract is created through signs such as allowing the lead apron to be put in place, inaction, or silence. Choices A, C, and D do not correctly reflect the statements.

87. Which of the following is the BEST example of a dental professional practicing nonmaleficence?

ANS: B
Attending required continuing education classes (B) is an example of a dental professional keeping skill current to provide a patient with the best possible care and to prevent nonmaleficence. Providing dental services regardless of age, race, and economic status (A) embodies the principle of justice. Diagnosing the correct classification of carious lesions found during an examination (C) upholds the principle of veracity. Explaining a treatment plan to a patient and allowing the patient to ask questions (D) upholds the principle of autonomy.

88. If a state's dental practice act prohibits a dental hygienist from using local anesthesia on patients, which branch of the government will enforce that statute against the hygienist if he or she decides to provide anesthetic services illegally to a patient?

ANS: D
The legislative (D) branch is responsible for enacting laws and statutes that prohibit activities within a state's outlined dental practice act. The judicial (A) branch is concerned with the rights and responsibilities of individuals subject to the laws of the state. The executive (B) branch plays a major role in the implementation and enforcement of the prescriptions and prohibitions enacted into law. There is no defined municipal (C) branch of government.

89. The primary purpose of the American Dental Hygienists' Association (ADHA) Code of Ethics is to guide decision making and encourage professional growth. The standards within this code are also defined by law.

ANS: C
The first statement is true, and the second statement is false (C). The first statement is true, as the ADHA Code of Ethics provides standards of care that hygienists should follow. The second statement is false because standards in the code are not regulated by the law. Choices A, B, and D do not correctly reflect the statements.

90. All of the following scenarios allow the dental professional to release confidential patient information EXCEPT one. Which one is the EXCEPTION?

ANS: C
The noncustodial parent of a minor child (C) does not have access to the child's confidential health information. Confidential patient information may be released in certain circumstances. Legislation in all 50 states mandates the reporting of suspected child abuse (A) to authorities, and many states also mandate the reporting of suspected elder abuse. Records must be released if subpoenaed in criminal cases (B). Knowledge of infection with certain reportable public health diseases (D) must be reported to the area public health department.

91. Which of the following statements BEST represents an example of due process?

ANS: B
According to due process laws, dental professionals have a right to notification of a violation and a hearing before a license can be suspended (B). Dental health care providers may be charged with civil suits (A), criminal suits, or both. The Statute of Limitations defines the state-specified amount of time (C) an individual has to initiate a lawsuit. Laws may not be enforced against a hygienist solely on the basis of race (D), which is an example of equal protection.

92. A patient can request copies of the dental records at any time. If the account balance is not paid in full, the dental office is not obligated to provide the dental records to the patient.

ANS: C
The first statement is true, and the second statement is false (C). The first statement is true, as the patient has a legal right to request dental records at any time. The second statement is false because it is illegal to deny a patient access to his or her records because of an outstanding account balance. Choices A, B, and D do not correctly reflect the statements.

93. During an employment interview, an applicant can be asked about all of the following EXCEPT one. Which one is the EXCEPTION?

ANS: D
It is unlawful to ask applicants questions about his or her financial status, which includes garnishment of wages (D), during an interview. An applicant can be asked about his or her background, including education, employment history, and skills (A). An applicant can be asked if he or she has ever been convicted of a crime (B) but cannot be asked about his or her arrest record. Although an applicant cannot be asked about citizenship, it is acceptable to ask if the applicant is authorized for work in the United States (C).

94. Which type of contract is created when a patient signs a consent form?

ANS: C
An expressed contract is entered through oral or written communication (C). An implied contract is entered through signs, inaction, or silence (A). An apparent contract is another term for implied contracts (B).

95. All of the following examples represent contractual duties of dental professionals to their patients EXCEPT one. Which one is the EXCEPTION?

ANS: B
Dental professionals are only required to complete procedures in a reasonable time frame, as there are unexpected events that occur during an appointment or with a treatment plan (B). Using standard techniques, medications, and products (A); providing adequate postoperative instructions (C); and referring patients who cannot be adequately treated by the general dentist (D) are all contractual duties of the dental professional.

96. A noncompliant patient may be dismissed before the treatment already started has been completed. If the office dismisses a patient in active treatment without proper notification, the office may be charged with abandonment.

ANS: D
The first statement is false, and the second statement is true (D). A patient must have all treatment already started completed before being dismissed, so the first statement is false. The second statement is true because a written notification of termination is necessary to protect against charges of abandonment. Choices A, B, and C do not correctly reflect the statements.

97. Which of the following is NOT a permissible reason to terminate a dental hygienist's employment under the at-will employment relationship?

ANS: B
A dental hygienist hired under the at-will employment relationship cannot be terminated because of his or her ethnicity (B). The hygienist who consistently has cancellations and does not maintain a full schedule (A), calls in sick because of a child's illness more than 2 to 3 days per month (C), or works for a practice that no longer has enough dentists to legally allow the current number of hygienists to practice (D), are permissible reasons for terminating the hygienist hired under the at-will employment relationship.

98. All of the following aspects of malpractice must be proven for the patient to initiate a lawsuit EXCEPT one. Which one is the EXCEPTION?

ANS: C
A patient's verbal accusation that a wrong act was committed (C) is not enough evidence required for the patient to initiate a lawsuit. For the patient to initiate a lawsuit, occurrence of injury to the patient must be proven (A), a contractual relationship between the patient and the dental professional exists (B), and the harm inflicted was caused by the actions of the dental professional (D).

99. Which of the following statements BEST represents the purpose of a dental practice act?

ANS: A
The primary purpose of a dental practice act is to prevent harm to the public (A). Dental practice acts are designed to regulate the practice of dentistry and dental hygiene, but protection of the dental hygienist (B) is not within the scope of the practice act. A dental practice act may regulate the length of time patient records are maintained by a dental office, but

does not maintain dental records for patients (D). A dental practice act does not control fee schedules for dental services (C).

100. Which regulatory body grants a dental hygiene license after successful completion of board examinations?

    ANS: B
    The State Board of Dental Examiners (B) has the legal authority to design and administer dental and dental hygiene licensing exams to graduates of approved schools. They are responsible for granting licenses to individuals to practice when they successfully pass the examination. The American Dental Association (A) is a professional association whose purpose it is to assist its members in providing the highest professional and ethical care and to advocate for the advancement of the profession. The American Dental Hygienists' Association (ADHA) (C) is a national organization of over 35,000 dental hygienists dedicated to advancing the art and science of dental hygiene. It is made up three levels: the Component level, the Constituent level, and the National level. The Joint Commission on National Dental Examinations (D) regulates the administration of credentialing examinations for the profession of dentistry.

101. Which of the following ethical values should a hygienist uphold if he or she finds a suspicious lesion during the intraoral examination?

    ANS: B
    The dental hygienist has the ethical responsibility to tell the patient about the lesion, which is practicing veracity or truth (B). Justice (A) refers to fairness and equality. Autonomy (C) refers to the patient's right to participate in treatment decisions. Nonmaleficence (D) refers to doing no purposeful harm to the patient.

102. A 12-month employment contract is an example of term employment. A hygienist hired as a term employee cannot be terminated without just cause.

    ANS: A
    Both statements are true (A) because a term employment relationship includes a contract of specified time, which means the dental hygienist cannot simply be terminated without just cause during the contracted term. Choices B, C, and D do not correctly reflect the statements.

103. All of the following are examples of individual risk management within a dental practice EXCEPT one. Which one is the EXCEPTION?

    ANS: D
    Verbally telling patients about credentials obtained (D) is appropriate but does not protect the dental professional against malpractice or other risks involved in treating patients. Compliance with statutes (A), maintaining dental licenses and certifications (B), and being knowledgeable about the state's dental practice act (C) are all ways to manage individual risk.

104. Which of the following scenarios represents the BEST example of "quid pro quo" sexual harassment?

    ANS: D
    "Quid pro quo" sexual harassment involves basing employment decisions on the return or rejection of sexual advances. A hygienist accepting higher pay in exchange for sexual favors with the dentist (D) is an example. The dental hygienist sending inappropriate emails to all employees (A), the dentist making derogatory remarks to all employees (B), or the dentist ordering female employees to wear provocative attire on Fridays (C) are examples of "hostile environment" sexual harassment.

105. Dental records are the ongoing documentation of all occurrences and encounters with the dental patient. It is not necessary for each entry to be signed as long as a date is included.

    ANS: C
    The first statement is true, and the second statement is false (C). The first statement is true because a dental record must include documentation of all occurrences and encounters with the dental patient, including treatment provided, missed appointments, recommendations, unexpected occurrences, medications, client education, and so on. The second statement is false, as all dental record entries must be signed and dated by the practitioner at the time of entry as legally defensible documents. Choices A, B, and D do not accurately reflect the statements.

106. Direct supervision requires that the dentist remain in the treatment room while the hygienist is performing procedures. General supervision allows the dental hygienist to perform procedures that have been authorized by the dentist, but the dentist need not be present in the facility.

    ANS: D
    The first statement is false, and the second statement is true (D). Direct supervision requires that the dentist be on the premises of the dental treatment, not within the treatment room. The second statement is true. General supervision allows the dental hygienist to

perform treatment procedures without the dentist on the premises, as long as the procedure has been authorized by the dentist. Choices A, B, and C do not accurately reflect by the statements.

107. Under which of the following circumstances is the release of protected health information allowed without violation of the HIPAA? (Select all that apply.)

ANS: A, C, D, E
Under certain circumstances protected health information (PHI) may be released without violation of the HIPAA. Provision of payment (A), treatment (C), facility operations such as accreditation (D), and release to governmental agencies (E) such as the military are all valid allowances for release of PHI. Releasing protected health information for the convenience of the family (B) is prohibited.

108. The Pregnancy Discrimination Act is an amendment to the

ANS: A
The Pregnancy Discrimination Act (A), which forbids discrimination based on pregnancy when it comes to any aspect of employment, is an amendment to Title VII of the Civil Rights Act of 1964. The Family Medical Leave Act (B) is federal law which requires covered employers to provide employees job-protected and unpaid leave for qualified medical and family reasons. The Americans with Disabilities Act (C) prohibits employment discrimination against qualified individuals with disabilities. The Equal Employment Opportunity Act (D) is the act which gives the Equal Employment Opportunity Commission (EEOC) authority to sue in federal courts when it finds reasonable cause to believe that there has been employment discrimination based on race, color, religion, sex, or national origin.

109. Which of the following BEST represents an assault?

ANS: B
Assault is considered any action that places someone in fear of bodily harm (B). Appropriation is using someone else's name for purposes of financial gain (A). Defamation is communication of an untrue statement about another person (C). Battery is intentional infliction of offensive or harmful bodily contact (D).

Community Health/Research Principles

## CHAPTER 14

Community Health and Research Principles

Christine French Beatty, Connie E. Beatty,
Elizabeth O. Carr

QUESTIONS

Questions 1 through 5 refer to information in the following testlet.

> A school district contracts with a local dental hygienist to begin a caries prevention program after a national report has indicated that the state had the highest tooth decay rate in the nation based on DMFS (decayed, missing, filled tooth surfaces) indices. The dental hygienist is asked to develop a pit and fissure sealant and fluoride varnish program in all the elementary schools in a rural district for children in grades K–5. This culturally diverse population consists primarily of children from lower socioeconomic status (SES) families. The only prior program in the schools is annual dental education conducted by the school nurses, based on their assessment that the oral hygiene of the school children is poor. The concentration of fluoride in the water is 0.3 parts per million (ppm), and a previous fluoridation campaign was unsuccessful. The DMFT (decayed, missing, filled teeth) and dft will be measured at the baseline with plans to repeat the measures annually to monitor the effectiveness of the program.

1. Which of the following is the FIRST data collection method needed for this program?
   A. Consult school nurse records
   B. Survey parents' oral health literacy
   C. Test the children's basic oral health knowledge
   D. Conduct sample DMFT and dft indices with the school children

2. Which of the following factors should be considered to determine the optimal level of water fluoridation for this community?
   A. SES of the population
   B. The brand of dentifrice used by the population
   C. The current level of fluoride in the water supply
   D. Children's decayed, missing, filled teeth (DMFT) scores
   E. Centers for Disease Control and Prevention (CDC) recommendation

3. All of the following are important risk factors for development of dental caries in this population EXCEPT one. Which one is the EXCEPTION?
   A. Children's poor oral hygiene
   B. Cultural diversity of the population
   C. Community water supply fluoride level
   D. Low SES of the population

4. Which change in the DMFT scores would indicate the most successful outcome 5 years after implementation of the program?
   A. Decrease in D, increase in F, and no change in M
   B. Decrease in D, decrease in F, and decrease in M
   C. Increase in D, decrease in F, and no change in M
   D. No change in D, increase in F, and decrease in M
   E. No change in D, increase in F, and increase in M

5. The "e" in the index used to assess this population indicates teeth that are (Select all that apply.)
   A. already exfoliated.
   B. extracted because of dental caries.
   C. surrounded by primate spaces.
   D. severely decayed and indicated for extraction.

Questions 6 through 11 refer to information in the following testlet.

A dental hygienist in a community clinic is working with the medical clinic staff to develop an interdisciplinary program to improve the oral care of pregnant women who are treated in the community clinic. The population of the community clinic is primarily Hispanic and of low SES. Approximately 30% of the pregnant women in this population develop gestational diabetes. When a woman first sees the nurse practitioner in the medical clinic for prenatal care, she is referred to the dental clinic for a dental examination and for routine dental treatment. Only 20% of the patients referred over the previous 6 months complied with the dental referral. As a result, the medical and dental staff collaborated to conduct a survey of the pregnant women served by this clinic. Results revealed that the women do not realize their risk for diabetes and are unaware of the relationship between oral health status and diabetes. The women

do not understand the benefits of an oral health assessment in relation to their overall health and the health of their babies. For the purpose of discussing the problem and possible solutions, the dental hygienist arranged a meeting of the medical clinic director, the dental clinic director, one of the nurse practitioners, a prominent leader of the Hispanic community, and a dental clinic staff member from the community.

6. Which of the following would be the MOST effective intervention to implement to increase compliance with the dental referral?
   A. Conducting oral health screening during prenatal care visits
   B. Developing written educational materials for distribution during prenatal visits
   C. Documenting the oral condition of the women who have complied and received a dental examination
   D. Planning an educational presentation about the relationship among oral health, systemic health, and the risks and consequences of diabetes for the pregnant women

7. Based on the results of the survey, which of the following health education theories would be the MOST appropriate to use as the foundation for an oral health education intervention to improve compliance with the dental referral?
   A. Learning Ladder
   B. Health Belief Model
   C. Social Cognitive Theory
   D. Theory of Reasoned Action
   E. Trans-theoretical Model or Stages of Change

8. Which of the following is a valid conclusion about the population from the results of the survey?
   A. They have low health literacy.
   B. They have no access to oral health care.
   C. They have other priorities higher than oral health care.
   D. They do not have access to care in private dental offices in the community.

9. Which characteristic of public health is exemplified by the dental referral by the medical clinic?
   A. Personal responsibility for oral health
   B. Community, rather than the individual, as the patient
   C. Application of biostatistics to analyze population health problems
   D. Multidisciplinary team approach to solving public health problems

10. The process of involving and activating members of the community in a meeting is an example of which theory of health promotion?
    A. Sense of Coherence
    B. Diffusion of Innovation Theory
    C. Community Organization Theory
    D. Organizational Change: Stage Theory

11. Lower-SES populations are identified as a high priority target populations in the United States because these populations are identified as having unmet oral health needs by the Surgeon General's Report.
    A. Both the statement and the reason are correct and related.
    B. Both the statement and the reason are correct but NOT related.
    C. The statement is correct, but the reason is not.
    D. The statement is NOT correct, but the reason is correct.
    E. NEITHER the statement NOR the reason is correct.

Questions 12 through 15 refer to information in the following testlet.

A dental hygienist is employed as a dental hygiene coordinator at a local, federally subsidized facility that provides assisted-living and full nursing home care. The hygienist's duties include (1) conducting initial assessments by utilizing a tongue blade and available light for new residents, (2) developing individual dental hygiene treatment plans, (3) planning educational and other oral health programs to meet residents' needs, (4) utilizing intermittent measurements of oral health status and oral hygiene for evaluation purposes, and (5) coordinating annual examinations. The dental hygiene coordinator arranges for another hygienist from the Health Department to help conduct annual epidemiologic examinations of oral health status and oral hygiene to monitor progress of the program. The O'Leary plaque index is used to evaluate oral hygiene. The dental hygiene coordinator and Health Department hygienist participate in a team calibration exercise prior to the annual examinations.

12. Which type of examination is used for the initial assessment of new residents?
    A. Type I
    B. Type II
    C. Type III
    D. Type IV

13. Which of the following BEST describes the purpose for calibrating the second dental hygienist before the team conducts the annual examinations?
    A. Increase the validity of the evaluation results
    B. Introduce objectivity into the evaluation process

C. Ensure the residents' cooperation with the screening process
    D. Increase the interexaminer (interrater) reliability of the evaluation results

14. In this testlet, the initial assessment of oral hygiene status performed by the dental hygiene coordinator is comparable with which component of private practice?
    A. Funding
    B. Diagnosis
    C. Treatment
    D. Evaluation
    E. Examination

15. Which of the following could be an effect of using a disclosant in the application of the O'Leary plaque index to measure plaque in this program? (Select all that apply.)
    A. Decrease validity
    B. Increase reliability
    C. Decrease sensitivity
    D. Decrease specificity
    E. Increase sensitivity

Questions 16 through 21 refer to information in the following testlet.

A dental hygienist is employed by the local health department and participates in a weekly school sealant program for children in kindergarten through sixth grade. The program is located in a lower and middle SES, multiethnic city with an adequately fluoridated community water supply. Although the community water supply is adequately fluoridated, DMF scores taken in the initial screening indicate much higher than expected caries rates. The hygienist's role is to place the sealants on the children's teeth and to provide classroom educational programs to teach proper oral hygiene. Children are screened at the beginning of the year to determine caries status and identify teeth to be sealed. Low-SES children who need treatment for active caries are referred to local dental offices for treatment. The program is evaluated by tracking the number of sealants placed, monitoring the participation level, and measuring the reduction in caries by comparing "D" in the DMF scores at baseline and at 1, 2, and 3 years.

16. What term correctly describes the rate of disease that is constant in a population?
    A. Endemic
    B. Epidemic
    C. Pandemic

17. Which of the following programs would be MOST recommended to provide safe and cost effective caries prevention, in addition to the sealant program for this high caries risk population?
    A. Application of fluoride varnish
    B. Weekly fluoride rinse program at school
    C. Distribution of over–the-counter (OTC) fluoride dentifrice at school
    D. Implementation of a fluoride supplement program
    E. Application of fluoride foam using the tray method

18. Which of the following are possible funding sources for this program? (Select all that apply.)
    A. Head Start
    B. State income tax
    C. Federal block grant
    D. Local school funding
    E. Local service organization

19. Which of the following is the MOST effective teaching strategy to evaluate learning for toothbrushing in the educational programs with these school children? (Select all that apply.)
    A. Lecture
    B. Role play
    C. Discussion
    D. Demonstration
    E. Games and activities

20. A public health problem is a condition that is widespread and has an actual or potential cause of morbidity or mortality. Using this definition, the school system has a public health problem based on the high DMF scores of the school children.
    A. Both the statement and the reason are correct and related.
    B. Both the statement and the reason are correct but NOT related.
    C. The statement is correct, but the reason is not.
    D. The statement is NOT correct, but the reason is correct.
    E. NEITHER the statement NOR the reason is correct.

21. If the DMF scores of the different SES groups are compared, which of the following would be the expected results?
    A. Lower rates of DMF in the lower-SES groups
    B. Higher DMF scores in the higher-SES children with more treated decay
    C. Higher DMF scores in the lower-SES children, with more treated decay
    D. Higher DMF scores in the higher-SES children, with more untreated decay
    E. Higher DMF scores in the lower-SES children, with more untreated decay

Questions 22 through 25 refer to information in the following testlet.

A dental hygienist employed by a children's hospital dental clinic is responsible for coordinating programs to serve medically compromised children in the service area. The population consists of a mix of diverse SES and ethnic groups. The dental hygienist's responsibilities include managing the clinic that provides dental and dental hygiene treatment for the children, training hospital staff in daily oral care of hospitalized children, serving as a resource to the hospital staff, conducting oral hygiene educational programs for clinic patients and their parents, and supervising the distribution of self-care fluoride products. The effectiveness of the educational programs is evaluated by comparing pretest and posttest scores of knowledge and oral health behaviors of the clinic patients.

22. Which of the following are the three characteristics that compose epidemiologic factors of disease? (Select all that apply.)
    A. Host
    B. Agent
    C. Multifactorial
    D. Environmental
    E. Interrelationship

23. Which type of evaluation involves comparison of the pretest and posttest scores?
    A. Formative and qualitative
    B. Formative and quantitative
    C. Summative and qualitative
    D. Summative and quantitative

24. The primary role of the public health dental hygienist is to provide direct patient treatment. The dental hygienist's role in this program is primarily coordination, training, and serving as a resource that fulfills the role of the public health hygienist.
    A. Both statements are true.
    B. Both statements are false.
    C. The first statement is true, and the second statement is false.
    D. The first statement is false, and the second statement is true.

25. Assessment data are collected from each pediatric patient to determine his or her dental experiences. Which of the following terms describes the children's annual visits to a dentist or dental hygienist?
    A. Access
    B. Demand
    C. Utilization
    D. Perceived need
    E. Normative need

Questions 26 through 30 refer to information in the following testlet.

> A dental hygienist consulted with a Head Start program to plan a program in a metropolitan community with optimally fluoridated water. The needs of the children are assessed with the Basic Screening Survey (BSS), including classification as treatment needed or having no treatment needs. Children who required treatment are classified as immediate treatment needed, treatment needed in the near future, and treatment that can be delayed. A fluoride varnish program is planned for the children along with oral health educational programs for children, parents, and staff.

26. What level of prevention is addressed by this program?
    A. Tertiary
    B. Primary
    C. Secondary

27. Which of the following is an appropriate instructional objective for the Head Start teachers in this program?
    A. After an instructional session, children will demonstrate correct brushing.
    B. After an in-service program, classroom teachers will be able to identify 75% of children with signs of early childhood caries in their classrooms.
    C. Parents will complete consent forms for fluoride varnish for 95% of the children.
    D. Parents will be able to select candies and gums made with noncariogenic sweeteners.

28. Which of the following types of data is represented by the classification of treatment needs?
    A. Ratio
    B. Ordinal
    C. Interval
    D. Nominal

29. Which of the following is the MOST appropriate use of the data generated by the screening? Select the *two* that are most applicable.
    A. Referral
    B. Research
    C. Program planning
    D. Calibration of examiners
    E. Baseline data for a funding request

30. Which of the following is the BEST fluoride program for this project?
    A. Fluoride rinse
    B. Fluoride varnish
    C. High fluoride dentifrice
    D. Fluoride tablet supplements

Questions 31 through 34 refer to information in the following testlet.

> A dental hygienist is interested in conducting an oral health program for a nursing home in her community. The intraoral screening reveals that out of 100 residents, 50 are fully edentulous (50%), and of those edentulous residents, 75% have dentures. The majority of residents require assistance with basic self-care. A program is planned to train the nurses' aides to provide daily oral care, including cleaning of dentures. The educational program for the aides includes their own personal oral care.

31. Which of the following is the purpose of including personal oral care for the nurses' aides?
    A. To motivate them to attend the educational program
    B. To prepare them to serve as role models for the residents
    C. To help them understand and appreciate the value of personal oral care
    D. To learn the skills that they will use to provide oral care for the residents

32. Which of the following actions should occur next in this program?
    A. Developing a lesson plan for the educational program
    B. Selecting teaching strategies for the educational program
    C. Requesting funding for supplies from the local dental hygiene society
    D. Contacting the local dental hygiene program to solicit student involvement in the program
    E. Meeting with the director and director of nursing to determine program goals and objectives

33. Which of the following is the BEST program to implement after the nurse aides are trained in personal oral care?
    A. Fluoride program for the residents
    B. Denture care instruction for the residents
    C. Denture care instruction for the nurse aides
    D. Oral hygiene education program for the residents

34. Who is the responsible party to contact if the dental hygienist identifies possible oral cancer lesions during the intraoral screening?
    A. The family
    B. The residents
    C. The nurse aides
    D. The director of nursing
    E. No one because of confidentiality issues

Questions 35 through 40 refer to information in the following testlet.

A group of students in a dental hygiene program conduct a study to determine the best method to increase periodontal patients' compliance with their periodontal maintenance schedule. The research question to be answered is, "What effect does modifying the scheduling procedure for a periodontal disease maintenance appointment have on patient compliance with their appointments?" A survey is administered to all patients at their final visit about their attitudes, beliefs, and opinions about the importance of periodontal maintenance.

The students divide the patient population into three groups, using sequential assignment based on the order that they appear for treatment in the clinic. One group is appointed for the next periodontal maintenance appointment prior to leaving the clinic. The other group is entered into the computer to be called for an appointment when due. The third group is not scheduled at all. In the process of assigning patients to their method of appointment scheduling, the groups are matched to ensure that each group is similar for periodontal case types and gender. The groups are given the same verbal and written instructions about the importance of complying with periodontal maintenance on a recommended schedule in relation to their treatment outcomes. Review of past research indicates that the strength of the relationship between periodontal health and periodontal maintenance is a coefficient correlation of 0.62.

35. For each variable in the study and listed below, select the MOST closely linked type of variable from the list provided.

Variable in the Study	Type of Variable
___ 1. Age	A. Dependent
___ 2. Compliance with periodontal maintenance	B. Extraneous
___ 3. Gender	C. Independent
___ 4. Instructions about the importance of periodontal maintenance	D. Relevant and controlled
___ 5. Method of appointment scheduling	
___ 6. Periodontal status	

36. Which of the following is the purpose of giving the same verbal and written instructions about periodontal maintenance to all groups of patients?
   A. Increasing the validity of the study
   B. Satisfying the ethical requirements
   C. Increasing the reliability of the study
   D. Making the teaching process easier
   E. Increasing compliance with periodontal maintenance

37. The entire dental hygiene faculty in the dental hygiene clinic uses the same standardized design of periodontal probe at all times to measure clinical attachment loss to classify patients' periodontal status and has calibrated with each other on the use of this probe. Select the *two* factors that are enhanced by using the same periodontal probe and calibration.
   A. Greater sensitivity
   B. Increased reliability
   C. Higher interrater reliability
   D. Higher intrarater reliability
   E. Increased statistical significance

38. If the survey had been conducted on a sample of the population, which of the following would have been the BEST sampling method to use?
   A. Random
   B. Judgmental
   C. Systematic
   D. Convenience
   E. Stratified random

39. On the basis of the correlation coefficient, which of the following types of relationship was found between periodontal health and compliance with periodontal maintenance?
   A. Weak and positive
   B. Strong and negative
   C. Strong and positive
   D. Moderate and negative
   E. Moderate and positive

40. Which of the following is the BEST graphing technique to depict the compliance of both groups when the results are presented to the professional and administrative staff of the clinic?
   A. Pie chart
   B. Bar graph
   C. Histogram
   D. Scattergram
   E. Frequency polygon

Questions 41 through 45 refer to information in the following testlet.

Local dentists, hygienists, and assistants join together with second-year dental hygiene students and their faculty to provide a sealant and fluoride varnish clinic for children of migrant workers; the workers are employed at a meat packing plant in a rural town in southwestern United States. The migrant families are primarily Spanish speaking. The program is conducted in the local elementary school, and portable dental equipment is used. There are 300 children attending the school at the time the clinic is held. The school nurse selects the children enrolled in free lunch program from first, second, and fifth grade levels to participate in the program and obtains the necessary consent forms signed by parents. Working in teams, a dentist, a hygienist, an assistant, and a dental hygiene student provide screening for sealant placement and referral to Medicaid providers for additional treatment needed. Some teams provide oral hygiene instruction, and some place sealants, and some apply the fluoride varnish.

41. Which of the following is the BEST group to target for an oral health in-service to continue ongoing oral health education after the program has been implemented?
    A. Parents
    B. School nurse
    C. Classroom teachers
    D. Dental hygiene students

42. All of the following are stakeholders of this program EXCEPT one. Which one is the EXCEPTION?
    A. Parents
    B. School nurse
    C. Dental personnel
    D. School administrators
    E. State health department

43. Which of the following is the BEST way to evaluate the outcomes of the sealant program?
    A. Evaluate the percentage of children served
    B. Screen the children with the OHI-S 6 months later
    C. Ask the children about their perceptions of the program
    D. Conduct a basic screening a year later to assess for incidence of decay
    E. Conduct parent focus groups to determine their satisfaction with the program

44. Which of the following is the MOST culturally sensitive procedure to use during the presentation of an oral health education program for parents?
    A. Hiring translators to interpret
    B. Presenting the program in English
    C. Using children to translate for their parents
    D. Hiring Hispanic school staff and dental personnel who can translate

45. The program exemplifies all of the following recommendations of the National Call to Action to Promote Oral Health initiative EXCEPT one. Which one is the EXCEPTION?
    A. Increase collaborations
    B. Change perceptions of oral health
    C. Overcome barriers by replicating effective programs
    D. Increase workforce diversity, capacity, and flexibility
    E. Build the science knowledge base and accelerate science literacy transfer

Questions 46 through 49 refer to information in the following testlet.

A public health dental hygienist coordinates an annual assessment of the oral health needs of a local preschool with an enrollment of 90 3- to 4-year-old children. The children are from Hispanic, African American, and non-Hispanic White families of low SES, and 85% qualify for Medicaid or the Children's Health Insurance Program (CHIP). The preschool is located in a city that is not optimally fluoridated. A consent form is required to participate in the oral health assessment survey. The results of the screening revealed an average dmfs score of 1.0. The children that were screened were referred to a dental facility. A summary report of the results of the assessment and referral was prepared for the children's parents.

46. The dmfs of this population indicates that the children suffer from early childhood caries. The dmfs is the appropriate index used for detection of early childhood caries.
    A. Both statements are true.
    B. Both statements are false.
    C. The first statement is true, and the second statement is false.
    D. The first statement is false, and the second statement is true.

47. After seeing the high levels of ECC in the children, the public health hygienist is motivated to organize a fluoridation campaign for this community. Which of the following would be the BEST first step?
    A. Organizing a debate between profluoridationists and antifluoridationists

B. Testifying before the city council to convince them to fluoridate the water

C. Having a referendum to allow the citizens to express their opinion about fluoridation

D. Making contacts with key community leaders to obtain a broad base of support for fluoridation

E. Organizing a massive community educational program about the benefits and safety of fluoridation

48. What other index could be used to screen these children for dental caries in public health settings?
A. Decayed and filled (df)
B. Basic Screening Survey (BSS)
C. Decayed, missing, and filled (DMF)
D. Decayed, extracted due to caries, and filled (def)

49. All of the following procedures fulfill the ethical obligations of community oral health practice EXCEPT one. Which one is the EXCEPTION?
A. Preparation of the report
B. Requirement of a consent form
C. Use of a valid index to measure caries
D. Speaking with each parent individually
E. Referral of children with caries to a dental home

Questions 50 through 54 refer to information in the following testlet.

A dental hygienist employed by the local health department is charged with providing educational programs for the Women Infants and Children (WIC) program. One of her first assignments is to present an educational program on basic oral health for culturally diverse pregnant teens in an alternative high school in the district. She conducts a pre-test to provide a baseline assessment of the teens' knowledge. Based on the results of the baseline assessment, the dental hygienist develops an educational program, and then gives a follow-up post-test to evaluate the program's effectiveness.

50. Which of the following study designs is used?
A. Factorial
B. Time-series
C. Posttest-only
D. Pretest–posttest

51. All of the following procedures would enhance the cultural characteristics of the population EXCEPT one. Which one is the EXCEPTION?
A. Utilizing consistent teaching methods with all students
B. Conducting a class discussion of the student's family health practices
C. Including instructional materials into the first language of the students
D. Developing an activity for students to identify noncariogenic ethnic foods

52. The local health department asks the dental hygienist to write a grant application based on the results of the educational program presented to the high school students. Which of the following statements could serve as a null hypothesis for future studies?
A. There will be an increase in the participants' scores from the pretest to the posttest after the educational presentation.
B. There will be no increase in the participants' scores from the pretest to the posttest after the educational presentation.
C. There will be a decrease in the participants' scores from the pretest to the posttest after the educational presentation.
D. There will be a large increase in the participants' scores from the pretest to the posttest after the educational presentation.

53. What type of control group is used?
A. Passive
B. Placebo
C. Positive
D. Standard
E. No control group is used

54. All of the following characteristics of an experimental study are present in the program evaluation EXCEPT one. Which one is the EXCEPTION?
A. Use of randomization
B. Measurement of the dependent variable
C. Manipulation of the independent variable
D. Placement of the independent variable before the independent variable in the design

Questions 55 through 59 refer to information in the following testlet.

A community fluoride varnish program is funded by Kaiser Permanente. Kaiser Permanente will also fund dental treatment for the children who are suffering from dental pain and provide an educational program for the parents. The program is a collaborative effort of Head Start, a community clinic, and a local dental hygiene program. The Head Start children are screened by a dental hygienist whose position is funded by the program. The urban community is not fluoridated, and the natural level of fluoride in the community water supply is 0.01 ppm. The state dental practice act does not require a dentist for the screening because the children will be referred to the community clinic for treatment and follow-up. The screening is accomplished with a tongue blade and available light. The children are then referred to a community dental clinic for fluoride varnish placement by dental hygiene students on rotation from a local dental hygiene program and for dental treatment, as needed. An education program is conducted with parents to increase compliance with the referral. The rate of compliance with the referral is determined to evaluate the effectiveness of the educational program.

55. Which of the following additional sources of funding would be available to provide dental treatment for the children in this program?
    A. Medicaid
    B. Medicare
    C. Private dental insurance
    D. CDC budget line item
    E. National Institute for Dental and Craniofacial Research (NIDCR) grant

56. The type of caries assessment used by the program is basic screening. Basic screening is appropriate assessment to determine dental treatment needs.
    A. Both statements are true.
    B. Both statements are false.
    C. The first statement is true, and the second statement is false.
    D. The first statement is false, and the second statement is true.

57. What type of practice supervision is used in this program?
    A. Direct
    B. General
    C. Indirect
    D. Independent

58. According to current CDC recommendations, what level of fluoride in parts per million (ppm) must be added to this community's water to bring the fluoride level to the optimum?
    A. 1.0
    B. 1.1
    C. 0.09
    D. 0.06

59. What type of data is generated by the summative program evaluation of the educational program?
    A. Discrete
    B. Qualitative
    C. Continuous
    D. Dichotomous

Questions 60 through 63 refer to information in the following testlet.

A dental hygienist who works in private practice also volunteers weekly in an elementary school sealant program that is funded for 3 years and conducted by

the regional health department in a nearby community of migrant farm workers. The community water supply is not fluoridated, and the children have a high rate of tooth decay. An oral health screening is conducted prior to sealing the children's teeth, and a caries index is recorded for each child on the basis of a visual examination of teeth. Children identified as needing dental treatment as a result of assessment throughout the program are referred to a local dentist. The total number of sealants placed during the 3-year funding cycle is used to evaluate the success of the program.

60. The SES and the rate of tooth decay make this community appropriate to target for this program. The expected distribution of the DMF in this population would be more D than F scores.
    A. Both statements are true.
    B. Both statements are false.
    C. The first statement is true, and the second statement is false.
    D. The first statement is false, and the second statement is true.

61. What is the optimal level of fluoride in the drinking water for this population?
    A. 0.7 ppm
    B. 3.0 ppm
    C. 0.7 to 1.2 ppm
    D. 1.2 ppm

62. What additional program would be the MOST cost effective fluoride delivery system for the community where the hygienist volunteers?
    A. Fluoride supplements
    B. Community water fluoridation
    C. School fluoride mouth rinse program
    D. No additional fluoride program is required

63. Which of the following caries indices is MOST appropriate for assessment in this program?
    A. def
    B. dmft
    C. dmfs
    D. DMFT
    E. DMFS

Questions 64 through 67 refer to information in the following testlet.

A research study is conducted in a dental school setting with 100 healthy, dentate adult patients who have been compliant with 6-month maintenance visits to determine if a new pyrophosphate formula dentifrice is more effective in controlling calculus formation in adults. Study participants *are screened using the Volpe-Manhold index to measure calculus at the initial examination. They receive a dental prophylaxis, oral hygiene instructions, toothbrush, and floss and are instructed to use no other oral hygiene aids or mouth rinses during the study period. The participants are randomly assigned to use either a dentifrice with 5% percent soluble pyrophosphate or a standard dentifrice with 3.3% soluble pyrophosphate. All other ingredients of both dentifrices are standard, including 0.05 mg sodium fluoride (NaF). The Volpe-Manhold index is used to measure calculus after 4 months. It is a double-blind study, with both study participants and examiners unaware of the group assignment. After 4 months of ad lib usage, the group using the 5% pyrophosphate formula exhibits significantly less dental calculus than the group using the 3.3% pyrophosphate formula using a probability level of ($p <0.05$). The t-test is used to analyze the differences between the means of the differences in calculus scores between the two groups. The conclusion was that that the 5% pyrophosphate formula is more effective than the 3.3% pyrophosphate formula to control calculus formation. The research results were presented at a poster session for dental educators at a national meeting.*

64. Which of the following is the FIRST step in the scientific method?
    A. Asking a question
    B. Drawing a conclusion
    C. Developing a hypothesis
    D. Collecting and analyzing data
    E. Verifying or rejecting the hypothesis

65. For each numbered research term or phrase listed below, select from the list provided the MOST closely linked description in relation to this study.

Research Term or Phrase	Description in Relation to this Study
___ 1. Assumption	A. Acceptance of only dentate adults compliant with 6-month maintenance to participate in the study
___ 2. Control of a variable	B. A weakness of a study; individual rate of calculus formation; an attempt to control the limitation in this study was performing a prophylaxis at the onset of the program
___ 3. Delimitation	C. Inclusion of 0.05 mg NaF in both dentifrices
___ 4. Ethical principle	D. Performing a prophylaxis on all patients to start with baseline calculus free status prior to starting the study
___ 5. Limitation	E. The use of a higher concentration of pyrophosphates resulting in reduction in calculus formation

66. Select the four items that describe the type of study represented.
    A. Analytic
    B. Clinical trial
    C. Double blind
    D. Experimental
    E. Pretest–posttest

67. For each numbered potential variation in study design, select from the list provided the MOST closely linked description of that study design variation in relation to this study.

Study Design	Study Description
___ 1. Cross-over	A. If all participants used both dentifrices, using the 5% formula on one side of the mouth and the 3.3% formula on the other side of the mouth
___ 2. Factorial	B. If brushing time were added as a second independent variable, resulting in four groups: (1) 5% formula with 1 minute of brushing, (2) 5% formula with 2 minutes of brushing, (3) 3.3% formula with 1 minute of brushing, and (4) 3.3% formula with 2 minutes of brushing
___ 3. Split-mouth	C. If calculus formation were measured each month during the 4 months of the study
___ 4. Time-series	D. If the study continued for an additional 4 months with each group switching to the other dentifrice formula for the second 4-month period

Questions 68 through 72 refer to information in the following testlet.

A split-mouth, randomized, repeated-measures clinical trial is conducted to test the effect of calcium hypophosphate as a desensitizing agent in postperiodontal-therapy patients with hypersensitive teeth. A dental examination has been performed to ensure that the hypersensitivity is not related to caries or pulpal pathology. This in vivo study is conducted on 22 sensitive teeth from eight female patients in a dental school clinic. The treatment is randomly assigned; on one side of the dentition, 11 teeth are treated with calcium hypophosphate, and on the other side of the dentition 11 teeth are treated with a placebo of distilled water. Two desensitizing treatments are performed 1 week apart. Patients' responses to cold and mechanical stimulation are elicited with cold water and a #23 explorer at baseline, 1 week, and 1 month. The patients indicate on a 1-to-5 scale the degree of pain response to the stimuli. The researchers conclude that calcium hypophosphate significantly decreases the patients' pain response (p=0.01).

68. Which of the following defines "in vivo" in this study design?
    A. The study is retrospective.
    B. The population is limited by specific criteria.
    C. The study is conducted on live study participants.
    D. Laboratory tests are conducted prior to this study.
    E. The purpose of the study is to test the effectiveness of a product.

69. All of the following are required ethical procedures for the study EXCEPT one. Which one is the EXCEPTION?
    A. Publishing participants' pain responses
    B. Informed consent from study participants
    C. Protection of study participants' anonymity
    D. Communication of research results to the profession
    E. Approval of a committee to assess the safety of the study design

70. For each numbered research term listed below, select the MOST closely linked description that reflects this study. Descriptions can be used more than one time.

Research term	Description that reflects this study
___ 1. Control group	A. 11 teeth treated with calcium hypophosphate
___ 2. Experimental group	B. 11 teeth concurrently treated with distilled water
___ 3. Population	C. 22 sensitive teeth used for the research study
___ 4. Sample	D. Measurement of pain by self-report at all measurement periods
	E. Postperiodontal therapy patients with sensitive teeth
	F. Solicitation of pain with cold and mechanical stimulation

71. There is a 1% chance that the results of this study have a type II beta (β) error. A type II beta (β) error occurs when treatment was not really effective and invalid results show a statistically significant difference occurred between the experimental and control treatments.
    A. Both statements are true.
    B. Both statements are false.
    C. First statement is true, and the second statement is false.
    D. First statement is false, and the second statement is true.

72. This study represents the highest level of evidence for evidence-based decision making. All research studies, regardless of the type of study, represent the same level of evidence for evidence-based decision making.
    A. Both statements are true.
    B. Both statements are false.
    C. The first statement is true, and the second statement is false.
    D. The first statement is false, and the second statement is true.

Questions 73 through 77 refer to information in the following testlet.

A study is conducted with a convenience sample of adults to compare the effectiveness of two types of dental floss, a new one on the market and a popular one already on the market that has been previously tested. Two randomly formed groups of adults each use a different type of floss. Group assignment is accomplished in such a way to ensure that both groups have an equivalent number of males and females and an equivalent number in each age group. Each study participant is supplied with the appropriate type of floss, given flossing instructions, is instructed to floss once a day, and is asked not to use any other type of floss for the duration of the study. Plaque scores are recorded by a single examiner trained in the use of the Plaque Index at baseline and again at 2 weeks, 4 weeks, and 6 weeks. Because of the nature of the products being tested, the study participants are aware of the identification of the floss they are using. However, the examiner is unaware of which dental floss is used by each participant examined. All study participants are given a new soft toothbrush (same type and brand) and asked to brush twice a day for

2 minutes each time for the duration of the study. At the end of the 6-week period, the study participants are given the other type of floss to continue flossing, and another new soft toothbrush of the same type and brand used previously. Their plaque scores are measured at 2, 4, and 6 weeks later. The research report describing the study and results are published in a peer reviewed dental hygiene journal.

73. Who reviewed the research report to approve its publication in the journal?
    A. The journal editor
    B. Professional writers
    C. Experts in the content area
    D. Professional associates of the author

74. All of the following should be examined to judge the quality of the journal in which the study is published EXCEPT one. Which one is the EXCEPTION?
    A. Sponsorship of the journal
    B. Technical quality of the journal
    C. Advertising policy of the journal
    D. Qualifications of the editorial review board
    E. Number of pictures, tables, and graphs in the publication

75. Which of the following methods of group assignment was used in this study?
    A. Random assignment
    B. Sequential assignment
    C. Randomized matching
    D. Use of a comparison group

76. Match the study types with their correct descriptions.

Study Type	Study Description
____1. Clinical trial	A. Characterized by presence of a control group, control of extraneous variables, randomization, control of errors in measurement, use of blind examiners, and measurement of the dependent variable multiple times, manipulation of an independent variable, measurement of a dependent variable, and occurrence of the independent variable before measuring the dependent variable in the study design
____2. Cross-over	B. A well-controlled experimental study or group comparison based on epidemiologic principles and designed to test a hypothesis of a clinical nature

____3. Double-blind C. Groups switched to the other treatment halfway through the study after measuring the dependent variable to test the effect of the independent variable on the other group

____4. Experimental D. Both examiners and study participants unaware of group assignment

____5. Posttest only E. Dependent variable measured, for comparison purposes, before and after the introduction of the independent variable

____6. Pretest–posttest F. Dependent variable measured several times at posttest to establish that the independent variable is effective over time

____7. Split-mouth G. Random assignment used to form groups

____8. Randomized H. Half of the dentition used for the experiment; the other half used for control

____9. Time-series I. Dependent variable only measured after the independent variable is introduced

77. If the participants had been assigned a 1-month period between the two flossing phases of the study and during which they did not floss; that period would be called a
    A. placebo.
    B. baseline.
    C. washout.
    D. cross-over.

Questions 78 through 82 refer to information in the following testlet.

The effectiveness of teaching personal home care to periodontal patients treated in a federal prison dental clinic is evaluated to determine if changes in patient education are warranted. Gingival bleeding and plaque percentage data are routinely scored in the patients' charts at each appointment using the Sulcus Bleeding Index (SBI) and O'Leary Plaque Control Record, respectively. The clinicians in the clinic that score the index have been trained and calibrated on the use of the index. The percentage of plaque scored at the assessment appointment is presented in the following table and graph for a sample of 24 patients reviewed for this evaluation.

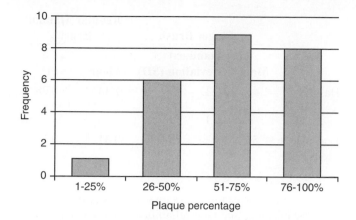

Plaque Percentage of Periodontal Patients at Assessment Appointment

Plaque %	Frequency	Percent
1–25%	1	4%
26–50%	6	25%
51–75%	9	38%
76–100%	8	33%
Total	24	100%

78. Which of the following is the number of intervals in the frequency distribution table?
    A. 100
    B. 24
    C. 8
    D. 4

79. The histogram is an appropriate way to present the frequency data because the data are continuous.
    A. Both the statement and the reason are correct and related.
    B. Both the statement and the reason are correct but NOT related.
    C. The statement is correct, but the reason is not.
    D. The statement is NOT correct, but the reason is correct.
    E. NEITHER the statement NOR the reason is correct.

80. According to the information presented in the table, what percentage of patients scored greater than 50% on the O'Leary Plaque Control Record at their first assessment appointment?
    A. 25%
    B. 29%
    C. 33%
    D. 38%
    E. 71%

81. Which type of curve does this distribution represent?
    A. Negatively skewed
    B. Positively skewed
    C. Symmetrical (bell)

82. Which of the following describes the reasons that the O'Leary Plaque Control Record and the SBI will be the only indices used at all appointments subsequent to the assessment appointment?
    A. It is more valid to compare measures from one index with those from another index because each index has different criteria.
    B. These are the only indices to measure oral hygiene and bleeding in a public health clinical setting.
    C. Use of these indices controls reliability, since the clinicians are trained and calibrated on them.
    D. Any valid oral hygiene and bleeding indices can be used; it is not necessary to use only these indices at each subsequent appointment.

Questions 83 through 87 refer to information in the following testlet.

> A national survey of dental hygienists is conducted to determine salaries and employment benefits. A 25% sample is formed by randomly selecting study participants from the list of 30,000 members of the American Dental Hygienists' Association (ADHA). During the random selection process, the sample is balanced to represent proportionally the number of members in each state. The results of the study indicate that increased age, and years in practice is strongly and positively associated with salary ($r=0.75$; $p < 0.05$).

83. What type of study is this?
    A. Case-control
    B. Longitudinal
    C. Retrospective
    D. Cross-sectional
    E. Statistical analysis

84. Which of the following would increase the return rate of the survey?
    A. Use of an electronic survey
    B. Including a self-addressed return envelope
    C. Establishing validity and reliability of the survey
    D. Eliminating the cover letter to reduce the reading time

85. What type of statistic is used to test the relationship of years in practice with salary?
    A. Parametric
    B. Correlation
    C. Descriptive
    D. Nonparametric

86. How can statistical significance of study results be determined?
    A. The results were statistically significant because the *p*-value was below 0.10.
    B. The results were statistically significant because the *p*-value was below 0.05.
    C. The results were not statistically significant because the *p*-value was below 0.01.
    D. The results were not statistically significant because the *p*-value was below 0.01.

	Finger Brush		Regular Manual Brush	
	Mean	Standard Deviation (SD)	Mean	SD
Baseline plaque scores	1.41	0.32	1.44	0.28
End-plaque scores	0.56	0.23	0.31	0.17

87. The results of this study establish a causal relationship between years in practice and salary. The sampling method used results in a representative sample for this heterogeneous population.
    A. Both statements are true.
    B. Both statements are false.
    C. The first statement is true, and the second statement is false.
    D. The first statement is false, and the second statement is true.

Questions 88 through 92 refer to information in the following testlet.

A blind study is conducted in a dental hygiene program to compare the plaque removal ability of a "finger brush" with an ADA-accepted regular manual toothbrush. Thirty-seven periodontally healthy dental hygiene student volunteers (11 male and 26 female) are recruited, trained in the use of both brushes, given written instructions to refer to, provided with a new finger brush and manual brush, and given a 3-week period to practice the use of both brushes throughout the mouth prior to taking baseline measurements. After the training period, participants return to have baseline plaque measured with the Plaque Index, are given a new finger brush and a new manual brush, and brush as assigned with supervision by other dental hygiene students. The first assigned toothbrush, the finger brush or the manual brush, is used in a randomly assigned half of the mouth. The other brush is used to brush the other half of the mouth. Participants brush without toothpaste for 2 minutes on each half of the mouth. After the participants brush, trained examiners measure plaque again using the same index, dental unit, and operating lamp. The null hypothesis of this study is that there is no difference in the plaque removal ability of the two devices. The mean and standard deviation (SD) of the baseline and end-plaque scores are presented in results of the study are that the manual toothbrush is 22% more effective in removing plaque compared with the finger brush (p <0.01). The research report is published in a national peer-reviewed dental hygiene journal dated 4 years prior to the current date.

88. Training the examiners is for the purpose of establishing interrater reliability. The procedures of giving a practice period for use of the toothbrushes, timing the toothbrushing, and withholding toothpaste during brushing are for the purpose of controlling the reliability of the study.
    A. Both statements are true.
    B. Both statements are false.
    C. The first statement is true, and the second statement is false.
    D. The first statement is false, and the second statement is true.

89. Examiner bias in this study is controlled. This is because the examiners are unaware of which brush was used in which area of the mouth by the research participants.
    A. Both statements are true.
    B. Both statements are false.
    C. The first statement is true, and the second statement is false.
    D. The first statement is false, and the second statement is true.

90. Using the information provided in the table, in which range of values did 95% of the baseline scores fall?
    A. 0.66 and 2.66
    B. 0.77 and 2.05
    C. 0.50 and 2.75

91. On the basis of the statistical results of this study, what decision should be made regarding the null hypothesis?
    A. Reject the null hypothesis; the manual toothbrush is more effective.
    B. Accept the null hypothesis; there is no difference in plaque removal ability of the two devices.
    C. Reject the null hypothesis; the finger brush is more effective.
    D. Accept the null hypothesis; the manual toothbrush is less effective.

92. The report is considered out of date according to the timing of its publication. The peer review of the journal is designed to provide quality assurance of published research.
    A. Both statements are true.
    B. Both statements are false.
    C. The first statement is true, and the second statement is false.
    D. The first statement is false, and the second statement is true.

Questions 93 through 97 refer to information in the following testlet.

A dental hygienist has been invited to speak to a group of women at the local Women Infants and Children (WIC) program about nutrition and oral health care, with an emphasis on influencing the oral health status of the family through the personal health choices that mothers make. The results of a brief verbal survey given to the group about dental utilization are given to the dental hygienist before the presentation to help in program focus. The results of the survey indicate that none of the participants has been to a dentist in the last 2 years because of the lack of financial resources and dental insurance. The population consists of expectant and recent post-partum women, all from low-SES backgrounds and representing a variety of ethnic groups. Their main interest in attending the session is to learn ways to raise a healthy baby.

93. All of the following would be goals of the dental hygienist's presentation EXCEPT one. Which one is the EXCEPTION?
    A. Describing the effects of dietary choices on oral health
    B. Providing information on orthodontic treatment in children
    C. Discussing the value of good oral health for the mother and the child
    D. Emphasizing the importance of caries transmission and prevention
    E. Highlighting dental providers in the area who accept Medicaid, have payment plans, or both

94. Which health behavior model addresses the dental hygiene focus of creating and increasing awareness of healthy choices through a process of change over time as individuals cycle through stages of awareness and readiness?
    A. Locus of Control
    B. Health Belief Model
    C. Social Cognitive Theory
    D. Stages of Change: Transtheoretical Model

95. Which stage of the community program development process is addressed by the verbal survey?
    A. Planning
    B. Diagnosis
    C. Evaluation
    D. Assessment
    E. Implementation

96. Focusing on regular dental visits for this population would be considered promotion of a health behavior. Increasing the participants' understanding of the infectious nature of dental caries would be considered an example of a health promotion strategy.
    A. Both statements are true.
    B. Both statements are false.
    C. The first statement is true, and the second statement is false.
    D. The first statement is false, and the second statement is true.

97. The expectant mothers express interest in receiving dental care. This is an example of potential demand because it represents an unmet need.
    A. Both statements are true.
    B. Both statements are false.
    C. The first statement is true, and the second statement is false.
    D. The first statement is false, and the second statement is true.

Questions 98 through 102 refer to information in the following testlet.

A dental hygienist working with the U.S. Public Health Service on a remote Indian reservation notices a large number of children coming into the school-based clinic with high levels of incipient decay and decay in some permanent molars. Her clinic recently received additional funding for dental public health programming, so the hygienist decides to create a school-based sealant program for the tribe. The hygienist must first secure approval for the project from the tribal leaders, who need to be educated regarding the necessity for the program. Once the hygienist receives their authorization, she begins by recording the children's current dental caries status.

98. Sealants are an effective dental public health strategy for this population because of their cost-effectiveness, regardless of SES. When used as a public health intervention, sealants are usually applied to 8- to 9-year-old children (third graders) and 12- to 13-year-old children (seventh grade) at risk for dental caries.
    A. Both statements are true.
    B. Both statements are false.

C. The first statement is true, and the second statement is false.
D. The first statement is false, and the second statement is true.

99. Which of the following indices would be the MOST useful to evaluate the long-term success of this program?
A. RCI
B. dmft
C. OHI-S
D. DMFT

100. The incidence of dental caries among this population is the number of carious lesions noted at the time of program inception. Monitoring of caries prevalence, filled teeth, and missing teeth because of nonrestorable caries that required extraction should continue throughout the program's duration to evaluate program outcomes.
A. Both statements are true.
B. Both statements are false.
C. The first statement is true, and the second statement is false.
D. The first statement is false, and the second statement is true.

101. All of the following are potential barriers to care for this program EXCEPT one. Which one is the EXCEPTION?
A. Shortage of providers to place sealants
B. Lack of consumer awareness of sealants
C. High cost of sealants compared with restorations
D. Lack of funding to provide necessary equipment

102. The necessity of educating the tribal leaders about the need for the sealant program characterizes which dental public health concept?
A. Supply
B. Demand
C. Utilization
D. Perceived need
E. Normative need

Questions 103 through 107 refer to information in the following testlet.

The director of a homeless shelter located downtown in a major metropolitan area has noticed an increase in demand for assistance in accessing basic medical and dental services. The director asks a dental hygienist who volunteers at the shelter for help in spearheading the organization efforts. On the basis of the perceived needs of the clients, the dental hygienist asks several organizations,

including the regional medical and dental schools, a faith-based group, a service club, and the local councilman's office to partner with the shelter and its clients. The proposed facility would provide initial screening services, referrals to appropriate providers, and health education. The assembly of organizations broadcasts a goal of creating a self-sustaining, on-site medical and dental clinic within the next 5 years. The natural fluoride content of the community water supply is 0.1 ppm.

103. All of the following are terms which could describe the formation of a relationship between the homeless shelter and the various organizations or institutions that are described EXCEPT one. Which one is the EXCEPTION?
A. Covenant
B. Networking
C. Partnerships
D. Collaboration
E. Coalition building

104. Which of the following is the role of the dental hygienist in this program?
A. Clinician
B. Advocate
C. Educator
D. Administrator or manager

105. What type of assessment tool would provide the BEST indication of the normative need of this population?
A. A survey
B. An index
C. A focus group

106. Which of the following forms the foundation of the success of the program?
A. Compliance of the clients
B. Cooperation of the community partners
C. Amount of needs assessment data collected
D. Formation of measureable program objectives

107. All of the following *Healthy People 2020* objectives are pertinent for this population EXCEPT one. Which one is the EXCEPTION?
A. Decrease untreated dental decay
B. Increase dental sealant utilization
C. Implement water fluoridation for the community
D. Increase early detection of oral and pharyngeal cancers
E. Increase the proportion of school-based health centers with an oral health center

Questions 108 through 112 refer to information in the following testlet.

The administration of a small municipal hospital has noted a slow but steady increase in oral and pharyngeal cancers in the surveillance data over the last decade. This change in the pattern of cancer cases prompts the administration to take action to address the issue. They would like the city council to implement a smoke-free ordinance for all the restaurants, bars, and eateries within the city limits. As part of the efforts to encourage public support, a dental hygienist schedules several presentations with the parent-teacher organizations of the local schools. He gives a pretest and posttest to measure parent and teacher awareness of the connection between smoking and oral diseases. The hygienist discusses the research connections between smoking and oral and pharyngeal cancers, as well as the scientifically proven association of smoking with periodontal disease. To support his points, he cites data from recent National Institutes of Health (NIH) correlation studies.

108. Which of the following is another descriptor for the increase in oral and pharyngeal cancer rates referred to in this example?
    A. Trend
    B. Epidemic
    C. Incidence
    D. Pandemic
    E. Prevalence

109. A parent in the audience would be correct in interpreting the cited studies as showing that smoking is the primary cause of oral and pharyngeal cancer because the studies cited were statistically significant.
    A. Both the statement and the reason are correct and related.
    B. Both the statement and the reason are correct but NOT related.
    C. The statement is correct, but the reason is NOT.
    D. The statement is NOT correct, but the reason is correct.
    E. NEITHER the statement NOR the reason is correct

110. What type of visual graphic would BEST reflect relationship data such as the type discussed in the research studies cited in the presentation?
    A. Pie chart
    B. Bell curve
    C. Histogram
    D. Scattergram
    E. Simple bar graph

111. To evaluate the parents' learning, which of the following evaluation outcomes would reflect successful results from the dental hygienist's presentation?
    A. High level of audience interaction
    B. A well-organized, accurately informed presentation
    C. Change in audience knowledge as measured by the posttest

112. Which of the following types of evaluation is used to determine the program outcome of implementing a smoke-free ordinance for all the restaurants, bars, and eateries within the city limits?
    A. Internal
    B. External
    C. Formative
    D. Summative

Questions 113 through 118 refer to information in the following testlet.

The people of an isolated rural region have almost no access to oral health care. In addition, their water supply from the closest river has 0.3 ppm of fluoride. These combined factors have historically led to poor oral health status. The members of a state dental hygiene society want to improve oral health for this isolated region. A team is commissioned to assess the five villages that compose the community. A comprehensive community oral health assessment is analyzed and reveals high rates of dental caries, existing dental pain, and missing teeth.

Assessment results include the oral health status information included in the following table:

	Southern Village	Northern Village	Eastern Village	Western Village	Village Central
# people screened	27	35	29	33	25
# of people who were not screened	10	15	12	10	14
# people who had seen a dentist in the last year	2	0	1	1	1
# people currently experiencing dental pain	10	14	17	15	14
# people missing 6 teeth or more	8	16	13	11	8
# people who have loose teeth	2	5	1	3	3

113. All of the following should be included as components of the assessment for this population EXCEPT one. Which one is the EXCEPTION?
    A. Identifying the oral health needs of the population
    B. Evaluating the determinants of health for this population
    C. Determining what brands of toothbrushes and floss are available
    D. Asking about the resources and assets available to the community
    E. Quantification of disparities and inequities among the population groups

114. For this population, which of the following assessment tools are MOST effective to provide authentic data?
    A. Personal interviews
    B. Oral health screenings
    C. Written questionnaire surveys

115. Which of the following is the mean of the distribution of the number of people currently experiencing dental pain across the five villages?
    A. 10
    B. 12
    C. 14
    D. 16
    E. 18

116. The mode is the most frequently occurring score or most repeated number in a distribution of scores. This distribution of scores is unimodal.
    A. Both statements are true.
    B. Both statements are false.
    C. The first statement is true, and the second statement is false.
    D. The first statement is false, and the second statement is true.

117. The hygienists should focus on all of the objectives as they start their program planning EXCEPT one. Which one is the EXCEPTION?
    A. Establishing referrals with health care providers
    B. Establishing preventive health care programs in the rural areas
    C. Increasing health literacy levels, especially pertaining to oral health
    D. Increasing overall literacy levels by collaborating with local educators

118. Which of the following statements represents the community dental hygiene diagnosis for this population?
    A. High rates of oral cancer are related to low health care literacy.

B. High rates of dental caries are related to lack of access to care.
    C. High rates of dental caries are related to low health care literacy.
    D. High rates of dental disease are related to the lack of access to care.
    E. High rates of periodontal disease are related to the lack of access to care.

Questions 119 through 122 refer to information in the following testlet.

A public health dental hygienist consulting for the WHO is assigned to a team of professionals to implement an ongoing system of tracking long-term data related to periodontal disease in the western African nation of Ghana. A comprehensive community profile is developed by the team. The intent is to use the data for dental public health programming and evaluation in this nation. The hygienist is fluent in French and easily establishes contacts with local public health officials, village leaders, and government workers. At the 2-year mark, the team's initial reports indicate the prevalence of the following levels of periodontitis for the region: 64% mild periodontitis, 12% moderate periodontitis, and 24% severe periodontitis.

119. Which of the following types of health data reporting is the dental hygienist developing?
    A. Screening
    B. Surveying
    C. Examining
    D. Surveillance

120. The periodontal disease summary data reported as a result of this epidemiologic surveillance may be described as the proportion of the population with that amount of disease because the data express the presence of each level of periodontitis in relation to the size of the population.
    A. Both the statement and the reason are correct and related.
    B. Both the statement and the reason are correct but NOT related.
    C. The statement is correct, but the reason is NOT.
    D. The statement is NOT correct, but the reason is correct.
    E. NEITHER the statement NOR the reason is correct.

121. Which of the following indices is MOST commonly used for gathering the data for this surveillance project?
    A. Periodontal Index (PI)
    B. Community Periodontal Index (CPI)
    C. Periodontal Screening and Recording (PSR)
    D. Community Periodontal Index of Treatment Needs (CPITN)

122. The following factors contribute to the dental hygienist's cultural sensitivity in relation to this project EXCEPT one. Which one is the EXCEPTION?
    A. Relationship with local leaders
    B. Fluency in the language of the country
    C. Familiarity with the customs of the country
    D. Previous experience as public health hygienist

Questions 123 through 127 refer to information in the following testlet.

A dental hygienist is employed by the health department of one of the largest unfluoridated cities in the country. Recently, the hygienist has been contacted by members of the school board because of an increase in school absence rates related to dental pain. Equipped with school absence data from the past 5 years, the hygienist meets with the school board and presents CDC data about the benefits of community water. The school board asks the dental hygienist and the health department to work with them to get public support for community water fluoridation.

123. Which of the following should be the hygienist's first step in meeting the goal for the school board?
    A. Identifying key community leaders to gain a broad base of support
    B. Conducting a referendum in the community to show public support
    C. Bringing the decision before the city council at an open meeting of the council
    D. Educating each of the city council members by meeting with them individually

124. Which of the following is the MOST recent CDC recommendation for the optimal level of fluoride in the community water supply of this city?
    A. 2.0 ppm
    B. 0.7 ppm
    C. 1.2 ppm
    D. 0.3 ppm

125. Which of the following is the LEAST complex governmental intervention for adoption of community water fluoridation?
    A. Referendum at the local level
    B. Passage of law at the state governmental level
    C. Passage of law at the federal governmental level
    D. Adoption by the city council or other local governmental entity

126. The hygienist can accurately educate the public that water fluoridation is considered the most

cost-effective population-based mechanism for prevention of dental caries. The community can expect that fluoridation will provide a 60% decrease in the caries rate of a community.
    A. Both statements are true.
    B. Both statements are false.
    C. The first statement is true, and the second statement is false.
    D. The first statement is false, and the second statement is true.

127. The initiative of the school district to contact the hygienist represents which step on the Learning Ladder Continuum health education theory?
    A. Action
    B. Awareness
    C. Self-interest
    D. Involvement
    E. Unawareness

Questions 128 through 132 refer to information in the following testlet.

A local health department is holding a health fair for their community as part of a back-to-school event for low-SES children and families. Among the participants providing oral health care and information are volunteers from the local dental hygiene society, local dentists, and dental and dental hygiene students from nearby professional programs. The dental hygiene society invites the dental hygiene school program to involve their students in the planning of the oral health component of the event as well as participating in the actual event. The dental hygiene faculty design their student involvement to meet course objectives and for extra course credit. The dentists and dental students provide basic oral health screenings using a light, a mirror, and a tongue blade. Any dental concerns noted are documented, patients are provided with a referral to a local dental clinic, and the importance of complying with the referral is explained to the parents. Volunteer hygienists apply fluoride varnish treatments and provide oral health education to the children and their parents. Contact information on participants is collected to follow up on compliance with referrals.

128. Decreasing which of the following factors would be the adverse effect of using this particular type of examination method?
    A. Validity
    B. Reliability
    C. Sensitivity
    D. Specificity

129. Which of the following is an appropriately stated outcome objective for this program?
    A. Treatment will be provided for referred children.
    B. Oral health status of the low-SES children will be improved.
    C. Parents of 90% of referred children will seek treatment for their children.
    D. Children will participate in the screening, education, and varnish program.
    E. Children will be referred for treatment based on the results of the basic screening.

130. Volunteer participation of dental and dental hygiene students in this program is an example of all of the following concepts EXCEPT one. Which one is the EXCEPTION?
    A. Peer sanction
    B. Professionalism
    C. Service learning
    D. Community service
    E. Ethics of pro bono work

131. This public health approach promotes better oral health in all of the following ways EXCEPT one. Which one is the EXCEPTION?
    A. Increases oral health literacy
    B. Provides preventive services
    C. Increases demand for oral health care
    D. Promotes utilization of dental services
    E. Provides oral health care for the aged through Medicare

132. Which of the following formats could the dental hygiene volunteers use to engage the GREATEST amount of participation by the community participants?
    A. Children's songs about dental concepts
    B. An educational video about dental caries
    C. Posters with colorful graphics depicting dental concepts
    D. A hands-on activity or craft simulating the process of dental caries

Questions 133 through 137 refer to information in the following testlet.

A dental hygienist who is a new graduate begins working at her first job as the director of the oral health program in a Federally Qualified Health Clinic (FQHC) in rural Mississippi. The dental hygienist's main responsibility is to establish an oral health program for underserved residents of the community with three goals: (1) promoting oral health and prevention of dental disease by educating the public; (2) utilizing an interdisciplinary approach involving community leaders; and (3) developing a program of oral health surveillance.

133. The dental hygienist uses an interdisciplinary approach involving community leaders to implement the oral health program. This is because support from other entities will assist the hygienist in changing the perceptions and values of the underserved residents of the community.
    A. Both statements are true.
    B. Both statements are false.
    C. The first statement is false, and the second statement is true.
    D. The first statement is true, and the second statement is false.

134. Which of the following is the target population that will be recipients of the benefits of the program the dental hygienist is organizing?
    A. The public
    B. Community leaders
    C. Underserved residents of the community
    D. Patients at the FQHC

135. All of the following are scenarios that are examples of an educational program that the dental hygienist could implement to achieve the program's goals EXCEPT one. Which one is the EXCEPTION?
    A. Hosting an ongoing event at the FQHC and offering seminars presented via lecture and discussion
    B. Sponsoring a free event held in the elementary school gymnasium and incorporating other professionals and community leaders as hosts of the event
    C. Providing educational information via brochures and personal discussion during each patient's visit to the FQHC
    D. Conducting a small group presentation to a Sunday school class in the church setting and making sure to give each participant a brochure about the importance of oral health
    E. Visiting private dental offices in the area and providing brochures and information to be distributed to the patients in the practice

136. Which of the following surveillance methods is MOST cost effective in providing necessary assessment data?
    A. DMFT or deft
    B. Radiographic imaging, as needed
    C. Complete periodontal charting for each patient
    D. Questionnaire evaluating reasons the patient has not received dental treatment

137. All of the following are components of the dental hygiene process of care EXCEPT one. Which one is the EXCEPTION?
    A. Assessment
    B. Diagnosis
    C. Prevention
    D. Implementation
    E. Evaluation

Questions 138 through 141 refer to information in the following testlet.

A dental hygienist has been asked to organize and implement a program to promote oral health for the players and coaches of the local public high school football team before football season begins in September. The team is made up of Hispanic, African American, and Caucasian players. After receiving the results from a preliminary questionnaire sent to a random sample of the coaches, parents, and football players, the dental hygienist begins the task of deciding the program's content. Results of the questionnaires are that the majority of coaches and parents (78%) report that the players do not use tobacco. Sixty-three percent of the surveyed players occasionally use either smokeless tobacco or smoke cigars in social settings. The players' responses reveal that 96% are aware that the use of tobacco is illegal at their age and is detrimental to their health. The results also reveal that the football players are required to wear mouth guards while on the field, and 47% of responding players answered that they were unsure of the reason for the rule. The results gathered from the coaches and parents' questionnaires show that they would like the importance of wearing mouthguards to be the focus of the presentation. After reading the questionnaire results, the dental hygienist decides to provide the group with a presentation utilizing presurvey and postsurvey findings, lecture, and discussion. The dental hygienist plans to use pictures of healthy and diseased mouths as well as a short question-and-answer segment.

138. Utilizing the Learning Ladder continuum health behavior model, which rung of the learning ladder are 78% of parents and coaches on in regards to the football players' use of tobacco products?
    A. Awareness
    B. Self-interest
    C. Involvement
    D. Unawareness

139. All of the following are examples of an appropriate presentation title for the football players and coaches EXCEPT one. Which one is the EXCEPTION?
    A. How to Quit Using Tobacco
    B. Correct Use of Mouth Guards
    C. The Importance of Brushing and Flossing for Athletes
    D. The Link between Oral Cancer and Tobacco Use in Athletes

140. All of the following are purposes of the survey that the dental hygienist administered to segments of the parents, coaches, and football players before the presentation EXCEPT one. Which one is the EXCEPTION?
    A. Determining the beliefs of the parents
    B. Avoiding unpleasant or controversial topics
    C. Evaluating the coaching staff's influence on the players
    D. Surveying the knowledge of the group and its influencers
    E. Tailoring the appropriate instruction methods for the audience participating in the event

141. After introducing herself to the players, the dental hygienist mentions that since she is of Hispanic descent, she knows that the Hispanic players will "get it" when she discusses the importance of tobacco cessation. Which of the following terms correctly describes what the dental hygienist is trying to convey?
    A. Ethnography
    B. Ethnocentrism
    C. Cultural diversity
    D. Cultural sensitivity
    E. Cultural competency

Answers and Rationales

1. Which of the following is the FIRST data collection method needed for this program?

   ANS: D
   Even though the state dental caries rates are high, it is important to document the caries status of the target population to have a baseline to which to compare future results for evaluation purposes (D). This assessment is also important to aid in the determining the type of programs needed. For example, if the survey shows that most decay has been treated (high filled score F versus high decayed score D), a treatment referral program is not as critical as primary prevention programs to prevent future decay. The survey of dental caries can be done with the DMFT or the DMFS, although the DMFS yields more detailed information. The school nurse records have already provided information in their assessment that the oral hygiene of the children is poor (A). It will be important to understand the children's and the parents' oral health literacy, but those surveys will be geared toward the results found from the caries survey (B, C).

2. Which of the following factors should be considered to determine the optimal level of water fluoridation for this community?

   ANS: E
   The CDC sets recommendations for the optimum fluoride level of community water (E). All SES groups benefit from fluoridation at the same optimal level (A). Most of the population in the United States uses fluoride dentifrice, and this has been taken into consideration by the CDC when setting the recommended level (B). The current level of fluoride in the community water supply is used to figure the amount of fluoride that needs to be added to bring the level to optimum, but it does not affect the CDC's recommendation for optimum fluoride level of community water (C). The optimal fluoride level is not affected by oral health status as reflected by DMFT scores (D).

3. All of the following are important risk factors for development of dental caries in this population EXCEPT one. Which one is the EXCEPTION?

   ANS: B
   Cultural diversity is not associated with dental caries when SES is held constant (B). Poor oral hygiene is associated with dental caries (A). At 0.3 ppm, the community water supply fluoride level is below the recommended CDC guidelines of 0.7 to 1.2 ppm, and

the suboptimal fluoride is a risk factor for dental caries (C). Low SES is a risk factor for dental caries (D).

4. Which change in the DMFT scores would indicate the most successful outcome 5 years after implementation of the program?

   ANS: B
   The most successful program will present as a decrease in the total DMFT with a decrease in D and M and F component (B). If the program results in treatment of decay, it may produce an increase in the F component of the DMFT (A). An increase in D, with a decrease in F, and no change in M indicates that dental caries rates are continuing to rise, without adequate treatment being received (C). No change in D and an increase in F, either with a decrease in M or an increase in M indicates that dental treatment needs are not being met (D, E). A successful program will also provide treatment primarily in the form of restorations rather than extractions, so the number of missing teeth caused by dental caries (M) should remain relatively constant. A slight increase in M may occur if the some of the population have severe caries prior to the beginning of the program.

5. The "e" in the index used to assess this population indicates teeth that are (Select all that apply.)

   ANS: B, D
   All designations with the different forms of DMF, including dmf, def, and df, indicate only effects of dental caries, either an active carious lesion, or extraction as a result of caries (B). The "e" of the def index indicates teeth that are so badly decayed that they are indicated for extraction (D). Teeth that are already exfoliated are not included in the DMF indices (A). Teeth extracted because of caries are indicted with m in the dmf. The dmf index is used before teeth begin to exfoliate, and the df index is used after exfoliation to avoid having to decide if a missing primary tooth has been extracted because of caries or has naturally exfoliated. Primate spaces are part of the natural spacing of primary teeth and are not related to the DMF indices (C).

6. Which of the following would be the MOST effective intervention to implement to increase compliance with the dental referral?

   ANS: D
   Results of the survey reveal the need for the educational program to bring the pregnant women's

risk to their attention (D). Oral health screenings during prenatal care visits would not help to bring the women's attention to the need for oral care throughout their pregnancy (A). Lower-SES populations tend to have lower literacy rates, and written educational materials may not be as effective as providing personal oral education (B). Documenting the oral condition of women who have participated in the dental referral and comparison with women who did not participate in the referral is useful for tracking and research purposes but will not help to improve compliance which is the goal of the intervention (C).

7. Based on the results of the survey, which of the following health education theories would be the MOST appropriate to use as the foundation for an oral health education intervention to improve compliance with the dental referral?

ANS: B
Results of the survey revealed that the women do not realize their risk for diabetes, are unaware of the relationship between oral health status and diabetes, and do not understand the benefits of an oral health assessment in relation to their overall health and the health of their babies. The Health Belief Model, a psychological model that attempts to explain and predict health behaviors, directly addresses these educational needs (B). Although other models may be useful in combination, especially to provide motivation for behavior change, this model is indicated from the results of the survey. The Learning Ladder Theory suggests learning takes place in sequential steps, beginning with ignorance and culminating with habit (A). The Social Cognitive Theory suggests that behaviors are learned through observation, modeling, and motivation (such as positive reinforcement) (C). The Theory of Reasoned Action suggests that behavior is determined by a person's intention to perform the behavior and that this intention is, in turn, a function of the person's attitude toward the behavior and his or her subjective norm (D). Trans-theoretical Model or Stages of Change assesses a person's readiness to act on a new healthier behavior and provides strategies to guide the person through the stages of change: precontemplation, contemplation, preparation, action, maintenance, and termination (E).

8. Which of the following is a valid conclusion about the population from the results of the survey?

ANS: A
The survey indicates lack of knowledge of health issues, which is a component of health literacy (A). The women have access to oral health care through the dental clinic that is associated with the medical clinic in this community facility (B). People tend to value what they understand, and lack of knowledge of health issues makes it unlikely that it will become a high priority (C). It is presumptuous to assume that people in a lower SES do not have access to care in private dental offices (D).

9. Which characteristic of public health is exemplified by the dental referral by the medical clinic?

ANS: D
The collaboration of the dental and medical clinic staff is a classic example of the multidisciplinary approach to solving public health problems (D). The concern of the medical and dental clinic staff to improve the compliance rates is an example of the social, not personal, responsibility for the oral health of the community they serve (A). Planning an educational intervention to reach the women as a group, rather than approaching each one individually, is an example of community rather than the individual as the patient (B). The analysis of the survey data to help identify a solution is an example of the public health principle of applying biostatistics to analyze this population health problem (C).

10. The process of involving and activating members of the community in a meeting is an example of which theory of health promotion?

ANS: C
The Community Organization Theory is the process of involving and activating members of the community in a meeting (C). In this testlet, the Community Organization Theory is exemplified through the dental hygienist's action to arrange a meeting with stakeholders to discuss the problem of noncompliance of pregnant women in utilizing dental services. Sense of Coherence is a method of seeing the world and one's place in it, cognitively, perceptually, and socially (A). By choosing participants who are willing to work together for the benefit of others, the dental hygienist who organized the meeting would be using a planning strategy that would help ensure the meeting was successful. The Diffusion of Innovation Theory helps in assessing how innovations are adopted or how new ideas, products, or services spread within a group (B). The Organizational Change: Stage Theory can be used during the meeting as stakeholders discuss the process of initiating change and how the changes will affect each entity or stakeholder (D).

11. Lower-SES populations are identified as a high priority target populations in the United States because these populations are identified as having unmet oral health needs by the Surgeon General's Report.

    ANS: A
    The Surgeon General's Report identified the oral health needs and related problems of the U.S. population (A). The report highlights the problem of oral health disparities among the lower-SES segments of the population and the need to prioritize dental public health programming to reach these population groups. Choices B, C, D, and E do not adequately reflect the statement and the reason.

12. Which type of examination is used for the initial assessment of new residents?

    ANS: D
    A type IV examination, which involves screening with a tongue depressor and available illumination, is commonly used in dental public health assessments such as the initial assessment of new residents (D). It is also known as the *Basic Screening Survey* and is the simplest, least comprehensive, and least valid type of examination, producing the most false negatives. Type I is the most comprehensive procedure and includes radiographic images, mouth models, and a complete clinical examination (A). Type II, called a *limited examination*, is less comprehensive and is accomplished with bitewing radiographic images, selected periapical radiographic images, and a complete clinical examination (B). This type of examination is the most commonly used in public health clinical settings where restorative treatment is provided. Type III, referred to as *inspection*, is even less comprehensive and is achieved with a clinical examination, using appropriate dental instruments and adequate illumination (C). This type is referred to as an *epidemiologic examination* and is used for research purposes such as the annual monitoring and program evaluation. A type III examination is also used for assessment in community-based sealant programs because radiographic images are not used in these programs.

13. Which of the following BEST describes the purpose for calibrating the second dental hygienist before the team conducts the annual examinations?

    ANS: D
    The purpose for training and calibrating the second dental hygienist before the team conducts the annual examinations is to increase the interexaminer reliability of the evaluation results (D). Reliability is the reproduction or consistent results when evaluations are repeated. Interexaminer (interrater)

reliability is consistency between multiple examiners and is increased by calibration. Calibration is a form of training where examiners work together to gain consistency of their measurements of variables. Validity is accuracy, assuring that the evaluation measures what it is intended to measure (A). Objectivity is not increased by calibration but can be increased by using random sampling (B). Calibrating will not ensure the residents' cooperation with the screening process (C).

14. In this testlet, the initial assessment of oral hygiene status performed by the dental hygiene coordinator is comparable with which component of private practice?

    ANS: E
    The steps in the process of care apply to both private practice and public health. Initial examination of the patient is comparable with the initial assessment in the community setting (E). Funding in public health is usually provided by governmental agencies, whereas funding in private practice may be provided by the private patient or third-party payors such as insurance companies (A). The dental hygiene diagnosis is applied to both the individual patient and the community, based on the results of the examination or community assessment, respectively (B). Provision of treatment for the patient is comparable with program implementation in the community setting (C). Evaluation of treatment outcomes in private practice is comparable with evaluation of program outcomes in dental public health practice (D).

15. Which of the following could be an effect of using a disclosant in the application of the O'Leary plaque index to measure plaque in this program? (Select all that apply.)

    ANS: B, E
    Using a disclosant in the application of the O'Leary plaque index to measure plaque in this program would increase reliability or reproducibility of assessment (B). Using a disclosant in the application of the O'Leary plaque index to measure plaque in this program will also increase the ability to see the plaque biofilm and will increase the sensitivity of the index (E). Using a disclosant would increase, not decrease, the validity or accuracy of assessing the effectiveness of home care (A). Using a disclosant will not decrease sensitivity but increase it (C). Using a disclosant will increase, not decrease, specificity, since specificity is the ability of an examination instrument to correctly identify the absence of a disease or condition (D). Use of a disclosant will allow the clinician to identify those teeth that do not have plaque.

16. What term correctly describes the rate of disease that is constant in a population?

    ANS: A
    Endemic is the constant, normal presence of disease in a population (A). Dental caries is a good example of an endemic condition. An epidemic occurs when new cases of a disease during a given period far exceed the expected occurrence based on recent endemic experience (B). Pandemic is an epidemic that has spread across a large region such as several continents or worldwide (C).

17. Which of the following programs would be MOST recommended to provide safe and cost effective caries prevention, in addition to the sealant program for this high caries risk population?

    ANS: A
    Application of fluoride varnish is the recommended program for groups at high risk for caries by the American Dental Association (ADA) and the Centers for Disease and Control Prevention (CDC) (A). Fluoride varnish programs are effective, safe, cost effective, and efficient. Varnish application can be done quickly, requires minimal equipment and supplies, and can be carried out by dental and medical personnel in some states, adding to its cost effectiveness and efficiency. Fluoride varnish only needs be administered every 3 to 6 months compared with weekly rinse programs. School weekly fluoride rinse programs are not as effective as fluoride varnish programs (B). Although the use of OTC fluoride dentifrice is safe and effective, it is not cost effective to distribute it at school (C). Fluoride supplements are not indicated or safe for this population (D). Since the community water supply is fluoridated, the addition of a second source of systemic fluoride would result in excess fluoride that would cause fluorosis if consumed during the late secretion to early maturation stage of enamel formation. Application of fluoride foam using the tray method is not practical or cost effective in a school setting (E). In addition, fluoride varnish is considered more effective.

18. Which of the following are possible funding sources for this program? (Select all that apply.)

    ANS: B, C, D, E
    State income tax is primarily used to support the state government; however, each state is responsible for how funding is spent, and preventive measures such as vaccines and sealant programs may receive funding from this source (B). Federal block grants are available to regional governments with general provisions with regard to how to spend the funds,

allowing states the flexibility necessary to respond to the top health priorities (C). These funds can be used for programs that address oral health issues identified as critical by public health officials. School funding is primarily used for educational purposes, but schools may choose to use their funding to provide health services (D). Local service organizations such as Kiwanis or Rotary support various preestablished health programs in the community (E). Head Start only provides funding for Head Start programs that target preschool age children (A).

19. Which of the following is the MOST effective teaching strategy to evaluate learning for toothbrushing in the educational programs with these school children? (Select all that apply.)

    ANS: B, C, D
    The purpose of the classroom education in this program is to teach oral hygiene, which involves psychomotor as well as cognitive objectives. This is best accomplished with a combination of role play, discussion, and demonstration (B, C, D). Role play is extremely effective with young children who tend to be very imaginative. Discussion can be used to stimulate group interaction and encourages active involvement, challenging cognitive development. Demonstration allows visualization and engagement in the activity. Lecture is effective to impart a large amount of information to a big audience to meet cognitive objectives and can be effective when combined with an activity (A). However, lecture is not always effective with young children and not the best choice for psychomotor objectives. Games and activities are useful for affective objectives and stimulate cognitive and psychomotor development through participation (E). Games and activities work well with young children.

20. A public health problem is a condition that is widespread and has an actual or potential cause of morbidity or mortality. Using this definition, the school system has a public health problem based on the high DMF scores of the school children.

    ANS: A
    Both the statement and the reason are correct and related (A). The definition of a public health problem is a condition that is widespread and has an actual or potential cause of morbidity or mortality. The higher than average DMF scores of the school children show a widespread or endemic condition of caries. Dental caries are a significant cause of illness or morbidity and, in rare cases, even morbidity and death. Choices B, C, D, and E do not accurately reflect the statement and the reason.

21. If the DMF scores of the different SES groups are compared, which of the following would be the expected results?

    ANS: E
    SES is a powerful predictor of dental caries experience, untreated caries, and low dental utilization. National survey data demonstrate that low-SES children, especially in ethnic minority groups, compared with higher-SES children, have greater dental caries experience, higher rates of untreated carious lesions, and lower dental utilization rates (E). Because of these disparities, about 75% to 80% of dental caries are said to be found in 25% of the children in the U.S. population, and these children are from low-SES families. This phenomenon is true regardless of ethnic group membership. Ethnic group membership is associated with dental caries only in relation to SES. When SES is held constant among ethnic groups, ethnicity is no longer associated with dental caries. The true association is between SES and dental caries, not between ethnicity and caries. Lower SES is associated with higher DMF scores, not lower DMF scores (A). Higher SES groups are more likely to have more treated decay because higher SES is associated with higher utilization, but compared with lower-SES groups, the DMF score would be lower (B). Choices C and D do not accurately reflect the statements.

22. Which of the following are the three characteristics that compose epidemiologic factors of disease? (Select all that apply.)

    ANS: A, B, D
    Epidemiology is the study of disease trends in populations and is a multifactorial approach to controlling disease. The three characteristics that compose the epidemiologic factor are categorized as host, agent, and environmental factors. The epidemiologic triangle depicts the interaction of these factors as they contribute to disease, injury, or disability. Host factors relate primarily to susceptibility and resistance to disease through immunity, anatomic or physiologic factors, knowledge, behavior modification, and personal power (A). The structure of tooth enamel and the flow and composition of saliva are host factors for dental caries. Agent factors are the biologic causes of disease, injury, or disability, for example, the bacteria that cause dental caries (B). Environmental factors include physical, sociocultural, sociopolitical, and economic components of the disease process (D). The interaction of these three characteristics makes the study of most diseases multifactorial, or related to the interaction of agent, host, and environment (C). The interrelationship of these factors may result in disease (E).

23. Which type of evaluation involves comparison of the pretest and posttest scores?

    ANS: D
    Summative evaluation provides data related to the end results, for example, the learning outcomes of these educational programs, and quantitative evaluation provides numerical data based on actual measurements of phenomena, for example, test scores (D). Formative evaluation occurs in the process of implementing the program, for example, tracking the number of children and parents that participate in the educational programs. Qualitative evaluation provides data that deal with descriptions of phenomena that can be observed but not measured numerically, for example, patient satisfaction or value placed on oral health (A). Choices B and C do not accurately reflect the statements.

24. The primary role of the public health dental hygienist is to provide direct patient treatment. The dental hygienist's role in this program is primarily coordination, training, and serving as a resource that fulfills the role of the public health hygienist.

    ANS: D
    The first statement is false, and the second statement is true (D). The primary role of the public health dental hygienist is rarely to provide direct patient treatment. The public health hygienist's primary role is to provide services that allow the community to be served as the patient rather than an individual. The second statement is true because the dental hygienist's role in this program is much broader than providing only patient treatment. In coordinating, training, and serving as a resource, this hygienist fulfills many of the roles of the public health hygienist. Choices A, B, and C do not correctly reflect the statements.

25. Assessment data are collected from each pediatric patient to determine his or her dental experiences. Which of the following terms describes the children's annual visits to a dentist or dental hygienist?

    ANS: C
    Utilization is defined as actual attendance at treatment facilities to receive care, expressed as the proportion of people who visit the dentist, usually within a year, or the average number of visits per person per year (C). Access is the ability of an individual to obtain care (A). Demand is the population's expression of a desire to receive dental care (B). Perceived need, which may be subjective or felt needs, are those determined by the individual or community (D). Normative need is the professionally determined oral health needs of the individual or population

through assessment (E). Factors such as education, cost, availability, and convenience often need to be addressed to meet the demand for dental care.

26. What level of prevention is addressed by this program?

ANS: B
Primary preventive strategies such as this fluoride and oral health educational program are designed to prevent the onset of disease (B). Tertiary preventive measures involve replacement of lost tissues and rehabilitation (A). Secondary preventive approaches consist of routine treatment methods to terminate a disease process, restore tissues, or both (C).

27. Which of the following is an appropriate instructional objective for the Head Start teachers in this program?

ANS: B
An instructional objective communicates what the student will be able to perform after learning has taken place. A well-written objective is specific, observable, and measureable and has the following components: the audience or target group, a performance verb that tells what the learner will be able to do, a condition that tells the relevant factors affecting the performance of the action, and the criterion that tells how to evaluate the level of achievement or acceptable performance. For the correctly stated objective in this question, "classroom teachers" are the audience, "identify children with signs of early childhood caries" is the action, an "in-service program" is the condition, and "75% of children" is the criterion for evaluation (B). This is a general outcome statement without the characteristics and components of an objective (A). This statement is an outcome objective, rather than an instructional objective (C). It possesses the required characteristics (specific, observable, measurable) but does not relate to action of the learner. This statement is a poorly written instructional objective, missing a condition and more importantly a criterion, which results in it not being specific and measureable (D).

28. Which of the following types of data is represented by the classification of treatment needs?

ANS: B
The ordinal scale organizes data into mutually exclusive categories that are rank ordered on the basis of some criterion, but the difference in ranks is not numerically equal, for example, ranking the children as no treatment needed, immediate treatment needed, treatment needed in the near future, and treatment that can be delayed (B).

Data can be classified by using the four scales of measurement: nominal, ordinal, interval, and ratio. The ratio scale has equal intervals between variables, plus an absolute 0 point (A). Examples of the ratio scale are height, weight, and age. The interval scale has numerically equal intervals, but no true zero. An example is degrees Fahrenheit in which the 0 point is arbitrary so that 100 degrees cannot be numerically interpreted as twice as hot as 50 degrees (C). The nominal scale organizes data into named categories, and there is no numeric relationship or ranking of data such as male and female or ethnic groups (D).

29. Which of the following is the MOST appropriate use of the data generated by the screening? Select the *two* that are most applicable.

ANS: A, C
The BSS, or type IV screening, is used to collect data in this program. This data collection instrument identifies and classifies dental caries. This survey is a screening versus an epidemiologic examination and is appropriate for referral and to assess the needs of a population for program planning (A, C). Caries research typically requires a more in-depth examination instrument such as the type III epidemiologic examination (DMF) (B). Calibration of examiners is required regardless of the instrument used, but this is not the purpose of baseline data collection (D). Funding requests usually require the more detailed or specific data that results from a DMF survey (E).

30. Which of the following is the BEST fluoride program for this project?

ANS: B
Fluoride varnish is recommended by both the ADA and the CDC for young children and should be used to supplement water fluoridation in high-risk populations (B). It can be applied easily in a school program. Fluoride varnish is more effective and safer because of minimal fluoride ingestion compared with other types of fluoride programs. Head Start is a program that serves preschool-age children from lower-SES families; these children are at high risk for caries. Management of caries in children with high risk requires the use of additional fluorides. Fluoride rinses are not recommended for children younger than age 6 years, as they are likely to swallow the rinse when they attempt to swish and expectorate it (A). High fluoride dentifrice is inappropriate in a community with an optimally fluoridated water supply (C). Fluoride tablet supplementation is inappropriate because the community is optimally

fluoridated (D). The addition of a second systemic fluoride system would result in excess fluoride consumption and fluorosis.

31. Which of the following is the purpose of including personal oral care for the nurses' aides?

    ANS: C
    The purpose of including their own personal oral care is to help the nurses' aides appreciate the importance of oral care (C). Unless they value oral care, nurse aides and others in a position of caring for the oral health of their clients do not appreciate its importance and are less likely to provide the necessary care. The inclusion of personal oral care in the presentation for nurses' aides would not serve as a strong motivator to attend the educational program (A). Role modeling does not apply because the residents are not performing self-care but depend on the aides for their care (B). The skills needed by the aides to provide oral care for the residents will differ from the skills needed for their personal oral care (D).

32. Which of the following actions should occur next in this program?

    ANS: E
    Meeting with key personnel such as the director and director of nursing to determine program goals and objectives is the next step and is necessary to proceed with other activities (E). After the goals and objectives are determined, a lesson plan for the educational program can be developed to meet the program goals and objectives, and appropriate teaching strategies for the educational program can be selected (A, B). Contacting the local dental hygiene program to solicit student involvement in the program and requesting funding for supplies can occur later (C, D).

33. Which of the following is the BEST program to implement after the nurse aides are trained in personal oral care?

    ANS: C
    Since the majority of the residents are edentulous and have dentures, and the majority of them require assistance with their oral care, the nurse aides need training in denture care (C). A fluoride program is a lower priority, since most residents are edentulous (A). In addition, the need for a fluoride program depends on the residents' level of risk for caries, which is unknown. Denture care and oral hygiene for the residents is a lower priority because most residents require assistance with basic self-care, which includes oral self-care (B, D).

34. Who is the responsible party to contact if the dental hygienist identifies possible oral cancer lesions during the intraoral screening?

    ANS: D
    The director of nursing has the responsibility to coordinate further care needed by the residents (D). The confidentiality of health data is important, even in community settings, but referral for treatment is an ethical obligation any time professionals are aware of disease that requires treatment. The director of nursing has the responsibility to coordinate further care needed by the residents. This type of confidential information should be reported only to the director of nursing and not the family, residents, or nurse aides (A, B, C). Failure to report possible pathology would be irresponsible, since it would lead to failure to take action that could potentially save a life or improve quality of life (E).

35. For each variable in the study, select the MOST closely linked type of variable from the list provided.

    ANS: 1B, 2A, 3D, 4D, 5C, 6D
    Relevant variables that are not controlled such as age are an example of an extraneous variable that decreases the internal validity and limits the value of the research results (1B). For example, failing to match the groups for age leaves the reader wondering if the difference in compliance might be a result of age rather than the method of appointment scheduling. Compliance with periodontal maintenance is a dependent variable, the one measured to determine if the manipulation of the independent variable affects it (2A). Gender; instruction about the importance of periodontal maintenance; and the periodontal status are relevant variables, which can influence how the independent variable affects the dependent variable (3D, 4D, 6D). These relevant variables should be controlled to increase the internal validity of the study. Method of appointment scheduling is an independent variable, the one manipulated in the study (5C).

36. Which of the following is the purpose of giving the same verbal and written instructions about periodontal maintenance to all groups of patients?

    ANS: A
    Validity is a measure of accuracy of the research methods, ensuring that the test, the instrument, or the study measures what it is intended to study (A). Controlling relevant variables increases the accuracy of the results. Presenting the same verbal and written instructions about periodontal maintenance to all groups of patients controls this relevant variable. Giving the same verbal and written instructions about

periodontal maintenance to all groups of patients does not satisfy any ethical requirement but does increase the internal validity of the study (B). Reliability refers to the consistency of a measure, which is affected by using a valid instrument or index and having trained and calibrated examiners (C). Although having consistent verbal and written instruction will make the teaching process easier, this is not the purpose in relation to this study (D). Giving the same verbal and written instructions about periodontal maintenance to all groups of patients will not increase compliance with periodontal maintenance (E).

37. The entire dental hygiene faculty in the dental hygiene clinic uses the same standardized design of periodontal probe at all times to measure clinical attachment loss to classify patients' periodontal status and has calibrated with each other on the use of this probe. Select the *two* factors that are enhanced by using the same periodontal probe and calibration.

ANS: B, C
Reliability is the consistency or reproducibility of a measure, which is important to obtain valid results. Reliability of measuring instruments and examiners ultimately affects the validity of a study. Training and calibration (the process of testing examiner consistency) helps ensure the reliability of the dental hygiene faculty, which is further increased by use of the standardized probes. Calibration and training of the faculty and use of standardized probe will increase interrater or interexaminer reliability or consistency across examiners (B, C). Sensitivity refers to having a positive measure of a condition when it is present and is not directly related to calibration and training (A). Intrarater or intraexaminer reliability refers to consistency within one examiner (D). Statistical significance is not directly related to calibration and training (E).

38. If the survey had been conducted on a sample of the population, which of the following would have been the BEST sampling method to use?

ANS: A
A simple random sample is effective to select a representative sample from a homogeneous population (all subjects being similar to each other such as this group). A random sample is one in which every study participant is selected independently and has an equal chance of being selected, resulting in an unbiased, representative sample. A random sample is considered the most valid sample (A). A judgmental sample is biased, since the clinician uses personal judgment to select patients to represent typical patients who would

best meet the purposes of the research. Judgmental samples are not appropriate for experimental research but are useful for action research that evaluates current community programs designed to improve health practices and behaviors by changing them (B). A systematic sample is one in which the first individual is selected randomly and then every *nth* individual is selected on the basis of the size of the population and the desired sample size (C). A convenience sample consists of individuals who are most readily available to be selected (D). Intact groups and volunteers are used because of the impracticality of using random or other samples for some studies, but these studies are not as valid as random samples. With a heterogeneous (diverse) population, the random sampling process must be adjusted by dividing the population into groups based on any relevant variables. These groups are called *strata*, and individuals are proportionately selected from the various groups to result in a sample that represents the characteristics of the population. The resulting sample is called a *stratified random sample* (E).

39. On the basis of the correlation coefficient, which of the following types of relationship was found between periodontal health and compliance with periodontal maintenance?

ANS: E
Correlation coefficient is represented as r; its value of 0.62 in this case indicates a positive (+) moderate (between 0.50 and 0.69) relationship (E). The results are interpreted by considering the numerical value, which indicates the strength of the association, and the sign + or −, which indicates the direction of the association. In addition, the nature of the variables and the numbers involved in the comparison are important to consider in addition to the correlation coefficient in determining the strength of the relationship. The numerical values used to gauge the strength of the association in the correlation coefficient are interpreted as follows: 0.00 to 0.25 is little or no association, 0.26 to 0.49 is a weak association, 0.50 to 0.69 is a moderate association, 0.70 to 0.89 is a strong association, and 0.90 to 1.00 is very strong. A positive sign represents a relationship when both variables move in the same direction. If one variable increases, the other also increases, or if one variable decreases, the other also decreases. In a negative relationship, the variables move in opposite directions. If one variable increases, the other decreases, and vice versa. The strength of the relationship is based on the numerical values, positive is not stronger than negative. Choices A, B, C, and D do not adequately reflect the statements.

40. Which of the following is the BEST graphing technique to depict the compliance of both groups when the results are presented to the professional and administrative staff of the clinic?

ANS: B
Compliance is a discrete variable on the nominal scale of measurement; that is, individuals are either compliant or noncompliant, and a numerical scale of compliance does not exist. Discrete data are data that are counted in whole numbers and cannot be expressed as fractions, for example, number of children or number of teeth. Continuous data have data points along a continuum and can be expressed as a fraction. Frequency data for discrete variables are depicted best with a bar graph (B). One bar would represent the compliance of one appointment-scheduling-method group, and the other bar would represent the compliance of the other group. A pie chart is used to represent parts of a whole. Although it could be used in this case, the professional presentation of data from a research study is given in a bar graph. Pie charts may be used in presentations to a variety of audiences (A). A histogram is a graphic display of frequency distribution used to represent intervals or ratio scaled continuous variables represented as a bar graph with bars touching (C). A frequency polygon is a line graph representing the same data as a histogram (E). A scattergram is used to plot the relationship between two variables. It would be appropriate to plot the association between periodontal health and compliance with periodontal maintenance, which was discussed in the previous question (D).

41. Which of the following is the BEST group to target for an oral health in-service to continue ongoing oral health education after the program has been implemented?

ANS: C
Classroom teachers have daily access to the migrant children and have preset curriculum that includes oral health, so are the most logical providers of ongoing oral health education (C). The parents would have to be trained in oral health education and access to the parents to provide the training could be problematic (A). The school nurse generally does not have access to groups of children at one time (B). Dental hygiene students could present further lessons but will have limited access to the children (D).

42. All of the following are stakeholders of this program EXCEPT one. Which one is the EXCEPTION?

ANS: E
A stakeholder is a person, group, organization, member, or system, who affects or can be affected by an organization's actions. In this scenario, the state health department is not a stakeholder because it is not directly involved and will not be directly affected by the program (E). However, these types of programs may fulfill a state requirement to receive federal funding for some areas such as Indian Health Service, remote villages in Alaska, and other designated sites. In this case, the parents of the children involved, the school nurse, the dental personnel involved in the program, and the school administrators, all have a stake in the success of the program (A, B, C, D).

43. Which of the following is the BEST way to evaluate the outcomes of the sealant program?

ANS: A
The projected outcome of a sealant program is a reduction in caries rates of the children targeted by the program. Because of the transient nature of the target population, the goal is to treat as many children as possible and to seal as many teeth as possible before the occlusal surfaces decay. Evaluating the percentage of children who received sealants is the best way to evaluate the program (A). Evaluation of outcomes must relate to the disease process that is impacted by the program, in this case dental caries, not oral hygiene (B). Both the children's perception of the program and the parents' satisfaction are important formative evaluation processes that provide valuable information that can be applied to ensure success of the program (C, E). Conducting a basic screening a year later to assess for incidence of decay is not practical in a migrant population where many of the children will be gone the following year (D).

44. Which of the following is the MOST culturally sensitive procedure to use during the presentation of an oral health education program for parents?

ANS: D
Ethnic groups respond best to individuals from their own culture with whom they are familiar; using Hispanic school staff provides a more personal approach than using outside translators (D). Hispanic dental personnel have the added advantage of knowing dental terminology to communicate about oral health issues. Hiring translators to interpret is an option, but it does not have the element of community familiarity (A). Presenting the program in English is insensitive and ineffective because it ignores the language of the audience (B). Using children as translators can be demeaning to the parents, put the children in an inappropriate parental role, and cause misinterpretation of the information being presented (C).

45. The program exemplifies all of the following recommendations of the National Call to Action to Promote Oral Health initiative EXCEPT one. Which one is the EXCEPTION?

ANS: E
Action 3 of the National Call to Action to Promote Oral Health initiative is to build the science base and accelerate science transfer to promote biomedical and behavioral research (E). The organizations working together to plan and implement this program address the recommendation to increase collaborations (A). One of the goals of educating the migrant children during the program is to change perceptions of oral health (B). This program overcomes barriers of access to care by replicating other sealant and varnish programs that have been effective in addressing the problem of childhood caries in this population (C). This program (D) is an example of a diverse workforce that uses creativity and flexibility to maximize health care provision.

46. The dmfs of this population indicates that the children suffer from early childhood caries. The dmfs is the appropriate index used for detection of early childhood caries.

ANS: A
Both statements are true (A). Early childhood caries (ECC) is defined as the presence of one or more dmfs in primary teeth of children age 71 months or younger. The second statement is also true; the dmfs is required to establish the prevalence of ECC and severe early childhood caries (ECC-S). ECC-S is defined as any smooth-surface caries in children younger than 3 years. In children over 3 years, ECC-S is the presence of one or more dmf smooth surfaces in primary maxillary anterior teeth or a dmfs score of 4 or greater at age 3 years, 5 or greater at age 4 years, or 6 or greater at age 5 years. Choices B, C, and D do not accurately reflect the statements.

47. After seeing the high levels of ECC in the children, the public health hygienist is motivated to organize a fluoridation campaign for this community. Which of the following would be the BEST first step?

ANS: D
Making contacts with key community leaders to obtain a broad base of support for fluoridation is the first step in organizing a fluoridation campaign (D). A debate with antifluoridationists is not recommended because they tend to appeal to emotions rather than deal with facts (A). Testimony at a city council meeting (B) would occur before the referendum.

A referendum or public vote should be avoided, if possible, because this action is susceptible to the actions of antifluoridationists (C). A massive community educational program is critical if a referendum is scheduled (E).

48. What other index could be used to screen these children for dental caries in public health settings?

ANS: B
The BSS, which uses a tongue blade and available light, is a screening instrument acceptable for this age group for needs assessment data on which to base program planning and implement referrals (B). The df and def are used to measure primary teeth in children with mixed dentition because of the problem of determining missing teeth caused by caries during the ages of exfoliation (A, D). The DMF is the caries index for permanent teeth which are not yet present in 3- to 4-year-old children (C).

49. All of the following procedures fulfill the ethical obligations of community oral health practice EXCEPT one. Which one is the EXCEPTION?

ANS: D
Speaking with each parent individually is not necessary to fulfill the ethical obligations of community oral health practice (D). Preparation of a summary report may facilitate the preschool director in assisting the parents with finding a dental home (A). The ethical obligation of informed consent requires that a consent form be required to provide any dental services for children in any community settings, including preschools and schools (B). Use of a valid index such as the BSS to measure caries in conducting the program is an ethical obligation to assure accurate results (C). There is an ethical obligation to provide referral of the children to a dental home to ensure follow-up and continuing care (E).

50. Which of the following study designs is used?

ANS: D
A pretest–posttest study design is one in which the dependent variable is measured before the independent variable is introduced and then repeated (D). In this program, the baseline measure of the teens' knowledge is the pretest. It is followed by introducing the educational program (the independent variable), and then their knowledge is measured again. The pretest and posttest are compared to determine if the educational program impacted the teens' knowledge. In a factorial design, a second independent variable is introduced to determine if different combinations of the two variables impact the

dependent variable differently (A). In a time-series design, the dependent variable is measured several times at posttest to see if the change in the dependent variable will hold over time (B). In this program, knowledge was measured only one time after the educational program was implemented, and only one independent variable was introduced, the educational program. In a posttest-only design, the pretest or baseline measure is not taken, and the posttest follows the introduction of the independent variable (C).

51. All of the following procedures would enhance the cultural characteristics of the population EXCEPT one. Which one is the EXCEPTION?

ANS: A
Teaching methods should be targeted to the needs of the audience, which will vary according to cultural characteristics (A). The other procedures are ways to discuss cultural health practices to acknowledge their value, tailor instructional materials into the first language of the students to enhance cultural characteristics of the audience, and develop an activity that will provide culturally relevant teaching materials (B, C, D).

52. The local health department asks the dental hygienist to write a grant application based on the results of the educational program presented to the high school students. Which of the following statements could serve as a null hypothesis for future studies?

ANS: B
The null hypothesis is a negative statement of the expected outcome of a study. The purpose of this program evaluation is to determine if the educational program increased the teens' information about oral health. The negatively stated expected outcome "There will be no increase in the participants' scores from the pretest to the posttest after the educational presentation" is the null hypothesis (B). The positively stated expected outcome "There will be an increase in the participants' scores from the pretest to the posttest after the educational presentation" is the research hypothesis (A). Choices C and D are not examples of a null hypothesis.

53. What type of control group is used?

ANS: E
All students received health education material; there was no control group used in this activity (E). The group that receives no treatment is called a *passive control* (A). A placebo is a control that is similar to the treatment without the active ingredient so that study participants cannot identify if they are in the treatment group or the

control group (B). A positive control group receives a standard treatment; this is used when it is unethical or unsafe to withhold treatment from the control group (C). There is no standard control group (D).

54. All of the following characteristics of an experimental study are present in the program evaluation EXCEPT one. Which one is the EXCEPTION?

ANS: A
These are intact groups; groups were not randomly assigned (A). Randomization means that study participants are assigned to groups randomly. The test of the teens' knowledge is the measurement of the dependent variable (B). Presentation of the educational program is the manipulation of the independent variable (C). The educational program was presented before the posttest was given to determine if knowledge increased, representing placement of the independent variable before the dependent variable (D).

55. Which of the following additional sources of funding would be available to provide dental treatment for the children in this program?

ANS: A
Head Start children are primarily low SES, and often qualify for Medicaid or CHIP, based on the level of family income (A). A lower income is required to qualify for Medicaid than for CHIP. Medicaid and CHIP are a source of funding for dental services provided by the dentists associated with this community clinic. In many states, the dentist must be an approved provider to receive reimbursement by these programs for dental services. Medicare is a federal program that funds health care (but not dental care) for older adults, not dental care for children (B). Low-SES populations are less likely than higher-SES populations to have private dental insurance (C). The CDC does not fund local programs but provides educational information and guidelines for local public health programs (D). NIDCR funding is available for research only (E).

56. The type of caries assessment used by the program is basic screening. Basic screening is appropriate assessment to determine dental treatment needs.

ANS: C
The first statement is true, and the second statement is false (C). The use of a tongue blade and available light is considered basic screening or a type IV examination, so the first statement is true. The second statement is false because this type of examination

is appropriate to assess needs of a community for program planning, to assess the need for immediate care, and to make referrals for complete examination and treatment. An epidemiologic examination (type III) is used to survey a population to determine disease levels and to qualify teeth for sealant placement in a community-based sealant program. A limited examination (type II) at least is required to assess dental treatment needs. Choices A, B, and D do not accurately reflect the statements.

57. What type of practice supervision is used in this program?

ANS: D
Independent (unsupervised, limited access) practice is the practice of dental hygiene without the need of a supervising dentist (D). In many states in the United States, independent or unsupervised practice is allowed in certain public health settings. Direct supervision requires the presence of the dentist in the dental office during dental hygiene treatment (A). General supervision does not require the dentist's physical presence, with restrictions varying according to the state's practice acts (B). In some states, the patient must be a patient of record for general supervision to be permitted, whereas in other states, the patient must be examined by the dentist within a specified period before or after dental hygiene treatment. Indirect supervision requires the presence of the dentist in the clinical facility although not in the treatment operatory (C).

58. According to current CDC recommendations, what level of fluoride in parts per million (ppm) must be added to this community's water to bring the fluoride level to the optimum?

ANS: D
The most current CDC recommendation, effective in 2012, is 0.07 ppm. Since the fluoride level of the water in this scenario is 0.01 ppm, the required additional fluoride to bring the level to optimum is 0.06 ppm (D). Adding 1 ppm, 1.1 ppm, or 0.09 ppm would cause the fluoride level in the community water to exceed the current CDC recommendations (A, B, C).

59. What type of data is generated by the summative program evaluation of the educational program?

ANS: D
The rate of compliance with the referral is the summative (end of program) evaluation of the educational program conducted for parents. This is measured as either complying or not complying

with the referral. Dichotomous data is categorical data that has only two groups, which is characteristic of this compliance data. Categorical data means that it has mutually exclusive categories but has no numeric scale, for example, ethnic groups and SES (D). Discrete data are numeric data that are expressed only in whole numbers, for example, number of children who received fluoride varnish treatment (A). Qualitative data are descriptive in nature only and cannot be expressed numerically; an example would be the reasons for noncompliance (B). Continuous data are numeric data that have points on the scale that fall between the whole numbers and can be expressed meaningfully as a fraction, for example, measurements such as height, length, and weight (C).

60. The SES and the rate of tooth decay make this community appropriate to target for this program. The expected distribution of the DMF in this population would be more D than F scores.

ANS: A
Both statements are true (A). Research has shown migrant population to traditionally have a low SES, high rates of dental caries, high rates of untreated decay, poor access to oral health care, and low utilization rates, making the population a high priority to target with preventive dental public health programs. As a rule, the migrant workers do not have access to dental insurance. The breakdown of the DMF (more D than F) reflects the pattern of untreated decay that has results from poor access to care. Choices B, C, and D do not correctly reflect the statements.

61. What is the optimal level of fluoride in the drinking water for this population?

ANS: A
The current CDC recommendation for fluoride level in community water supplies is 0.7 ppm (A). At 3.0 ppm, the Environmental Protection Agency (EPA) would recommend defluoridation or removal of high levels of naturally occurring fluoride from the water, following EPA recommendations for defluoridation for water fluoridation levels of 2.0 to 4.0 ppm (B). When the water fluoridation level is above 4.0 ppm, defluoridation is required. The CDC recommendation has been adjusted from the previous recommendation of 0.7 to 1.2 ppm because of the increase in availability of fluorides from other sources (C). Levels of 1.2 ppm now exceed the current CDC recommendation for fluoride level in community water supplies (D).

62. What additional program would be the MOST cost effective fluoride delivery system for the community where the hygienist volunteers?

ANS: B
Community water fluoridation is the most cost effective means of delivering fluoride to a population. Water fluoridation meets the criteria for an ideal public health program: safe, effective in reducing the targeted disease or condition, easily and efficiently implemented, potency maintained for a substantial period, attainable regardless of SES, quickly effective, relatively inexpensive, and affordable to the community (B). Fluoride supplements are an effective means of delivering systemic fluoride, but delivery and compliance are more difficult to accomplish than community water fluoridation (A). A school fluoride mouth rinse program has some benefit but does not have the same caries reduction benefits, especially in a high-risk population such as this (C). Increasing the percentage of communities with optimally fluoridated water supplies is a *Healthy People 2020* goal, making water fluoridation an important public health goal for caries reduction making this option invalid (D).

63. Which of the following caries indices is MOST appropriate for assessment in this program?

ANS: D
The program description includes the measurement of the DMF on permanent molars based on an epidemiologic examination to qualify the teeth for sealants. Public health sealant programs target only permanent molars. DMF (with capital letters) indices denote measurement of permanent teeth (D). A surface index is not required for the purpose of the assessment in this program (E). Choices A, B, and C are indices for primary teeth, which would not be used for elementary school children.

64. Which of the following is the FIRST step in the scientific method?

ANS: A
The first step in the scientific method is to ask the research question (A). The sample study describes the question: What effect does an increase in pyrophosphates in tarter control toothpaste have on calculus formation? A review of the existing literature for background research helps develop a hypothesis: There will be no difference in calculus formation between the 5% formula and the 3.3% pyrophosphate formula (C). The hypothesis will be tested by conducting research, collecting data, and analyzing the data (D). Analysis of the data will verify or reject the hypothesis, allowing the researcher to draw a conclusion and communicate the results to the scientific community (B, E).

65. For each numbered research term or phrase, select from the list provided the MOST closely linked description in relation to this study.

ANS: 1E, 2D, 3A, 4C, 5B
An assumption is anything that is a given or that can be taken for granted. In this case the assumption is that the higher dosage of soluble pyrophosphates will be more effective in controlling calculus formation (1E). Variables are controlled to prevent extraneous variables that would limit the validity of the results; some of the variables that are controlled are providing prophylaxis and oral hygiene instructions, giving toothbrushes and restricting use of other oral hygiene aids, and choosing healthy, dentate participants (2D). Delimitations establish the boundaries of the population under study; dentate status and healthy adults compliant with 6-month maintenance are delimitations of this study (3A). One of the ethical principles of conducting research is that risk of participation should be minimized; the idea that study participants are not deprived of treatment that is the standard of care such as the inclusion of fluoride in the dentifrices exemplifies this ethical principle (4C). Study limitations are elements over which the researcher has no control and produce weaknesses in a study that reduce its validity and limit the usefulness of the results. Limitations are prevented by controlling variables and sources of error; providing a prophylaxis and oral hygiene instruction are a way of controlling the amount of calculus present at the beginning of the study, preventing preexisting calculus from limiting the accuracy of the study, and increasing its internal validity (5B).

66. Select the four items that describe the type of study represented.

ANS: B, C, D, E
A clinical trial is a well-controlled experimental study or group comparison based on epidemiologic principles and designed to test a hypothesis of a clinical nature. It is conducted on clinical patients and tests that a particular agent or procedure favorably alters the natural progression of a disease or condition. This study meets these characteristics (B). In this study, both the examiners and the study participants were unaware of group assignment; it is a double-blind study (C). Experimental studies are conducted with small representative samples, are longitudinal in nature, and use specific methods to test hypotheses. An experimental study is characterized by presence

of a control group (the 3.3% pyrophosphate group), control of extraneous variables (adult, periodontal maintenance compliance, prophylaxis provided, oral hygiene instructions), randomization (random assignment of study participants to the experimental and control groups), control of errors in measurement (use of a valid index to measure calculus, use of examiners unaware of which group is the experimental group, and measurement of the dependent variable after an appropriate length of time for calculus to form). Experimental studies are based on manipulation of the independent variable (the pyrophosphate formula toothpaste). In this study, measurement of the dependent variable (calculus formation) was taken before and after use of the independent variable to determine the effect of the pyrophosphate dentifrice after four months (D). In a pretest–posttest design, such as this one, the dependent variable is measured before and after the introduction of the independent variable, for comparison purposes (E). This study is not an analytical, case history, cohort, descriptive, or survey type of study; rather, it is experimental. Analytical studies are nonexperimental (A).

67. For each numbered potential variation in study design, select from the list provided the MOST closely linked description of that study design variation in relation to this study.

ANS: 1D, 2B, 3A, 4C
In a cross-over design, the groups are switched to the other treatment half way through the study after measuring the dependent variable to test the effect of the independent variable. The dependent variable is measured again after the study runs with the switched groups (1D). In a split-mouth design, one treatment is assigned to one half of the mouth, and the other treatment is assigned to the other half. Both cross-over and split-mouth designs control for all subject relevant variables and produce twice as much data (3A). In a factorial design, more than one independent variable is manipulated in the same study by forming multiple groups that have various combinations of the independent variables present (2B). In a time-series design, the dependent variable is measured multiple times at posttest to determine if the change in it will hold over time (4C).

68. Which of the following defines "in vivo" in this study design?

ANS: C
"In vivo" is the Latin term for "within the living." This term is used to describe studies that are conducted on live animals or people versus laboratory studies (C).

A retrospective study uses data collected in the past; also termed an *ex post facto* study (A). Choices B, D, and E do not accurately answer the question.

69. All of the following are required ethical procedures for the study EXCEPT one. Which one is the EXCEPTION?

ANS: A
Publishing participants' pain responses violates the ethical procedure of keeping all data collected from study participants confidential. Individual responses are destroyed after a specified time after study completion, and results are reported as group data only (A). Informed consent is required to protect the safety of study participants. It is the responsibility of the principal investigator to obtain informed consent. Informed consent consists of a formal written consent form that study participants read and sign prior to starting the study (B). Study participants' identity must be kept anonymous unless the participant has chosen otherwise. Special provisions must be made if this is a choice (C). It is the researcher's professional responsibility to report research results to the professional community to make new information available (D). Research studies within institutions must be approved by a review committee, frequently called an *institutional review board* or *institutional review committee*, to ensure that the proposed procedures are safe and ethical. This review committee is part of the organization that sponsors, and funds the research (E).

70. For each numbered research term listed, select the MOST closely linked description that reflects this study. Descriptions can be used more than one time.

ANS: 1B, 2A, 3E, 4C
The control group is the group that concurrently (at the same time) receives the control treatment; in this case was the 11 teeth treated with distilled water, the placebo (1B). The experimental group receives the experimental treatment being studied; the 11 teeth treated with calcium hypophosphate (2A). The population is the group to which the results of the research can be applied; this is defined by the population delimitations or boundaries described by the researcher (postperiodontal-therapy patients with sensitive teeth) and is also represented by the sample (3E, 4E).

71. There is a 1% chance that the results of this study have a type II beta (β) error. A type II beta (β) error occurs when treatment was not really effective and invalid results show a statistically significant difference occurred between the experimental and control treatments.

ANS: B

Both statements are false (B). The probability value of p=0.01 indicates that there is a 1% chance that the results of this study have a type I alpha (α) error, rather than a type II beta (β) error. A type I alpha (α) error is an error in judgment on the part of the researcher. In a type I alpha (α) error, the researcher falsely accepts the results or effect of the treatment as being accurate when in reality the results are caused by chance. A type I alpha (α) error occurs when the researcher mistakenly rejected the null hypothesis. The second statement is false: A type II beta (β) error is a researcher or statistical decision error, like the type I alpha (α) error. With the type II beta (β) error, the researcher mistakenly concludes that a treatment has no effect when, in fact, it has an effect. A type II beta (β) error is when the researcher mistakenly accepts the null hypothesis. This type of error may occur when the group size is too small. Choices A, C, and D do not accurately reflect the statements.

72. This study represents the highest level of evidence for evidence-based decision making. All research studies, regardless of the type of study, represent the same level of evidence for evidence-based decision making.

ANS: B

Both statements are false (B). The highest level of evidence is systematic reviews, preferably with meta-analysis. This is trailed by the following evidence, listed in their order on the hierarchy: one or more randomized controlled clinical trials, well-designed cohort studies, well-designed case control studies, cross-sectional studies without concurrent controls and uncontrolled experiments, opinions of respected authorities based on clinical experience, descriptive surveys, case reports, reports of expert committees, and finally nonhuman (animal) research. This study is a randomized controlled clinical trial, which is below systematic reviews on the hierarchy of evidence. Choices A, C, and D do not accurately reflect the statements.

73. Who reviewed the research report to approve its publication in the journal?

ANS: C

According to the description given, the sample study report is published in a peer-reviewed journal. Peer review is a juried process of experts in the content area to ensure the quality of published research. By definition, manuscripts submitted to a peer reviewed journal are reviewed by experts in the content area of the manuscript. Most dental hygiene journals have a group of dental hygienist content experts available to review submitted manuscripts (C). The journal editor

coordinates the reviews and makes final decisions about publication of manuscripts based on the recommendations of the reviewers (A). Professional writers are on staff of publishing companies to assist in the process of editing (B). Authors may consult with professional associates in the process of preparing a manuscript for submission and revising it based on the reviewers' comments (D).

74. All of the following should be examined to judge the quality of the journal in which the study is published EXCEPT one. Which one is the EXCEPTION?

ANS: E

The number of pictures, tables, and graphs is not a criterion to judge a journal but will be a result of the types of articles published (E). The following criteria are used to judge the quality of a journal: sponsorship by a learned society, professional organization, or reputable scientific publisher (A); high technical quality (B); adherence to a strict advertising policy (C); presence of a reputable editorial review board (D); and publication of unbiased, objective articles.

75. Which of the following methods of group assignment was used in this study?

ANS: C

With randomized matching, the groups are matched in the process of random assignment. The groups in this study are randomly assigned but also matched for gender and age (C). With simple random assignment, the study participants are randomly assigned to groups (A). Sequential assignment is used when study participants are assigned in the order as they appear (B). Sometimes an already existing group is used for comparison purposes, rather than actually assigning participants to groups, in which case random assignment does not occur (D).

76. Match the study types with their correct descriptions.

ANS: 1B, 2C, 3D, 4A, 5I, 6E, 7H, 8G, 9F

A clinical trial is a well-controlled experimental study or group comparison based on epidemiologic principles and designed to test a hypothesis of a clinical nature (1B). A cross-over study has groups that are switched to the other treatment halfway through the study after measuring the dependent variable to test the effect of the independent variable on the other group (2C). A double-blind study is one in which both examiners and study participants are unaware of group assignment (3D). An experimental study is characterized by presence of a control group, control of extraneous variables, randomization, control of errors in measurement, use of blind examiners, and measurement of the dependent variable multiple times, manipulation of an independent variable, measurement of a dependent variable, and occurrence of the independent variable before measuring the dependent variable in the study design (4A). The posttest-only study design is one in which the dependent variable is only measured after the independent variable is introduced (5I). In the pretest–posttest study design, the dependent variable is measured, for comparison purposes, before and after the introduction of the independent variable (6E). The split-mouth study design uses half of the dentition for the experiment; the other half is used for control (7H). Randomized studies use random assignment to form the groups (8G). In time-series studies, the dependent variable is measured several times at posttest to establish that the independent variable is effective over time (9F).

77. If the participants had been assigned a 1-month period between the two flossing phases of the study and during which they did not floss; that period would be called a

ANS: C
A washout period is a period for the two groups in a cross-over study to return to baseline levels before starting the other intervention. The purpose of the washout period is to allow time for the effects of the first treatment assignment to wear off before introducing the next treatment intervention (C). A placebo is an inactive drug or treatment given instead of one with a known effect (A). The baseline is the initial reading or measurement against which later treatment or interventions are measured for effect (B). A cross-over design that during which study participants receive no treatment before the independent variable is switched for the two groups (D).

78. Which of the following is the number of intervals in the frequency distribution table?

ANS: D
The interval is the difference between one tick-mark to the next along the axis of a graph. On a frequency distribution table, it is the grouping of scores. There are four intervals: 1%–25%, 26%–50%, 51%–75%, and 76%–100% (D). There are 24 data points (total frequency is 24; there are 24 in the patient sample) denoted by the total frequency on the frequency distribution table and on the *y* axis of the graph (B). There are 8 scores in the interval of 76%–100% (C). A total of 100% of scores reported (A).

79. The histogram is an appropriate way to present the frequency data because the data are continuous.

ANS: A
A histogram, a bar graph with the bars touching each other that presents frequency data such as the one illustrated, is an appropriate graph to communicate continuous data. Continuous data are numeric data that have points on the scale that fall between the whole numbers and can be expressed meaningfully as a fraction (A). Choices B, C, D, and E do not accurately reflect the statement.

80. According to the information presented in the table, what percentage of patients scored greater than 50% on the O'Leary Plaque Control Record at their first assessment appointment?

ANS: E
Both a frequency and a percentage are reported for each interval. The frequencies or percentages are added to determine how many are in a combination of intervals: 38% and 33% (38% in the interval 51%–75% and 33% in the interval 76%–100%) are added to determine the percentage in the combined interval of 51%–100% (71%) (E). Choices A, B, C, and D do not accurately answer the question; the percentages are all too low.

81. Which type of curve does this distribution represent?

ANS: A
A nonsymmetrical curve is called a *skewed curve*. A negative skew occurs when the majority of the scores are high and there are some extreme scores on the low end. When it is plotted on a graph, the curve "leans" to the right and the "tail" is to the left (A). A positive skew is the opposite; the majority of scores are low, and there are some extreme high scores, producing a curve than "leans" to the left with the "tail" to the right (B). A bell-shaped curve is a normal distribution in which the mean, median, and mode are the same value in the middle of the curve. When it is plotted on a graph, it is symmetrical in shape (C).

82. Which of the following describes the reasons that the O'Leary Plaque Control Record and the SBI will be the only indices used at all appointments subsequent to the assessment appointment?

ANS: C
Clinicians should be trained and calibrated on any index that is used to measure an oral disease or condition, including plaque biofilm and bleeding (C). It is invalid to compare scores measured with different indices because each index has different

criteria (A). There are several indices that can be used to measure plaque biofilm in a dental public health setting (B). Regardless of the index selected to measure a variable, the same index must be used to measure it throughout the program to yield comparable data for evaluation purposes (D).

83. What type of study is this?

ANS: E
This study is a survey with specific statistical analysis comparison between uncontrolled variables (E). A case-control study, or case history, is a retrospective, analytic study that compares two groups, one with a disease or condition and one without it, to determine possible associated factors in the history of those with the disease or condition (A). In longitudinal and prospective studies, a group is observed from one point forward to detect exposure, which requires multiple measures of the disease or condition being researched; cohort studies are longitudinal and prospective studies (B). Retrospective studies look backward to determine exposure in the past; case control (case history) studies are retrospective studies (C). A cross-sectional study is an analytical study that uses a representative cross-section of the population (one group) to assess a condition at one point in time and associate other variables with each other as well as describe the prevalence of the condition (D).

84. Which of the following would increase the return rate of the survey?

ANS: A
Use of an electronic survey instrument such as Survey Monkey increases the return rate of the survey because response to e-surveys is higher than traditional mail surveys (A). Including a self-addressed return envelope makes it easier for individuals to respond; they do not have to find an envelope or incur any cost; however, this method is less effective than electronic surveys (B). Establishing validity and reliability of the questionnaire are important to ensure validity of research results but is not directly related to the response rate (C). A cover letter is usually included to explain the purpose of the research, which is an ethical requirement, but a well-designed survey with questions that are clearly explained would not require a cover letter (D).

85. What type of statistic is used to test the relationship of years in practice with salary?

ANS: D
Nonparametric inferential statistics are used to compare the actual distributions of data (rather

than mean scores) that do not meet the assumptions required for parametric data. Chi square is a common nonparametric statistic used in oral health research. It is used in this example to test the statistical significance of the various relationships of salary and employment benefits with age and years in practice (D). Parametric inferential statistics are used when the data include interval or ratio scales such as data from a large randomized sample and normally distributed data. The t-test is used to compare two mean scores and determines statistical significance of the difference between these two means; it may be used to compare treatment and control sample groups or pretest and posttest mean scores of the same group (A). Correlation is used to associate the dental hygienist's years in practice with his or her salary (B). Descriptive statistics summarize data, and correlation statistics demonstrate the relationship or association among variables. In this case, a descriptive study would be used to summarize how many dental hygienists have been practicing for different periods, and how many are earning salaries of different ranges (C).

86. How can statistical significance of study results be determined?

ANS: B
Statistical significance is established by a *p*-value of 0.05 or lower (B). The *p*-value indicates what percentage of the results is from chance and not from sound research methodology. A *p*-value of 0.05 indicates that there is a 5% error or that 95% of the results are valid. Although there was not a null hypothesis in this case, the *p*-value is used to accept or reject the null hypothesis. If the *p*-value is 0.05 or below, the null hypothesis is rejected; if the *p*-value is greater than 0.05, the null hypothesis is accepted. A smaller *p*-value denotes greater statistical significance. Choices A, C, and D do not accurately answer the question.

87. The results of this study establish a causal relationship between years in practice and salary. The sampling method used results in a representative sample for this heterogeneous population.

ANS: D
The first statement is false, and the second statement is true (D). This testlet is reporting a survey with specific statistical analysis comparison between uncontrolled variables. There is no cause-and-effect in this testlet information. Causality cannot be inferred by descriptive studies or other types of analytic studies. The second statement is true. The sampling method is stratified random sampling, which results in a representative sample for a heterogeneous

(different from each other) population. The population is heterogeneous based on the inclusion of dental hygienists from all states in the United States. Choices A, B, and C do not accurately reflect the statement.

88. Training the examiners is for the purpose of establishing interrater reliability. The procedures of giving a practice period for use of the toothbrushes, timing the toothbrushing, and withholding toothpaste during brushing are for the purpose of controlling the reliability of the study.

ANS: C
The first statement is true, and the second statement is false (C). Reliability refers to the consistency of the measuring instruments and examiners. Interrater (interexaminer) reliability is the consistency among multiple examiners. The second statement is false. The procedures of giving a practice period for use of the toothbrushes, timing the toothbrushing, and withholding toothpaste during brushing are for the purpose of establishing validity, rather than the reliability, of the study. Validity is the accuracy of a measure or a study. Procedures that control variables and the accuracy of the measurement of the dependent variable help establish validity. Internal validity is the accuracy of the results of a study and is affected by controls in the conduct of the study such as those described in this question and includes the reliability of a measure. Reliability affects internal validity but internal validity does not affect reliability. External validity is the accuracy of generalizing or applying to the population the results of the study carried out in a sample. This type of validity is affected by the representativeness of the sample. The more representative the sample, the higher is the external validity. Choices A, B, and D do not accurately reflect the statement.

89. Examiner bias in this study is controlled. This is because the examiners are unaware of which brush was used in which area of the mouth by the research participants.

ANS: A
Both statements are true (A). The study is designated a blind study. This means that the examiner is unaware of group assignment. The examiner does not know which study participants are using the finger brush and which are using the regular manual toothbrush, to prevent examiner bias. If examiners have an expectation of the outcome, it may subconsciously affect their measurements. Choices B, C, and D do not accurately reflect the statement.

90. Using the information provided in the table, in which range of values did 95% of the baseline scores fall?

ANS: B
According to the empirical rule of the normal (bell-shaped) curve, there is a naturally occurring distribution of scores around the mean of the distribution of scores: 68% of the scores fall between plus and −1 standard deviation (SD) from the mean score, 95% of the scores fall between plus and −2 SDs from the mean score, and 99% of the scores fall between ±3 SDs from the mean score. Knowing the mean and the SD, the percentage of scores within a range of scores can be determined. The mean baseline score of the finger brush group is 1.41. Adding and subtracting two SDs from the mean results in a range of scores of 0.77 to 2.05 ($1.41 - [2 \times 0.32] = 0.77$ and $1.41 + [2 \times 0.32] = 2.05$) (B). Choices A and C do not accurately reflect the statement.

91. On the basis of the statistical results of this study, what decision should be made regarding the null hypothesis?

ANS: A
Reject the null hypothesis; the manual toothbrush is more effective. The null hypothesis of this study is that there is no difference in the plaque removal ability of the two devices. The decision is based on the p-value of the statistical results. The null hypothesis is rejected when the p-value is equal to or less than 0.05 ($p < 0.05$). The results of this study are a p-value of 0.01 (less than 0.05); the null hypothesis is rejected. Comparison of the baseline and posttest or end scores of the two groups demonstrates that the regular manual toothbrush removed more plaque compared with the finger brush. The manual toothbrush is more effective, voiding the null hypothesis (A). Choices B, C, and D do not accurately answer the question.

92. The report is considered out of date according to the timing of its publication. The peer review of the journal is designed to provide quality assurance of published research.

ANS: D
The first statement is false, and the second statement is true (D). In general, scientific literature published within 5 years is considered current. It is important to note, however, that epidemiologic research—the knowledge base of the causes, prevention, and treatment of diseases—may change quickly, and the literature may become outdated sooner than 5 years. The researcher must make an effort to stay current with the literature. The second statement is true as peer review is the process by which manuscripts

that are submitted to journals for publication are reviewed by experts in the field prior to publication. The reviewers for a journal make recommendations about whether to accept a manuscript for publication, accept it with revisions, or reject it. The purpose of this juried process is to ensure the quality of the research articles published in the journal. Textbooks and other materials published by professional and scientific publishers go through the same peer review process. Responsible professionals use peer-reviewed materials to search for information for the purpose of evidence-based practice. Choices A, B, and C do not accurately reflect the statements.

93. All of the following would be goals of the dental hygienist's presentation EXCEPT one. Which one is the EXCEPTION?

ANS: B
Providing information on orthodontic treatment in children would not be an appropriate goal for the presentation to this group. WIC provides services for pregnant and breastfeeding low-SES women, and infants and children up to 5 years of age who are at nutritional risk. As a general rule, children should have an orthodontic referral when the first permanent molars are fully erupted, around age 6 to 7 years, so this information is not relevant to this group (B). Describing the effect of dietary choices on oral health encourages healthy behavior because making good choices involves taking a physical action (A). Discussing the value of good oral health for the mother and the child affects the participant's ideas and beliefs in a way that would hopefully prompt the mother to choose healthy behaviors (C). Emphasizing the importance of caries transmission and prevention may be considered health promotion because it is informing and motivating individuals to incorporate positive behaviors (D). Highlighting dental providers who make their services accessible to this population is a form of health education because it is imparting facts or knowledge; it could also be classified as promoting a healthy behavior because it encourages a specific action such as visiting a dental provider for routine care (E).

94. Which health behavior model addresses the dental hygiene focus of creating and increasing awareness of healthy choices through a process of change over time as individuals cycle through stages of awareness and readiness?

ANS: D
Creating and increasing awareness of a problem, in this case health choices, directly reflects the Stages of Change: Transtheoretical Model (D). This model proposes the theory that change must develop as a

process over time while individuals cycle through different stages of awareness and readiness. The cycle starts by raising awareness of a problem, progresses to contemplating change, deciding to change, acting on a specific plan, and finally follows up with maintenance of that desired action or behavior. Locus of Control is an extension of the Social Learning Theory and deals with one's perception of personal control over the elements described in that theory (A). The Health Belief Model addresses perceived susceptibility and severity of a disease as well as perceived effectiveness of the preventive intervention and perceived ability to overcome barriers to change (B). The Social Cognitive Theory (also known as the *Social Learning Theory*) is based on how environment, knowledge, and behavior interact to affect one's lifestyle choices and the idea that people learn through personal experience as well as by observing the experiences of others and the resulting outcomes (C).

95. Which stage of the community program development process is addressed by the verbal survey?

ANS: D
Part of the assessment process involves collecting data or information; that includes verbal and written surveys, interviews, focus groups, oral examinations, and more (D). Planning builds on the diagnosis of the population's needs and creates a plan of action for a public health intervention (A). Diagnosis is the process of taking the information gathered and making a determination about the needs of the population (B). Evaluation or analysis of the success of the program follows implementation (C). Implementation is the actual execution of the plan (E).

96. Focusing on regular dental visits for this population would be considered promotion of a health behavior. Increasing the participants' understanding of the infectious nature of dental caries would be considered an example of a health promotion strategy.

ANS: A
Both statements are true (A). Health promotion has been defined by the World Health Organization (WHO) as "the process of enabling people to increase control over their health and its determinants, and thereby improve their health." This includes activities that provide people with the knowledge and resources to make changes as well as sociopolitical actions that support change. Health education is one aspect of health promotion, the process of increasing people's awareness of health and disease for the purpose of enabling them to make healthy decisions. Focusing on regular dental visits for this population may be classified as promoting a healthy behavior

because it encourages a specific action (visiting a dental provider for regular care). Emphasizing the importance of dental caries transmission and prevention may be considered health promotion because it is informing and motivating individuals to incorporate a behavior. Choices B, C, and D do not accurately reflect the statements.

97. The expectant mothers express interest in receiving dental care. This is an example of potential demand because it represents an unmet need.

ANS: A

Both statements are true (A). Based on the scenario, we know that none of the participants has received dental care for the past 2 years, which represents an unmet need. The reason stated by the participants for the unmet need is lack of financial resources and dental insurance, which are access to care issues. Potential demand is defined as the desire for dental care that is unmet because of lack of access. Choices B, C, and D do not accurately reflect the statements.

98. Sealants are an effective dental public health strategy for this population because of their cost-effectiveness, regardless of SES. When used as a public health intervention, sealants are usually applied to 8- to 9-year-old children (third graders) and 12- to 13-year-old children (seventh grade) at risk for dental caries.

ANS: C

The first statement is true, and the second statement is false (C). Dental sealants are a resin-based material applied to the pits and fissures of the occlusal, buccal, and lingual surfaces of teeth to prevent dental decay. Sealant programs are a cost-effective public health intervention for preventing caries among populations at risk for caries. Public health sealant programs are timed in conjunction with the eruption of permanent first and second molars, teeth at risk for dental caries because of their deep pits and fissures. In public health settings, sealants are placed most commonly on 6- to 7-year-old children, soon after the eruption of the first permanent molar. That age usually aligns with the period a child is in the second grade. Sixth graders, or 11- to 12-year-old children, are also an appropriate age group for sealant intervention in public health settings because of the eruption of the second permanent molars. Choices A, B, and D do not accurately reflect the statements.

99. Which of the following indices would be the MOST useful to evaluate the long-term success of this program?

ANS: D

Programs are evaluated according to their success in impacting the specific disease or condition targeted by the program. The long-term success of a sealant program is measured by the lowering the incidence of dental caries in the population. The DMFT measures caries prevalence on permanent teeth by recording the number of decayed, missing, and filled teeth. This index is appropriate for this population because the teeth being assessed are permanent teeth (D). The root caries index or RCI measures caries on root surfaces where recession is present, which is uncommon in children (A). Even though this population is in the mixed dentition period, long-term success is measured by the caries rate on permanent teeth, disqualifying the dmft index, which is used only for primary teeth (B). The OHI-S index is a means of evaluating oral hygiene and cannot be used to measure caries (C).

100. The incidence of dental caries among this population is the number of carious lesions noted at the time of program inception. Monitoring of caries prevalence, filled teeth, and missing teeth because of nonrestorable caries that required extraction should continue throughout the program's duration to evaluate program outcomes.

ANS: B

Both statements are false (B). Incidence is defined as the number of new cases of disease in a population over a given period. Prevalence is the amount of cases present when measured at one specific point in time. In this program, prevalence of dental caries is represented by the DMFT scores noted at the time of the initial assessment. Prevalence may be monitored over time to establish a trend, but this monitoring of prevalence over a sustained period does not establish incidence because it is not measuring new disease in the same group. Choices A, C, and D do not accurately reflect the statement.

101. All of the following are potential barriers to care for this program EXCEPT one. Which one is the EXCEPTION?

ANS: C

Sealants are far more cost effective compared with dental restorations (C). The cost of a one-surface restoration is higher than the cost of a sealant placement. Shortage of providers is an issue in community programs and may be a potential barrier to care (A). Lack of consumer awareness continues to be an issue for community sealant programs, highlighting the need to provide education for the target population to promote participation (B). Lack of funding to provide necessary equipment is a potential barrier to care (D).

102. The necessity of educating the tribal leaders about the need for the sealant program characterizes which dental public health concept?

ANS: D
Perceived need is the individual's or community's perception of the need for care, based on their understanding of their health status. The tribal leaders are unaware of the need for and the potential benefits of the program. Education is a means of changing these perceptions to match the normative needs, so they will approve of and promote the program for their community (D). Supply defines the amount of dental services available (A). Demand is the desire of the population for care (B). Utilization reflects the number of dental services actually used or consumed, reported as the actual attendance at a treatment facility to receive care (C). Normative need is the need of the individual or group established through professional judgment by examination (E).

103. All of the following are terms which could describe the formation of a relationship between the homeless shelter and the various organizations or institutions that are described EXCEPT one. Which one is the EXCEPTION?

ANS: A
Covenant is a term for formal promises made under oath; no formal promises have been made in this scenario (A). Networking, or the sharing of resources, to reach a goal, may be one type of relationship between the homeless shelter and the various groups (B). Partnerships may be formed in between the shelters and groups to forge a deeper association and work together regularly to achieve a common objective. Partnerships usually have affiliation agreements or contracts to delineate the responsibilities of each party (C). Collaboration, often the entry point of relationships, is the process of working cooperatively with others toward a common goal (D). Coalitions are alliances, usually temporary, between individuals or groups cooperating in joint action, for a common cause. Essential to the success of any coalition is the involvement of the stakeholders, which include the community of interest (the homeless shelter clients), community opinion leaders (the faith-based group, service club, and medical and dental schools), and public policy makers (the councilman's office) (E).

104. Which of the following is the role of the dental hygienist in this program?

ANS: D
The role of administrator or manager involves managing the operation of a program, which is the role the dental hygienist in the program has agreed to perform in spearheading organizational efforts (D). The role of the clinician is to deliver clinical services to the members of the target population (A). Advocates work to champion a specific cause or change in public policy. Advocates see the bigger picture of promoting health and preventing disease on a community level and work to influence the minds and hearts of the community, public opinion leaders, and policy makers (B). The role of the educator is to conduct educational programs for the purpose of encouraging change in health behaviors (C).

105. What type of assessment tool would provide the BEST indication of the normative need of this population?

ANS: B
Dental indices are objective instruments used to assess actual disease and disease related conditions, and they may be used by oral health professionals to determine normative need (B). Normative need is recognized when a professional judgment is rendered, indicating oral health status and need for care. Surveys and focus groups are methods used to collect data from the members of the population (A, C). The resulting data reflect the characteristics, knowledge, opinions, beliefs, and values of the population rather than their actual oral health status.

106. Which of the following forms the foundation of the success of the program?

ANS: D
The success of a program is based on the measurable program objectives or outcomes related to the condition (creating a clinic) being targeted by the program. The purpose of this program is to be able to create a self-sustaining, on-site clinic within the next 5 years. Specific program objectives will provide a framework to evaluate extent to which the program meets its goal. Objectives must be specific and measureable to be effective (D). Cooperation of the community partners also reflect successful processes of community programming and may be a supplemental objective measured through formative evaluation in the process of planning and conducting a program for this population (B). Client compliance and the amount of needs assessment data collected are not related to the achievement of the goal of building a self-sustaining clinic (A, C).

107. All of the following *Healthy People 2020* objectives are pertinent for this population EXCEPT one. Which one is the EXCEPTION?

     ANS: E
     The *Healthy People 2020* objective to increase the proportion of school-based health centers with an oral health center is not pertinent for this population (E). The rate of untreated dental decay is higher in lower-SES groups and especially high in a homeless population without access to care (A). Increasing dental sealant utilization is relevant to all populations (B). The natural fluoride level of the community water is below the recommend level of 0.7 ppm, so water fluoridation would be a cost-effective means of delivering fluoride to this population (C). Many individuals are homeless because of alcohol or drug abuse, putting them at risk for oral and pharyngeal cancers (D).

108. Which of the following is another descriptor for the increase in oral and pharyngeal cancer rates referred to in this example?

     ANS: A
     Trend (A) refers to the long-term changes in disease patterns and health-related conditions as identified by surveillance data. Epidemic (B) refers to the occurrence of disease that spreads very rapidly in excess of normal expectancy in a community. Incidence (C) records the number of new cases over a period of time. Pandemic (D) references the spread of disease over very wide areas; affecting a large proportion of the population. Prevalence (E) is the amount of disease present in a single snapshot of time.

109. A parent in the audience would be correct in interpreting the cited studies as showing that smoking is the primary cause of oral and pharyngeal cancer because the studies cited were statistically significant.

     ANS: E
     NEITHER the statement NOR the reason is correct (E). Analytical and correlation studies do not establish causality, or cause and effect; they only demonstrate associations or relationships among variables, providing evidence for risk. Both statistical significance (*p* value) and the correlation coefficient (*r* value) must be present in studies to enable one to interpret the association of variables and their statistical significance for evidence-based decision making, and this testlet does not contain that information. Choices A, B, C, and D do not accurately reflect the statement and the reason.

110. What type of visual graphic would BEST reflect relationship data such as the type discussed in the research studies cited in the presentation?

     ANS: D
     A scattergram, also known as a *scatter plot*, is the best choice of graph for relationship studies because it plots the two variables (tobacco use and cancer, smoking and periodontal disease) to visually show the relationship or association (D). A pie chart is an esthetically pleasing, easy-to-understand chart; it depicts parts of a whole. The pie chart is used to represent categorical data and should not be used to depict scientific results (A). The bell curve is the normal curve created by depicting the distribution of population data and forms the foundation of probability theory and its application to statistical procedures (B). A histogram is a horizontally-oriented bar graph that displays the frequency of interval or ratio data, and sometimes ordinal data if they are being used as continuous data (C). A simple bar graph functions in the same way as a pie chart in that it represents simple categorical data (E).

111. To evaluate the parents' learning, which of the following evaluation outcomes would reflect successful results from the dental hygienist's presentation?

     ANS: C
     Successful results from the presentation are the summative outcomes of this strategy or intervention, in this case the change in knowledge as a result of the presentation (C). The levels of audience participation and the organization of the presentation are principles that will add to a successful presentation and are assessed through formative evaluation, but they are not the measures of an increase in knowledge (A, B).

112. Which of the following types of evaluation is used to determine the program outcome of implementing a smoke-free ordinance for all the restaurants, bars, and eateries within the city limits?

     ANS: D
     Summative evaluation measures the outcomes of a program after it is complete. The successful implementation of a smoke-free ordinance for all the restaurants, bars, and eateries within the city limits would be an example of summative evaluation (D). Internal evaluation is a process of quality review within an organization to ensure standards are being maintained (A). External evaluation comes from outside agencies such as accrediting or credentialing agencies and is intended to uphold standards of that discipline (B). Formative evaluation is ongoing

during program implementation and may lead to adjustments for the purpose of improvement. An example of formative evaluation would be observing the audience's body language or level of participation, which may lead to adjusting the delivery style of the presentation if necessary (C).

113. All of the following should be included as components of the assessment for this population EXCEPT one. Which one is the EXCEPTION?

    ANS: C
    Determining what brands of toothbrushes and floss are available does not influence the health of the population (C). Various types of information are necessary to consider when conducting a comprehensive community oral health assessment. A community profile such as this includes identifying the oral health needs of the population (A), evaluation of the determinants of health (B), asking about the resources and assets available to the community (D), and quantification of disparities and inequities among the population groups of the community (E). Another factor to be measured is the rate of preventable disease, injury, disability, and death in the community.

114. For this population, which of the following assessment tools are MOST effective to provide authentic data?

    ANS: B
    Oral health screenings use indices to measure actual diseases and disease-related conditions, resulting in a description of the oral health status of a population, and will give the most complete data (B). Personal interviewing allows the interviewer to interact directly with the patient; however, it does not provide as much assessment data as oral health screenings (A). Written questionnaire surveys require reading comprehension; and it may not be possible to administer them to every person (C).

115. Which of the following is the mean of the distribution of the number of people currently experiencing dental pain across the five villages?

    ANS: C
    The mean is a measure of central tendency used to identify the central value or average of distribution of scores in a sample. The mean is the arithmetic average score, or the sum of the scores divided by the total number of scores. The mean is the most commonly used statistic and is reliable for normal distributions. In this question, the mean of the number

of people currently experiencing dental pain in the five villages is 14 ($[10 + 14 + 17 + 15 + 14] \div 5 = 14$) (C). Choices A, B, D, and E do not accurately answer the question.

116. The mode is the most frequently occurring score or most repeated number in a distribution of scores. This distribution of scores is unimodal.

    ANS: C
    The first statement is true, and the second statement is false (C). The mode is the most frequently occurring score or most repeated number in a distribution of scores. A distribution may have no mode when all scores occur only once. A distribution may have only one mode (unimodal), two modes (bimodal), or multiple modes (multimodal). For this group of score distributions, the number 14 occurs twice, whereas all other scores occur only once, making the distribution bimodal. Choices A, B, and D do not accurately reflect the statements.

117. The hygienists should focus on all of the objectives as they start their program planning EXCEPT one. Which one is the EXCEPTION?

    ANS: D
    Although increasing the overall literacy levels of the population may be a worthy goal, it is not within the scope of this project and does not directly relate to improvement of oral health status (D). Establishing referrals with health care providers will promote health and will increase access to health care (A). Establishing preventive health care programs in the rural areas will help promote oral health care (B). Increasing the oral health literacy of the population is vital because it lays the foundation for the communication of risk, which is the understanding of one's susceptibility to oral diseases. Communicating risk, in turn, contributes to the public's demand for, and hopefully their utilization of, oral health services (C).

118. Which of the following statements represents the community dental hygiene diagnosis for this population?

    ANS: D
    The community dental hygiene diagnosis for this population would be that high rates of dental disease related to the lack of access to care (D). The comprehensive community oral health assessment revealed high rates of dental caries, existing dental pain, and missing teeth, which are all indicators that adequate health care is not readily available. Choices A, B, C, and E do not accurately answer the question.

119. Which of the following types of health data reporting is the dental hygienist developing?

ANS: D
The hygienist is working with a team to monitor the frequency of a condition or disease (periodontology) in a given population in an ongoing process. This is an accurate description of the epidemiologic term *surveillance*, also called *syndromic surveillance* (D). Screening refers to a basic clinical examination of individuals during the assessment and evaluation stages of a program used to detect or rule out a condition or disease (A). Surveying is a method of collecting quantitative information from the population and is used in a surveillance system but does not describe the type of data that result (B). Examination is a more comprehensive clinical procedure than screening, compiling data for purposes of assessment, diagnosis, and treatment (C).

120. The periodontal disease summary data reported as a result of this epidemiologic surveillance may be described as the proportion of the population with that amount of disease because the data express the presence of each level of periodontitis in relation to the size of the population.

ANS: A
Both the statement and the reason are correct and related (A). Prevalence data are reported in the scenario. Prevalence is defined as the proportion of a population found to have a condition. It is calculated by dividing the number of people found to have the condition by the total number of people surveyed. Although the total number of persons surveyed is not disclosed, the ratio or percentage of persons with periodontal disease indicates the portion of the population affected with the disease. Prevalence may be expressed as a ratio, a percentage (as in this scenario), or the number of cases per 10,000 or 100,000 people. Choices B, C, D, and E do not accurately reflect the statement and the reason.

121. Which of the following indices is MOST commonly used for gathering the data for this surveillance project?

ANS: B
The CPI was adapted by the WHO from the CPITN to measure the periodontal status of populations. The CPI includes measures of gingival health, gingival bleeding, supragingival or subgingival calculus, periodontal pockets (4 to 5 mm and 6 mm or more), and loss of attachment (LOA), which is the same as clinical attachment loss (CAL) (B). The PI is a classic periodontal index that historically was used for periodontal research. It does not reflect LOA or CAL, nor does it provide separate measures of the various parameters of periodontal diseases; so it is not widely used today to measure periodontal diseases (A). The PSR was developed by the American Dental Association (ADA); it is similar to these indices but is primarily used for periodontal assessment of individual patients in a clinical settings (C). The CPITN measures treatment needs rather than periodontal status (D).

122. The following factors contribute to the dental hygienist's cultural sensitivity in relation to this project EXCEPT one. Which one is the EXCEPTION?

ANS: D
Previous experience as a public health hygienist would not contribute to the dental hygienist's cultural sensitivity in relation to this project because every culture is unique (D). The ability to build a relationship with local leaders helps establish rapport and acceptance in the community (A). The hygienist's fluency in French helps promote understanding with the participants in the surveillance study (B). Familiarity with the customs of the country would help the hygienist be respectful and observant of the customs of the country (C).

123. Which of the following should be the hygienist's first step in meeting the goal for the school board?

ANS: A
Promoting a community water fluoridation program is accomplished by following a series of steps. The hygienist must be well informed on fluoridation information to gather support for the program. The hygienist needs to identify, educate, and get endorsement from key community leaders for a broad base of support (A). A referendum or public vote should be avoided, if possible, because it presents an opportunity for antifluoridationists to oppose water fluoridation. Referendums are frequently unsuccessful because antifluoridationists appeal to emotions rather than use facts and are more vocal than supporters of fluoridation (B). The decision makers (members of the city council or similar governmental structures) are presented with the endorsements and educated about the issue (D). After the council has individually endorsed the issue, the dental hygienist will bring the decision before the council for a vote, attending the council meeting to show public support for the issue when it is formally presented and voted upon (C).

124. Which of the following is the MOST recent CDC recommendation for the optimal level of fluoride in the community water supply of this city?

ANS: B
The most recent CDC recommendation for optimal level of fluoride in the community water supply is 0.7ppm (B). The CDC recently changed its recommendation from 0.7 to 1.2ppm fluoride on the basis of the climate of the area and to 0.7ppm fluoride for all areas of the country. The change was precipitated by the increase in water fluoridation and multiple other sources of fluoride in the U.S. population (C). Community water fluoride levels of 2.0ppm will produce fluorosis in large enough numbers that the EPA recommends defluoridation of water with 2 to 4ppm of fluoride. In levels over 4ppm, the EPA requires communities to defluoridate the municipal water supplies (A). Community water fluoride levels of 0.3ppm are too low to produce consistent caries protection, and supplementation is recommended (D).

125. Which of the following is the LEAST complex governmental intervention for adoption of community water fluoridation?

ANS: D
Adoption by the city council or other local governmental entity is the simplest governmental intervention for adoption of community water fluoridation. Local governments are most familiar with the needs of their citizens, and keeping the issue at this level avoids the complex legislative process (D). A referendum should be avoided, if possible, to avoid opposition from antifluoridationists (A). Most states prefer to leave the decision to the local government to provide each locale a choice (B). In the United States, public health issues such as this are researched at the federal level, with implementation occurring at the local level (C).

126. The hygienist can accurately educate the public that water fluoridation is considered the most cost-effective population-based mechanism for prevention of dental caries. The community can expect that fluoridation will provide a 60% decrease in the caries rate of a community.

ANS: C
The first statement is true, and the second statement is false (C). Fluorides have been shown to be highly effective in preventing and controlling dental caries, and water fluoridation is considered the most cost-effective means of delivering fluoride to the population. In the early history of water fluoridation, a 60% to 65% reduction of caries was recorded in some populations. With the increase in multiple sources of fluoride, adding fluoride to a community water supply will not result in these same high caries reductions for the population of that community. This is called the *diffusion effect*. Reports indicate 18% to 35% reductions of dental caries with water fluoridation today, which is still considered significant and cost effective. Choices A, B, and D do not accurately reflect the statements.

127. The initiative of the school district to contact the hygienist represents which step on the Learning Ladder Continuum health education theory?

ANS: B
In this case, the school board members take action to contact the dental hygienist for strategies to reduce the incidence of dental caries within their district after they become aware of the problem of school absences because of dental pain. The Learning Ladder Continuum depicts the natural progression from knowledge absorption to value adoption, following a series of steps. These order of these steps are unawareness of the problem (E); awareness (B), which occurs when knowledge is gained through education or other means; self-interest (C), representing the recognition of the advantage of personal involvement in relation to the problem; involvement (D), which occurs when the individual becomes involved in the learning process; and action (A) which is taking steps to make a change, as well as habit in relation to self-care health practices. This theory is typically applied to an individual's progression through the learning process to the development of an oral health habit.

128. Decreasing which of the following factors would be the adverse effect of using this particular type of examination method?

ANS: D
Screening with a light, a mirror, and a tongue blade is a type IV examination, a screening instrument with low specificity. Specificity is the ability to determine if a patient without signs and symptoms is truly free of the condition (a true negative), and has the lowest level of validity (D). Validity is the ability to accurately measure the test (A). Reliability is the consistency of a measure and is not affected by the type of examination. Reliability can be improved by training or calibrating the examiners and using valid instruments in the examination process (B). Sensitivity is the ability to recognize disease that is present (true positive) and is a component of validity (C). Both specificity and sensitivity are reduced by using the type IV examination because disease may be overlooked or a nonexistent disease diagnosed.

129. Which of the following is an appropriately stated outcome objective for this program?

ANS: C
A *goal* is a general statement of purpose for the program, and an *objective* is a specific and measurable statement of the anticipated outcome of the program. Objectives must be specific and measurable to provide a basis for program evaluation. A well-constructed objective includes the audience, an action or behavior (parents comply with referral), and a criterion of measurement (percentage of compliance with referral). "Parents of 90% of referred children will seek treatment for their children" is an outcome objective that reflects all three of these components (C). Objectives (A, D, and E) do not have a criteria of measurement. "Oral health status of the low-SES children will be improved" is a goal statement (B).

130. Volunteer participation of dental and dental hygiene students in this program is an example of all of the following concepts EXCEPT one. Which one is the EXCEPTION?

ANS: A
Peer sanction or review is the process of a group of professionals reviewing the actions of another professional for appropriate behavior or for failure to uphold the standard of care. Peer review is often used by professional associations in cases of substance abuse to safeguard the health of the public or if there has been a complaint of professional misconduct (A). Volunteering for this event demonstrates ethical commitment to professionalism, or acting in a manner that upholds the standards of the profession (B). Service learning occurs when a service received by the community is combined with and equal to the learning that occurs for the students who deliver the service (C). Community service focuses more on the service received by the community and is not balanced by learning by the students (D). *Pro bono* means professional work undertaken voluntarily and without payment or at a reduced fee. In this case, the professional members of the dental hygiene and dental societies volunteered by offering their services pro bono (E).

131. This public health approach promotes better oral health in all of the following ways EXCEPT one. Which one is the EXCEPTION?

ANS: E
This public health approach will not be able to provide better oral health for the aged through Medicare because Medicare is a federal program that does not provide oral health care (E). The

educational component of this program is designed to increase oral health literacy of this target population and provide preventive services (A, B). A desirable program outcome will be increases in demand for oral health care along with promoting utilization of dental services (C, D).

132. Which of the following formats could the dental hygiene volunteers use to engage the GREATEST amount of participation by the community participants?

ANS: D
Hands-on activities or crafts promote the greatest amount of participation by community participants, and participation promotes learning (D). Children's songs are a good way to reinforce learning; however, they do not provide an explanation of the concepts, which is required for new learning to occur (A). An educational video is effective as part of a formal presentation but lacks audience participation and may be more difficult to incorporate into a health fair format such as this (B). Posters and other mass media formats serve to reinforce prior learning, but they do not effectively promote new learning (C).

133. The dental hygienist uses an interdisciplinary approach involving community leaders to implement the oral health program. This is because support from other entities will assist the hygienist in changing the perceptions and values of the underserved residents of the community.

ANS: A
Both statements are true (A). The dental hygienist is using an interdisciplinary approach involving community leaders to implement the oral health program. Having the support of several entities lends credibility to the program and will assist the hygienist in changing the perceptions and values of the underserved residents of the community. The values and perceptions of the public are influenced by community leaders. Involvement of community leaders usually helps the underserved residents of the community to be more receptive to adopting positive oral health changes. Choices B, C, and D do not accurately reflect the statements.

134. Which of the following is the target population that will be recipients of the benefits of the program the dental hygienist is organizing?

ANS: C
The testlet states, "The dental hygienist's main responsibility is to establish an oral health program for underserved residents of the community." A *target*

population is defined as a clearly identified segment of the population. Even though the hygienist is working as a public health dental hygienist, her main responsibility is to the underserved residents of the community (C). The public is not a homogeneous underserved group, although portions may fit into that category (A). The hygienist is eliciting help from community leaders to achieve her main goal of assisting the underserved residents of the community. Community leaders provide support and funding for the program but are not the target population (B). Part of the dental hygienist's assignment is to develop a surveillance program that may involve patients at the FQHC, and the patients at the FQHC may be underserved residents. However, the hygienist's responsibility is to reach out to the underserved residents regardless of location (D).

135. All of the following are scenarios that are examples of an educational program that the dental hygienist could implement to achieve the program's goals EXCEPT one. Which one is the EXCEPTION?

ANS: E
Visiting private dental offices in the area and providing brochures and information to be distributed to the patients in the practice is not an example of strategies that the dental hygienist could implement to achieve the program's goals. Patients who are seen in a private practice are not classified as underserved and already have access to oral health care (E). The underserved population in the community may not have the opportunity to visit the FQHC or be aware of the services offered at that facility (A). Sponsoring a multidisciplinary free event held in an easily accessible location supported by community leaders is most likely to assist the hygienist in achieving her program goals (B). Providing educational information via brochures and personal discussion during each patient's visit to the FQHC is too time intensive to adequately reach the underserved members of the community (C). Conducting a small group presentation to a Sunday school class may or may not include the target population (D).

136. Which of the following surveillance methods is MOST cost effective in providing necessary assessment data?

ANS: A
The decayed, missing, or filled teeth (DMFT (for permanent teeth) or deft (for primary teeth) provides a simple and versatile survey of an individual's dental history (A). Providing radiographic imaging would be cost and time prohibitive for surveillance of a population (B). To provide surveillance of a population, full-mouth periodontal charting would be too time intensive (C). Knowing the reasons that the patient has not received dental treatment is important, but the caries index information is more critical to the success of the program (D).

137. All of the following are components of the dental hygiene process of care EXCEPT one. Which one is the EXCEPTION?

ANS: C
Components of the dental hygiene process of care include all of the choices except prevention (C). The correct components in the dental hygiene process of care, also known as the *ADPIE model*, include Assessment (A), Diagnosis (B), Planning, Implementation (D), and Evaluation (E).

138. Utilizing the Learning Ladder continuum health behavior model, which rung of the learning ladder are 78% of parents and coaches on in regards to the football players' use of tobacco products?

ANS: D
The stages of learning begin with unawareness. The parents and coaches of the football players are unaware that 63% of their children occasionally use tobacco products (D). Awareness is having knowledge of the issue but not applying that knowledge to one's self (A). Self-interest is the realization that the issue might have consequences to the individual, but no action is being taken (B). Involvement is the active participation in changing the issue or behavior (D).

139. All of the following are examples of an appropriate presentation title for the football players and coaches EXCEPT one. Which one is the EXCEPTION?

ANS: C
The Importance of Brushing and Flossing for Athletes would not be an appropriate presentation title for the football players and coaches because it was not a topic chosen on the presurvey needs assessment (C). How to Quit Using Tobacco and The Link between Oral Cancer and Tobacco Use in Athletes are appropriate topics because 96% of the football players believe that tobacco use is detrimental to their health. A presentation outlining the steps to quit would be effective and would allow the dental hygienist to discuss tobacco cessation (A, D). Football players are required to wear mouth guards, but 47% of the football players were unsure of the reason that they were mandated. Correct use of mouth guards and the rationale behind mouth guard use would be an appropriate presentation (B).

140. All of the following are purposes of the survey that the dental hygienist administered to segments of the parents, coaches, and football players before the presentation EXCEPT one. Which one is the EXCEPTION?

ANS: B
Avoiding unpleasant or controversial topics is not a valid reason for administering a survey, especially if a discussion on these topics could prevent harm (B). Determining the parents' beliefs, evaluating the coaches' influence over the players, surveying knowledge of the group and its influencers are all reasons to implement the questionnaire (A, C, D). Tailoring the appropriate instruction methods for the audience participating in the event is another valid reason for using a survey (E).

141. After introducing herself to the players, the dental hygienist mentions that since she is of Hispanic descent, she knows that the Hispanic players will "get it" when she discusses the importance of tobacco cessation. Which of the following terms correctly describes what the dental hygienist is trying to convey?

ANS: B
The definition of *ethnocentrism* is the belief that one's own culture or traditions are better than other cultures (B). *Ethnography* is the science that deals with the origin of human races, their origins, relations, and cultures (A). The definition of *cultural diversity* is the integration of an individual's or populations' socio-ethno-cultural background into dental hygiene care. The dental hygienist was excluding the other cultures represented on the football team by singling out her culture (C). *Cultural sensitivity* is defined as awareness and understanding of cultures different from one's own. The dental hygienist was assuming that her Hispanic counterparts would understand her information more readily than the other cultures represented on the team (D). *Cultural competency* is defined as awareness and understanding of cultural difference. The dental hygienist's statement was not indicative of understanding the other cultures represented on the football team (E).

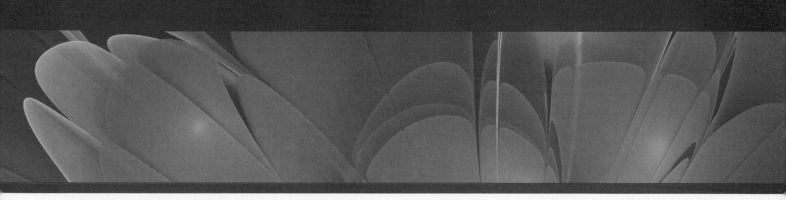

Additional Resources

The Anatomical Basis of Dentistry
The Anatomical Basis of Dentistry helps you master the essentials of gross anatomy. Complete, accurate coverage highlights the regions of the head and neck that are of clinical relevance.

Anatomy of Orofacial Structures: A Comprehensive Approach
A combined text and student workbook, *Anatomy of Orofacial Structures* makes it easy to understand oral histology and embryology, dental anatomy, and head and neck anatomy.

Applied Pharmacology for the Dental Hygienist
Applied Pharmacology for the Dental Hygienist provides an understanding of the basic principles of pharmacology. It covers the most common drugs that you will encounter in clinical practice—the drugs a patient may already be taking, and the drugs prescribed by the dentist.

Carranza's Clinical Periodontology
Carranza's Clinical Periodontology provides both print and online access to basic procedures as well as the latest in advanced procedures and techniques in reconstructive, esthetic, and implant therapy.

Community Oral Health Practice for the Dental Hygienist
Community Oral Health Practice for the Dental Hygienist helps you acquire the understanding to improve the oral health care of people throughout various communities and build a successful career in the public health sector.

Dental Anatomy Coloring Book
Featuring an array of coloring and labeling activities, *Dental Anatomy Coloring Book* provides an easy, fun, and effective way to memorize the structures of the head and neck region, as well as the basic body systems affecting dentistry.

Dental Hygiene: Theory and Practice
Comprehensive and up to date, *Dental Hygiene* offers complete coverage of today's dental hygiene skills and theories—all based on the Human Needs Model for better hygienist/patient communication.

The Dental Hygienist's Guide to Nutritional Care
The Dental Hygienist's Guide to Nutritional Care is specifically tailored to address relevant nutritional concerns for practicing hygienists and dental hygiene students.

Dental Instruments: A Pocket Guide
Dental Instruments: A Pocket Guide is a portable, visually-detailed resource that pairs thorough descriptions with high-quality photographs and illustrations in a convenient, pocket-sized format to help you quickly and accurately identify dental tools.

Dental Materials: Clinical Applications for Dental Assistants and Dental Hygienists
Dental Materials uses step-by-step procedures to show how to mix, use, and apply dental materials within the context of the patient's course of treatment.

Dental Materials: Properties and Manipulation
Dental Materials covers the tasks that dental assistants and dental hygienists typically perform. It shows the most current materials, how to mix and apply them in a clinical setting, and how to educate patients about them.

Dental Radiography: Principles and Techniques
Providing essential coverage of dental radiography principles and complete technical instruction, *Dental Radiography* is a combination of a textbook and a training manual, guiding you step-by-step through common procedures.

Essentials of Oral Histology and Embryology: A Clinical Approach
Essentials of Oral Histology and Embryology covers all areas of oral histology and embryology pertinent to clinical dental practice. Introductory material includes a complete discussion of the structure and function of the body's cells, as well as the stages of orofacial development from conception to birth. It also covers developmental problems.

Ethics and Law in Dental Hygiene
Ethics and Law in Dental Hygiene is written in the context of "real-world" situations that you will encounter on a regular basis in dental hygiene practice.

Exercises in Oral Radiology and Interpretation
An effective study tool for mastering radiography, this valuable question-and-answer book reinforces integral skills, including film handling, exposures, and clinical technique. A comprehensive review for national and state board examinations is also provided.

Handbook of Local Anesthesia
A practical "how-to" guide to safe anesthesia practices in dentistry, *Handbook of Local Anesthesia* covers all the latest advances in science, instrumentation, and pain control techniques. This book provides in-depth, full-color coverage of key anesthesia topics.

Handbook of Nitrous Oxide and Oxygen Sedation
Handbook of Nitrous Oxide and Oxygen Sedation is an invaluable resource for this method of sedation. It provides step-by-step administration techniques and responses to frequently asked questions that provide practical information for everyday use of N_2O/O_2, information on current equipment in analgesia delivery, and in-depth discussion of recovery from N_2O/O_2.

Infection Control and Management of Hazardous Materials for the Dental Team
Infection Control and Management of Hazardous Materials for the Dental Team covers everything from basic concepts in microbiology to protocols for clinical asepsis. Clear, step-by-step instructions make it easy for you to perform safety procedures and use the supplies and equipment needed to prevent the spread of infectious disease.

Illustrated Anatomy of the Head and Neck
Featuring a robust collection of full-color illustrations and photographs, *Illustrated Anatomy of the Head and Neck* provides a complete look at head and neck anatomy with an emphasis on the specific anatomy of the temporomandibular joint (TMJ).

Illustrated Dental Embryology, Histology, and Anatomy
Illustrated Dental Embryology, Histology, and Anatomy provides a complete look at dental anatomy, combined with dental embryology and histology and a review of dental structures. Going beyond an introduction to anatomy, this book also covers developmental and cellular information in depth.

Little and Falace's Dental Management of the Medically Compromised Patient
Learn how common medical conditions can affect the course of the dental treatment a patient receives. *Little and Falace's Dental Management of the Medically Compromised Patient* provides the information you need to provide appropriate dental care to any patient, regardless of existing medical conditions.

Local Anesthesia for the Dental Hygienist
Written by a dental hygienist for dental hygienists, *Local Anesthesia for the Dental Hygienist* helps you learn the safe and effective administration of local anesthesia. Coverage is tailored to fit the role and needs of the dental hygienist and promotes patient-centered care.

Medical Emergencies in the Dental Office
Medical Emergencies in the Dental Office prepares dental professionals to promptly and proactively recognize and manage medical emergencies that may occur in the dental office. It details how to anticipate potential emergencies and what resources must be on hand to deal effectively with these situations.

Mosby's Comprehensive Review of Dental Hygiene
Mosby's Comprehensive Review of Dental Hygiene offers a total of 2,500 review questions, including four online, timed practice exams—all with answers and rationales for remediation. It provides in-depth coverage, an easy-to-use outline format, expert authorship, and case studies.

Mosby's Dental Dictionary
Mosby's Dental Dictionary defines over 12,000 terms covering all areas of dentistry. Definitions include specialties (such as endodontics, periodontics, and surgery) and commonly used medical terms.

Mosby's Dental Drug Reference
Mosby's Dental Drug Reference provides the current, concise, *dental-specific* drug information you need at the point of care. More than 850 drug monographs make it easy to find indications and dosages, contraindications, interactions, side effects, serious reactions, and dental considerations.

Oral Anatomy, Histology and Embryology
Oral Anatomy, Histology and Embryology provides dental students with all of the information required to ensure a complete understanding of oral anatomy, histology, and embryology as they relate to dental practice. It contains useful "clinical application" boxes to clearly show relevance of subject area to routine dental practice.

Oral Pathology: Clinical Pathologic Correlations
Oral Pathology: Clinical Pathologic Correlations uses an atlas-style format to help you identify, diagnose, and plan treatment for oral disease presentations. Two-page spreads include clinical photos of common conditions on one side while the facing page lists the central features, causes, and significance of each specific disease. Each chapter is organized by clinical appearance.

Oral Pathology for the Dental Hygienist
This user-friendly, atlas-style text offers the ideal combination of clinical photographs, radiographs, and discussion to help you identify, understand, evaluate, and document the appearance of normal and disease states.

Periodontology for the Dental Hygienist
With an emphasis on recognizing periodontal problems and suggesting appropriate treatment, *Periodontology for the Dental Hygienist* covers the information that dental hygienists need to provide effective client care, from initial patient evaluation to patient education.

Practice Management for the Dental Team
Practice Management for the Dental Team provides step-by-step instructions for performing essential dental office skills, from managing patients to running the business. It covers all aspects of law and ethics, technology, communications, and business office systems.

Radiology for the Dental Professional and Study Guide
A complete guide to radiology principles and techniques, *Radiology for the Dental Professional* helps you develop imaging skills through practical application. Detailed step-by-step procedures demonstrate proper techniques; photos and illustrations improve comprehension and readability. The *Study Guide* will help you assess your comprehension with a wide range of engaging activities, exercises, and test questions.

Saunders Review of Dental Hygiene
Saunders Review of Dental Hygiene reflects the case-based format of the national exam along with content that covers new guidelines, especially in the areas of infection control and pharmacology. You will find multiple ways to study with over 60 clinical case studies and more than 1,500 questions.

Sedation
Sedation combines essential theory with "how-to" technical instruction and is the leading reference for basic techniques in sedation and anxiety control in the dental office. The latest guidelines from the ADA and the American Society of Anesthesiologists keep you up-to-date with the latest medical standards.

Ten Cate's Oral Histology: Development, Structure, and Function
Understand oral histology and learn to apply your knowledge in the clinical setting with this definitive reference. *Ten Cate's Oral Histology* provides insight on contemporary research and trends in oral histology, embryology, physiology, oral biology, and postnatal growth and development that is essential to your success in oral health.